Nursing Guide for Pediatric Neuroscience Patients

Kentlee Battick • Nir Shimony
George I Jallo
Editors

Nursing Guide for Pediatric Neuroscience Patients

Springer

Editors
Kentlee Battick
Hough Family Institute for Brain Protection Sciences
Johns Hopkins All Children's Hospital
St Petersburg, FL, USA

George I Jallo
Hough Family Institute for Brain Protection Sciences
Johns Hopkins All Children's Hospital
St Petersburg, FL, USA

Nir Shimony
St. Jude Children's Research Hospital
Le Bonheur Children's Hospital,
Semmes-Murphey Clinic, University of Tennessee Health Science Center, Johns Hopkins University School of Medicine
Memphis, TN, USA

ISBN 978-3-032-22663-1 ISBN 978-3-032-22664-8 (eBook)
https://doi.org/10.1007/978-3-032-22664-8

This Springer imprint is published by the registered company Springer Nature Switzerland AG
The registered company address is: Gewerbestrasse 11, 6330 Cham, Switzerland

Endorsement

AANN has reviewed this publication and recognizes it as a valuable educational resource. Endorsement does not imply that AANN independently verified every statement or recommendation contained within the text.

Foreword

This is a timely book written for nurses caring for children with medical and surgical disorders of the nervous system. It contains a wealth of information about the diagnosis and treatment of a wide variety of conditions presented in a clear and easy-to-read fashion. Each chapter is co-authored by a nurse and physician to provide unique practical pearls for professionals and trainees managing patients on the front lines. The topics are covered succinctly but comprehensively, beginning with the neurologic evaluation across age groups ranging from neonates to adolescents and ending with poignant discussions of brain death, palliative care, and medical ethics.

These internationally respected authors have assembled a pragmatic resource about the state-of-the-art management of children with neurological and neurosurgical illnesses. It will be a valuable read for years to come.

Chief of Pediatric Neurosurgery, Professor of Neurosurgery Oncology and Pediatrics
Carson-Spiro Professor of Pediatric Neurosurgery
The Johns Hopkins University School of Medicine
Baltimore, MD, USA

Alan R. Cohen

Foreword

Pediatrics encompasses a broad spectrum of patient ages and developmental stages, ranging from neonates to adolescents, which presents unique challenges in clinical care. Nurses caring for children with neurological disorders must possess the expertise to understand what is normal, anticipate changes in patient condition, and intervene promptly and appropriately. These changes can often be rapid, requiring nurses to recognize deviations from baseline and determine when escalation of care is warranted. The authors of *Nursing Guide for Pediatric Neuroscience Patients* have created a concise reference guide tailored for bedside nurses caring for this population. The chapters are presented in a clear and accessible format, covering fundamental topics such as pediatric neurological assessment, hydrocephalus, shunt management, craniosynostosis, Chiari malformation, infection control, patient transport, neuroimaging, epilepsy management, palliative care, and more. The chapters address pre- and postoperative nursing care, patient monitoring, criteria for escalating care, and education for patients and families. The comprehensive overview is further enhanced by case scenarios and video resources designed to facilitate the application of knowledge in clinical practice. Significantly, every chapter reflects a collaborative approach, co-authored by a nurse and a pediatric neurosurgeon, integrating pathophysiology and surgical considerations with nursing assessment, surveillance, and bedside interventions.

The book, *Nursing Guide for Pediatric Neuroscience Patients*, serves as a valuable resource for nurses who care for children.

Advanced Practice Provide Education and Training
University of Missouri Healthcare
Columbia, MO, USA

Cathy Cartwright

Preface

This textbook was conceived to meet a persistent gap in pediatric neuroscience nursing: a single, practical resource that speaks simultaneously to the neuroanatomy, pathophysiology, diagnostics, and procedures that define pediatric neurosurgery and to the moment-to-moment bedside care that sustains children and families through these conditions. Organized around common neurosurgical and neurocritical problems of childhood, it is designed for nurses and advanced practice providers who care for infants, children, and adolescents in settings ranging from intensive care units and operating rooms to general wards, clinics, and radiology suites. Each chapter pairs a pediatric neurosurgeon with a nurse or advanced practice nurse author, reflecting the team-based, interprofessional nature of contemporary pediatric neurosurgical care and the conviction that optimal outcomes arise when surgical decision-making and nursing expertise are fully integrated. Across topics—from neonatal and infant neurologic assessment, hydrocephalus and shunt management, craniosynostosis and Chiari malformation, to trauma, tumors, epilepsy, spasticity, infection, inflammatory disorders, ethics, and palliative care—the goal is to connect pathophysiology and operative strategy directly to nursing assessment, surveillance, and intervention at the bedside.

To support learners at different stages, the chapters follow a consistent structure that emphasizes practical clinical application. Readers will find succinct overviews of relevant neuroanatomy and pathophysiology; descriptions of neurosurgical and medical management (including neuroimaging basics, transport considerations for the critically ill child, and principles such as the Monroe–Kellie doctrine); case presentations; and explicit guidance on what to anticipate, monitor, and communicate in daily practice. Each chapter highlights when to contact a provider, how to educate patients and families during hospitalization and at discharge, and how to recognize complications early, thereby promoting safe, high-quality care across units and transitions.

As children requiring neurosurgical or complex neurologic care are never "just patients," the members of families must absorb frightening information, make difficult decisions, and reimagine futures in the face of uncertainty. Throughout this book, contributors emphasize patient- and family-centered care, including honest and developmentally appropriate communication, shared decision-making, and partnership with parents and caregivers in both acute and long-term management. The dual-author model underscores the importance of interprofessional collaboration—between nurses, neurosurgeons, neurologists, intensivists, anesthesiologists, rehabilitation specialists, child life, palliative care, and others—and is aligned with the broader movement toward interprofessional education and practice as a means of improving teamwork and outcomes in high-acuity environments.

This volume is intended primarily for bedside nurses, advanced practice nurses, and nurse leaders caring for pediatric neurosurgical and neurology patients, but it will also serve trainees and colleagues in neurosurgery, neurology, critical care, rehabilitation, and other disciplines who seek a clearer window into nursing perspectives and priorities. It may be used as a reference on busy units, as a foundation for orientation and competency development, and as a framework for interprofessional teaching conferences and simulation activities focused on pediatric neurocritical care. Above all, the hope is that the collective experience and wisdom of the nurse–neurosurgeon author teams will support readers in providing technically excellent, compassionate, and family-centered care to children with neurologic and neurosurgical disease.

St. Petersburg, FL, USA Kentlee Battick
Memphis, TN, USA Nir Shimony
St. Petersburg, FL, USA George I Jallo

Contents

Neurologic Assessment Neonatal, Infant, Toddler and Pediatric

Jennifer Coffman and Christopher Inglese

Introduction

The nursing neurological assessment is arguably the most critical component of care for children with neurological conditions. The ideal neurological assessment is systematic, repeatable, and conducted in a consistent manner across individuals and time. This assessment serves several fundamental purposes:

1. Establishes the child's baseline neurological function
2. Identifies changes in neurological status
3. Allows timely escalation of care
4. Evaluates the efficacy of interventions

The nursing neurological assessment should be conducted at regular intervals. The utility of the assessment becomes apparent as we compare results across time. Every patient, regardless of diagnosis, should have a neurological assessment at least once per shift as a part of their overall head-to-toe nursing physical assessment. Many patients without primary neurological diagnoses have conditions that can provoke secondary neurological sequelae. Those with underlying neurological conditions will often have neurological assessments or "neuro checks" ordered more regularly such as every 4 h, every 2 h, or even every hour. In addition to regularly scheduled neurological assessments, additional assessments should be

J. Coffman (✉)
Department of Neurosurgery, University of Colorado, Children's Hospital Colorado, Aurora, CO, USA
e-mail: Jennifer.Coffman@childrenscolorado.org

C. Inglese
Pediatric Neurology Hough Family Institute for Brain Protection Sciences Johns Hopkins All Children's Hospital Saint Petersburg, St. Petersburg, FL, USA
e-mail: cingles2@jhmi.edu

K. Battick et al. (eds.), *Nursing Guide for Pediatric Neuroscience Patients*,
https://doi.org/10.1007/978-3-032-22664-8_1

conducted when a neurological change is suspected, after an intervention aimed at impacting neurological function, and anytime there is a hand-off between nurses.

Components of a neurological assessment, depending on the purpose, can vary greatly. An assessment used for diagnostic purposes will be extremely detailed and would include elements intended to identify the anatomic location of specific neurological dysfunction. These more detailed assessments are usually reserved for providers with diagnostic and treatment responsibilities. The nursing neurological assessment should include, at a minimum, the following:

1. Mental status including the level of consciousness, orientation, and memory
2. Cranial nerves including pupillary response and facial symmetry
3. Speech or cry
4. Motor function
5. Vital signs
6. Cranium including fontanel, sutures, and head circumference for infants

The successful performance and interpretation of a pediatric neurological assessment is reliant upon understanding age-associated development, as well as the child's individual baseline level of development. Another unique aspect of the pediatric neurological assessment is the reliance on the caregiver's input and participation. The examination of the newborn, infant, toddler, and preschool child is best accomplished by abiding by three principles. First, "stop, look and listen", meaning time spent watching, using toys, "stand there and do nothing" and patiently watch.

Many organizations have adopted standardized neurological nursing assessments. This ensures the neurological assessment is administered consistently by all nurses and allows a more objective comparison of changes over time with the hope that even subtle changes will be identified earlier. Examples of commonly adopted standardized assessments include the following:

1. Glasgow Coma Scale (GCS)—Originally described in 1974, the GCS is one of the most widely used assessments to understand neurological injury severity. The scale considers and scores three major neurological domains: eye opening, verbal response, and motor function. It has been criticized in its use in the pediatric population due to its inability to account for age and development [1], as well as inconsistent application [2]. As a result, many variations of the GCS have been adapted to the pediatric population.
2. Full Outline of Un-Responsiveness Scale (FOUR Score)—Developed by researchers at the Mayo Clinic and published in 2005 [3], the FOUR Score was developed in response to the limitations of the GCS. This assessment is more detailed than the GCS. It evaluates and scores eye response, motor response, brainstem reflexes, and respiration. Originally validated in the adult population, like the GCS, it has been modified to accommodate pediatric patients [4].
3. Serial Neurological Assessment in Pediatrics (SNAP)—Developed by the Children's Hospital of Philadelphia and first described in 2021 [5], the SNAP assessment is one of the most recent attempts to standardize the nursing pediatric

neurological assessment. This assessment is a modified GCS accounting for patient age and development. Unlike the GCS and FOUR score, the individual scores that are relied upon for predictive value, the SNAP is dependent on the trending of scores across time. A score in isolation is less meaningful. Three different scales are used, based on age, to score mental status, cranial nerves, communication, and motor function.

Newborn

Mental status, resting level of alertness, postures, and tone are contingent upon gestational age and influenced by the circadian rhythms of sleep and sleep stages.

A. Important Definitions
   1. Post Menstrual Age: The time from the first day of the last menstrual period to the present, including the time spent in the womb and after birth.
   2. Gestational Age (GA): The time from the first day of the last menstrual period to the day of birth.
   3. Chronological Age: The time from birth usually described in days, weeks, months, or years.
   4. Corrected Age: The chronological age minus the number of weeks the baby was born early; this term is generally used up to the age of 3.

B. Mental Status: Level of arousal and attention
   1. Alertness is assessed by gently unswaddling the baby and observing the response to the examiner's soft and gentle voice first, followed by steadily increasing the volume as needed, to fully awaken and engage the child (and hopefully not provoke irritability and crying!). This part of the exam can be difficult to evaluate, especially if the newborn is very ill.
   2. As a rule, it is important to examine or observe the child serially over time before one concludes that tone is abnormal as it can be influenced and vary by quiet relaxed drowsing or quiet sleep, the relationship to feeding, or the administration of medications, nursing care, procedures, or temperature.

C. Cranial Nerves
   1. Cranial nerves V, VII, IX, X, and XII subserve suck and swallow, and a vigorous suck and normal swallowing of formula provide sufficient information.

D. Cry
   1. The child's cry provides much information; a lusty strong cry suggests intact glossopharyngeal and vagus nerves. Full and symmetric facial movement with crying is a seventh cranial nerve function.

E. Motor Function
   1. Resting tone varies considerably in newborns, A frog-legged supine posture is normal up until 26 weeks' gestation, and progression to the normal antigravity flexor tone, arms flexed, hips adducted, and legs flexed at the knees should appear at 34 to 36 weeks.

2. Upper and lower limb tone is tested with passive range of motion of each arm individually first. The arms are flexed and extended together at the elbows, and then each arm separately is tested by gentle traction of the extended arm, such that the ipsilateral shoulder comes off the mat or bed. The arms are then flexed at the elbows, and while holding the baby's wrists, simultaneously adducted and abducted across the chest. The wrists are then held and hands shaken for flappability.
3. Arm recoil consists of extending the flexed arms at the elbow, extending them fully for a moment and then releasing them to see if the previous slightly flexed arm posture returns.
4. These maneuvers are repeated in the same manner and order as the arms, for the range of motion of each leg, passive movements of legs in extension and flexion, and then while flexed at the knees, the hips are adducted and abducted. Leg traction is assessed with each extended leg first, followed by the feet for flappability as they are shaken while held at the ankles.
5. The extent to which the hands are tightly fisted or not is an important characteristic relative to the presence or absence of normal tone.
6. Myelination is most rapid in the first 2 years of life and continues for some time through the beginning of the third decade. Myelination begins with the posterior frontal lobes, followed by the parietal, occipital, and then frontal cortices, and is completed by the second year of life, except for the association cortices following a year later. This preferential sequence favors motor sensory roots, special senses, and the brainstem facilitating essential reflexes and earlier development of functions contributing toward survival from an evolutionary point of view. The shorter corticospinal axons myelinate first, hence, the earlier development of the upper limbs, followed by trunk and subsequently the legs which are innervated by longer nerves.

F. Vital Signs
1. Apnea
2. Bradycardia
3. Desaturations

G. Developmental Considerations
1. Primitive Reflexes
   (i) Palmar Grasp Birth to 2 Months: Place index finger in the infant's palm; the child grasps the examiner's finger
   (ii) Rooting Birth to 3 Months: Lightly stroke the cheek on both sides of the mouth and above and below the midline of the lip (at 12-3-6-9 o'clock or the four cardinal points, directions north east south west). The child turns their head, opens their mouth, and turns their head toward the stimulus.
   (iii) Placing Reflex Birth to 6 Weeks: The bottom of the foot is lowered and placed on the edge of the examining table; flexion of the legs at the hips and knees causes the lifting of the foot.
   (iv) Stepping: Birth to 4 months—Hold infant up and place the feet on the exam table; automatic quick stepping walking movements are noted.

(v) Moro: Birth to 6 months—In supine position, lift the head up and then allow a quick drop backward of 30 degrees below the level of trunk. Symmetrical abduction and flexion of the upper extremities should occur. Explain to parents what you are doing and why to avoid a misunderstanding about being overly rough.

(vi) Babinski: Birth to 2 years—Stimulating the lateral aspect of the sole from heel toward the ball of foot, flexion of the great toe, and fanning of the toes is a noted physiologic response.

Birth to 2 months	Birth to 3 months	Birth to 4 months	Birth to 2 years
Palmar Grasp	Placing Reflex Rooting	Stepping	Babinski

H. Cranial Sutures

1. The skull or cranium consists of four cranial base endochondral bones and three pairs of membranous bones that make up the cranial vault. Fibrous connective tissue unites the membranous bones of the cranium and face; these skull joints are called synarthrosis. They unite the large flat bones of the skull and are called sutures; the large fibrous nonossified membranes are called fontanels. The sutures and fontanels are pliant and are necessary to accommodate the rapid growth of the brain within the skull during infancy. The large boney plates comprising the skull are the frontal, parietal, and occipital bones. The four sutures are frontal or metopic, coronal or frontoparietal, sagittal, lambdoidal, or parieto-occipital
   (i) Metopic: Separates the two frontal bones and ends at the anterior margin of the anterior fontanel
   (ii) Coronal: Demarcates the frontal from the parietal bones
   (iii) Sagittal: Lies between the parietal bones
   (iv) Lambdoidal: Divides the occipital from the parietal bones

I. Fontanels: Normally concave and not flat. It can be depressed or more concave than normal with dehydration. A bulging fontanel properly examined is an important sign of increased intracranial pressure. If associated with frontal bossing, prominent scalp veins, and a rapidly enlarging OFC, be concerned about increased intracranial pressure.

1. Anterior Fontanel: Its margins are the frontal suture, coronal sutures, and the frontal and parietal bones. The fontanels permit up and down movements of the skull as opposed to the limited hinged movement of the sutures. Anterior fontanel closes at 1.5 years (range 3–27 months).
2. Posterior fontanel closes at birth to 2 months and not palpable after 6 weeks.
   (i) A crying infant may have a full or tense fontanel; the fontanel should be examined, with the baby sitting or held upright.
   (ii) Abnormal Head Shapes—See chapter on Craniosynostosis.

J. Head Circumference

1. Measure with a nonstretchable tape across the occiput and the supraorbital ridges halfway between the eyebrows and the hairline.

2. A newborn's and infant's head grows fastest during the first 3 months of life, and brain growth is approximately 80% of its eventual adult size by 2 years. Head circumference should be carefully measured and plotted routinely during the first 3 years of life.
   (i) 0–3 months: 2 cm per month
   (ii) 3–6 months: increases by 1 cm per month
   (iii) 6–9 months: increases by 2 cm generally
   (iv) 1–5 years: increases by 5 cm
3. Average Adult Head Circumference
   (i) Males 57 cm
   (ii) Females 55 cm
4. Can vary by ethnicity; larger head circumferences have anecdotally been described in Northern Europeans and can vary in accordance with height and weight.
5. Excessive head growth (crossing of percentiles) is more likely to be associated with the underlying pathology than a large head increasing in size appropriately and parallel to the percentiles.
6. When to Worry:
   (i) Excessive rate of head growth
   (ii) Marked separation of sutures, bulging fontanels
   (iii) Lethargy, persistent unexplained vomiting, sunsetting of eye position
   (iv) Paralysis of upward gaze
   (v) Focal neurologic signs associated with macrocephaly
   (vi) Developmental stagnation incoordination associated with macro-crania
7. Microcephaly: An occipitofrontal circumference that is significantly less than that of typically developing children of similar sex, age, and ethnicity:
   (i) It is a clinical sign and not a diagnosis, providing an estimate of brain size.
   (ii) Defined as either 2 or 3 SD below the mean or below the 0.4th centile, i.e., 2.67 SD below the mean.
   (iii) Primary: Brain growth is reduced during pregnancy.
   (iv) Secondary: Acquired, in other words, when OFC is within the limits of normal at birth but fails to grow typically thereafter
   (v) When to Worry:
      1. Associated with epilepsy
      2. Associated with focal neurological signs on examination
      3. Associated with stagnation or regression of development
      4. Downward crossing of centiles on successive measurement and plotting of OFC
      5. Dysmorphic features

Infant—3 Months

A. Mental Status: Alert and socially interactive and aware; social smile.
B. Cranial Nerves: Vestibular–ocular reflex, eye movements are full and conjugate, can track visually fully 180 degrees. Horizontal and vertical Doll's eyes can be elicited.
C. Motor Function:
   1. Hands to mouth.
   2. Decreasing flexor tone of upper extremities.
   3. Passive ROM still met with some resistance.
   4. Scarf sign; arm still not extended beyond shoulder.
   5. Bears weight on forearms while prone.
   6. Some brief transient wobbling of head while sitting supported.
   7. The child at this time is ready to start front to back roll; if done earlier, it can be falsely reassuring as a positive acquisition. Examine for other signs of upper motor neuron abnormalities for age, spasticity, dystonia, weakness, hyperreflexia, and pathologic and persistent primitive reflexes.

Infant—6 Months

A. Mental Status: Attentive and socially aware, quick clear orienting responses to visual and auditory stimuli.
B. Cranial Nerves:
   (a) Can track vertically and horizontally.
   (b) Facial movements permit testing of the seventh cranial nerve.
   (c) The presence of normal sucking and swallowing and the absence of pooled oral pharyngeal secretions or excessive drooling, and normal phonation permit a general sense of the integrity of lower cranial nerves.
C. Motor Function:
   (a) The infant is able to reach out and grasp objects, bring them to midline and in mouth.
   (b) Can grasp a cube; whole hand grasp.
   (c) Passive range of motion: lower extremities should be flexible enough to bring the foot to infant's mouth.
D. Developmental Considerations
   (a) Smiles, laughs, jabbers, dada, mama, baba
   (b) Stranger danger

Toddler

A. Mental Status: The period of "toddlerhood" beginning somewhat arbitrarily at 12 months can present challenges to the examiner. The parent can become a valuable coconspirator, using toys or even instruments instead of (replacing) the clinician, as reaching and grasps are observed as well as the presence or absence of early or normal handedness. The child, once comfortable, may imitate gestures or movements such as "so big", pat a cake or wave goodbye or follow simple instructions if the requested action is first done by the examiner or parent/caregiver
B. Motor Function: Tone is assessed, as performed with legs with infants by first flexing and extending each arm at the elbow and adducting each arm at the shoulder and again flexing and extending the limb across the chest.
   1. At 12 months, a fine pincer grasp should be established as small objects are grasped neatly between the thumb and index finger. Crossing the midline to consistently grasp a small object closer to the contralateral hand again is suggestive of hemiparesis, early handedness, or both. Beyond 12 months, the child should easily crawl into and out of sitting positions.
   2. The toddler typically begins to walk between 11 and 15 months; concern regarding the absence of walking begins at 16 to 17 months. Pulling to stand, along furniture with brief periods of standing, and "not holding on" are followed by cruising, then walking with increasingly less support and contact guarding.
C. Developmental Considerations: Indicates wants by pointing, gestures, and vocalizing:
   1. Has a vocabulary of 10 or more words
   2. Uses single words to indicate wants
   3. Has more complex social interactions; rich laughs vocalize thier wants
   4. Understands the use of objects
   5. Follows simple commands; still needs reinforcement and demonstration
   6. Points to pictures, cat, bird, dog; at least two on Denver II; repeats names of the pictures
   7. Names two body parts by 18 months and 6 of 8 body parts by 18 to 30 months
   8. Stranger danger

Child/School Age (6–12)

Assessing the neurological status of the school age child becomes easier as they are generally more cooperative. They are at an age and developmental stage where they can understand complex instructions, assess their environment, and make independent decisions regarding their safety and thus their willingness to participate. Use of a family member or caregiver to assist in the assessment is often not needed.

A. Mental Status—Assessing mental status consists of understanding the child's level of awareness and response to their surrounding environment. Start by assessing their responsiveness and then move on to a more detailed assessment of their orientation and memory.
   1. Responsiveness measures the least amount of stimulus needed to elicit a response, either motor or vocal. Start with the least intrusive means of stimuli and work your way to the most.
      (i) Voice—With a soft voice, expect the child to turn their attention and focus to the voice. This is often all that is needed for an awake patient and can often be observed by just walking in the room. If no response, move to light touch.
      (ii) Touch—With a gentle moving contact, touch an extremity while using a soft voice. If there is still no response, move onto more vigorous nudging with a louder voice. If there is still no response, noxious stimuli may be necessary.
      (iii) Noxious stimuli—Unpleasant stimuli may be necessary to elicit a response for patients who are neurologically compromised or pharmacologically sedated. Noxious stimuli can consist of pressure to nail beds (either fingers or toes) or more central stimulation such as a trapezius pinch or orbital notch pressure. If you do not get a response on one side, apply the stimulus to the other side. Due to reports of harm, a sternal rub is no longer recommended.

      Observe the type and level of response you receive to the above stimulation—does the child turn their attention fully to you, do they open their eyes, stir in the bed, or only withdraw from the noxious stimuli? A child with severe brain injury or who is heavily sedated may have no response, even to noxious stimuli.
   2. Orientation—If the child is awake and attentive to their surroundings, you may further assess their mental status by asking them some simple questions. Quiz them to understand their orientation to person, place, and time. School-age children may not have a firm grasp on their current situation or events.
      (i) Person—Often asking the child who the caregiver at the bedside is, is the most straightforward way to assess a "person". If they attend school, you can also ask the name of their teacher.
      (ii) Place—Ask them if they know, in general, where they are. A school-age child will most likely not know the formal name of the hospital or clinic they are in, but "hospital", "doctor's office", or something similar should suffice. They may even respond with the city they are currently in.
      (iii) Time—A young school-age child may not know the exact date but may be able to respond with the year, the season, or their birthday.

B. Cranial Nerves—There are 12 nerves that emanate from the brainstem and serve the head and neck. Some are sensory, some are purely motor, and some are mixed. While testing each cranial nerve is imperative for a thorough neurological assessment aimed at providing diagnostic insight, understanding and assessing a few can be valuable to a nurse attempting to understand acute intracranial changes in a patient.

1. Facial symmetry—Facial movement is controlled by cranial nerve VII (Facial). Close observation of a patient as they interact with their environment is often enough to identify an overt facial weakness; however, weakness of these small muscles can be subtle. Facial movement can be separated into upper and lower facial movements. To actively assess facial movement and symmetry, assess both. Ask the patient to raise their eyebrows (surprised look) and then request them to squeeze their eyes shut. Observe for equal movement. To assess the lower facial movement, a combination of several movements can be requested—puff the cheeks out like when blowing up a balloon, smile, and show your teeth. Again, assess for equal movement from both sides of the face.
2. Pupillary response—Cranial nerve III (oculomotor) controls the pupil's ability to expand and contract in response to changes in light.
   (a) First, looking at both eyes simultaneously, assess the size of each pupil and assess if they are equal. Size is often described in millimeters. The condition of unequal pupils is known as anisocoria.
   (b) Second, assess the pupil's ability to react to light. Assessing pupillary response is best done in low light. While the eye is open (either voluntarily or with help), move the light source from just lateral of the eye (at the temple) to the pupil. Observe the pupil's ability to briskly constrict when the light hits the pupil. Duplicate this movement in the same eye and assess the ipsilateral pupil. Even though the light is not shining on that side, the opposite pupil should equally react with consensual response. Pupillary response is often described as brisk, sluggish, or nonreactive.
   (c) Assessing pupil response can be very subjective with poor interrater reliability [6]; thus, many nursing units, especially critical care, have begun utilizing pupilometers. These handheld devices can be very useful in providing objective data; however, they can be very challenging to use in an uncooperative patient, such as an awake child.
   (d) There are other factors, beyond cranial nerve dysfunction, that can impact pupil size and reactivity—medications, congenital anisocoria, eye conditions, and conditions such as Horner's syndrome [7].
   (e) "Blown pupils" or pupils that are fully dilated and nonreactive to light, in an unresponsive patient, can be ominous and an indication of cerebral herniation.

C. Speech—Assessing speech can reflect the functions of specific cranial nerves as well as language centers within the brain. Because of this, it is important to assess the motor function associated with speech, as well as receptive and expressive speech.

1. Motor Function—Movement of the tongue is controlled by cranial nerve XII (hypoglossal). When this is impaired, word choice and expression may be appropriate, but the sound quality may be affected. Speech may sound

garbled, muffled, or slow. Children with cranial nerve XII impairment may also have trouble swallowing.

2. Receptive—The ability to understand and process words that are being spoken to you is known as receptive language. Receptive language is controlled by Wernicke's area which is in the posterior section of the superior temporal gyrus. To assess receptive language, request the child follow specific instructions. Compound instructions, or those that include at least two steps, are most helpful in assessing receptive language. For example, ask the child to touch their nose and then point to the TV.
3. Expressive—The ability to convert thoughts into spoken words is known as expressive language. Expressive language is controlled by Broca's area in the frontal lobe. Expressive language can be assessed by simply engaging in social conversation with the child, keeping in mind the child's age and development. Age-appropriate word choice/sentence structure, cadence, and fluency should all be observed.

D. Motor Function
  1. Extremity Strength—The child's ability to move extremities equally with full strength is reflective of healthy cortical (motor strip) as well as corticospinal tract function. Strength can be characterized in relation to the forces that are overcome to elicit movement—such as "against resistance", "antigravity", "within the plane of the bed", or "flicker movement". Each extremity should be independently assessed for movement. Ideally, proximal and distal movements of each should be checked.
     (a) Upper Extremities—Request that the child raise arms from the shoulder; then, apply consistent and equal pressure to the upper arm, just proximal to the elbow, and see if the child can overcome this pressure. Placing two fingers in their hands bilaterally, request that they squeeze. Pay attention to both the strength of the squeeze and its equality.
     (b) Lower Extremities—Request that the child lift each leg independently off the bed. Apply consistent pressure just above the knee to assess their ability to overcome gentle resistance. Request that the child push down with their feet against your hands (plantar flexion), again applying slight consistent and equal pressure. Then, ask them to pull them up (dorsiflexion), again applying counterpressure.
  2. Gait—When able, observe the child walking. Pay attention to any instability, imbalance, or wide-set stance that could indicate ataxia. Also attend to any inequality of movement between lower extremities that may hint at unilateral muscle weakness.

E. Vital Signs—Vital signs are underrated, yet important elements of the neurological exam. An understanding of the normal range of vital signs is imperative. For school-age children, a heart rate between 70 and 110 beats per minute, a systolic blood pressure between 80 and 120 mmHg, and a respiratory rate from 20 to 30 breaths per minute would be within normal parameters.

   Abnormal vital signs can be an indication of current or impending neurologic decompensation. A combination of bradycardia, widening pulse pressure

Table 1 Developmental Milestones for Child/School Age (6-12)

Gross motor	Fine motor	Self-help	Problem-solving	Social/emotional	Receptive language	Expressive language
Heel-to-toe walking	Draws diamond Writes first and last name Forms and writes short sentences Copies a drawing	Ties shoes Brushes hair Looks when crossing the street	Basic addition/subtraction Knows seasons Sounds out common words	Has best friend of same sex Plays board games Understands pretend play from reality Wants to be like friends and make them happy	Asks what unfamiliar words are Can determine which words do not belong in a group	Lists events in order Can state days of the week

Adapted from Scharf, Scharf and Stroustrup [9]

(increased systolic and decreased diastolic), and irregular respiration, known as Cushing's Triad, is an ominous sign of severe neurological decompensation and should be treated emergently. Increasing blood pressure can be an early sign, while irregular respiration is a late sign [8].

F. Developmental Considerations
   1. Developmental Milestones—Failure to gain milestones or loss of those already achieved can be a sign of neurological dysfunction. It is important to understand milestones for each age. At age 6, the following milestones should be met (Table 1):

      Appreciating these milestones can also aid in structuring and completing the neurological assessment—tailoring it specifically for the child's current developmental level.
   2. School Performance—While usually not an indication of acute changes in neurological status, decline in school performance can be an indication of a more insidious neurological process. This becomes an important data point in the school-age child. Asking parents about recent changes in school performance can clarify the nature of neurological dysfunction over time.

Teens/Adults

Like school age children, assessing the teenage or adult patient can be more straightforward. Most teenagers lack inherent anxiety around strangers and demonstrate better situational awareness as it relates to their medical condition and the healthcare milieu.

A. Mental Status—Assessing mental status consists of understanding the teen's level of awareness and response to their surrounding environment. Start by assessing their responsiveness and then move on to a more detailed assessment of their orientation and memory.

1. Responsiveness measures the least amount of stimulus needed to elicit a response, either motor or vocal. Start with the least intrusive means of stimuli and work your way to the most.
   - (i) Voice—With a soft voice, expect the teen to turn their attention and focus to the voice. This is often all that is needed for an awake patient and can often be observed by just walking in the room. If no response, move to light touch.
   - (ii) Touch—With a gentle moving contact, touch an extremity while using a soft voice. If there is still no response, move onto more vigorous nudging with a louder voice. If there is still no response, noxious stimuli may be necessary.
   - (iii) Noxious stimuli—Unpleasant stimuli may be necessary to elicit a response for patients who are neurologically compromised or pharmacologically sedated. Noxious stimuli can consist of pressure to nail beds (either fingers or toes) or more central stimulation such as a trapezius pinch or orbital notch pressure. If you do not get a response on one side, apply the stimulus to the other side. Due to reports of harm, a sternal rub is no longer recommended.

   Observe the type and level of response you receive to the above stimulation—does the teen turn their attention fully to you, do they open their eyes, stir in the bed, or only withdraw from the noxious stimuli? A teen with severe brain injury or who is heavily sedated may have no response, even to noxious stimuli.
2. Orientation—If the teen is awake and attentive to their surroundings, you may further assess their mental status by asking them some simple questions. Quiz them to understand their orientation to person, place, time, and current situation or events.
   - (i) Person—Often asking the teen who the caregiver at the bedside is, is the most straightforward way to assess the "person". They may also be asked to identify siblings, friends, or teachers.
   - (ii) Place—Ask them if they know, in general, where they are. A teen may know the formal name of the hospital or clinic they are in, but "hospital", "doctor's office", or something similar would suffice. They may even respond with the city they are currently in, depending on the specificity of your question.
   - (iii) Time—Depending on the circumstances, a teen may not know the specific date but should be aware of the year and even the month.
   - (iv) Current situation or events—A teen or adult should have at least a general understanding of their current situation and/or recent events that pertain to their healthcare. Ask the teen to describe why they are hospitalized or what events took place that day during their stay.

B. Cranial Nerves—There are 12 nerves that emanate from the brainstem and serve the head and neck. Some are sensory, some are purely motor, and some are mixed. While testing each cranial nerve is imperative for a thorough neurological assessment aimed at providing diagnostic insight, understanding and assessing a few can be valuable to a nurse attempting to understand acute intracranial changes in a patient.

1. Facial symmetry—Facial movement is controlled by cranial nerve VII (facial). Close observation of a patient as they interact with their environment is often enough to identify an overt facial weakness; however, weakness of these small muscles can be subtle. Facial movement can be separated into upper and lower movements. To actively assess facial movement and symmetry, assess both. Ask the patient to raise their eyebrows (surprised look) and then request they squeeze their eyes shut. Observe for equal movement. To assess the lower facial movements, a combination of several movements can be requested—puff the cheeks out like when blowing up a balloon, smile, and show your teeth. Again, assess for equal movement from both sides of the face.
2. Pupillary response—Cranial nerve III (oculomotor) controls the pupil's ability to expand and contract in response to changes in light.
   (a) First, looking at both eyes simultaneously, assess the size of each pupil and check if they are equal. Size is often described in millimeters. The condition of unequal pupils is known as anisocoria.
   (b) Second, assess the pupil's ability to react to light. Assessing pupillary response is best done in low light. While the eye is open (either voluntarily or with help), move the light source from just lateral of the eye (at the temple) to the pupil. Observe the pupil's ability to briskly constrict when the light hits the pupil. Duplicate this movement in the same eye and assess the ipsilateral pupil. Even though the light is not shining on that side, the opposite pupil should equally react with a consensual response. Pupillary response is often described as brisk, sluggish, or nonreactive.
   (c) Assessing pupil response can be very subjective [6]; thus, many nursing units, especially critical care, have begun utilizing pupilometers. These handheld devices can be very useful in providing objective data; however, they can be very challenging to use in an uncooperative patient, such as a concussed teen.
   (d) There are other factors, beyond cranial nerve dysfunction, that can impact pupil size and reactivity—medications, congenital anisocoria, eye conditions, and conditions such as Horner's syndrome [7].
   (e) "Blown pupils" or pupils that are fully dilated and nonreactive to light, in an unresponsive patient, can be ominous and an indication of cerebral herniation.

C. Speech—Assessing speech can reflect the function of specific cranial nerves as well as language centers within the brain. Because of this, it is important to assess the motor function associated with speech, as well as receptive and expressive speech.

1. Motor function—Movement of the tongue is controlled by cranial nerve XII (hypoglossal). When this is impaired, word choice and expression may be appropriate, but the sound quality may be affected. Speech may sound

garbled, muffled, or slow. Teens with cranial nerve XII impairment may also have trouble swallowing.

2. Receptive—The ability to understand and process words that are being spoken to you is known as receptive language. Receptive language is controlled by Wernicke's area located in the posterior section of the superior temporal gyrus. To assess receptive language, request the teen follow specific instructions. Compound instructions, or those that include at least two steps, are most helpful in assessing the receptive language. For example, ask the teen to touch their nose and then point to the TV.
3. Expressive—The ability to convert thoughts into spoken words is known as expressive language. Expressive language is controlled by Broca's area in the frontal lobe. Expressive language can be assessed by simply engaging in social conversation with the teen, keeping in mind the teen's age and development. Age-appropriate word choice/sentence structure, cadence, and fluency should all be observed.

D. Motor Function
1. Extremity Strength—The teen's ability to move extremities equally with full strength is reflective of healthy cortical (motor strip) as well as corticospinal tract function. Strength can be characterized in relation to the forces that are overcome to elicit movement—such as "against resistance", "anti-gravity", "within the plane of the bed", or "flicker movement". Each extremity should be independently assessed for movement. Ideally, proximal and distal movements of each should be checked.
   (a) Upper extremities—Request that the teen raise arms from the shoulder; then, apply consistent and equal pressure to the upper arm, just proximal to the elbow, and see if the teen can overcome this pressure. Placing two fingers in their hands bilaterally, request that they squeeze. Pay attention to both the strength of the squeeze and the equality of it.
   (b) Lower extremities—Request that the teen lift each leg independently off the bed. Apply consistent pressure just above the knee to assess their ability to overcome gentle resistance. Request that the teen push down with their feet against your hands (plantar flexion), again applying slight consistent and equal pressure. Then, ask them to pull them up (dorsiflexion), again applying counterpressure.
2. Gait—When able, observe the teen walking. Pay attention to any instability, imbalance, or wide-set stance that could indicate ataxia. Also attend to any inequality of movement between lower extremities that may hint at unilateral muscle weakness.

E. Vital Signs—Vital signs are underrated, yet important elements of the neurological exam. An understanding of the normal range of vital signs is imperative. For school-age children, a heart rate between 60 and 100 beats per minute, a systolic blood pressure between 90 and 120 mmHg, and a respiratory rate from 12 to 18 breaths per minute would be within normal parameters.

Abnormal vital signs can be an indication of current or impending neurologic decompensation. A combination of bradycardia, widening pulse pressure (increased systolic and decreased diastolic), and irregular respiration, known as Cushing's Triad, is an ominous sign of severe neurological decompensation and should be treated emergently. Increasing blood pressure can be an early sign, while irregular respiration is a late sign [8].

F. Developmental Considerations
   1. School Performance—Like school-age children, decline in school performance for a teen or young adult can be an indication of an insidious neurological process. Asking teens/adults that attend school about recent changes in school performance can clarify the nature of neurological dysfunction over time.
   2. Social Engagement—Maintaining productive peer relationships is important in developing social skills. These relationships and skills lead to healthy psychological development, academic success, and successful relationships later in life [10]. Like school performance, while not an indicator of acute neurological decline, changes in social engagement over time can mark an underlying subtle process.

Assessment in the Developmentally Delayed Child

A. Ask the parents/guardians about the child's developmental milestones, if and/or when they began rolling over, walking, talking, etc. Parents are key into knowing any deviations from their baseline
   1. The history will establish the patient's baseline to determine if and when there is a deviation which could be an indicator of a neurologic change or neurological emergency.

B. It is very important to be mindful that the term developmental delay has a large spectrum; by definition, it is delay in achieving one or more developmental milestones in comparison with their peers.

C. Developmental delay can have significant long-term sequelae, impacting subsequent cognitive, psychosocial, and academic attainments and adaptations.

D. Early screening and persistent surveillance importantly contribute, by virtue of timely referrals to appropriate remedial providers and resources, to a more positive influence on the trajectory of the acquisition of adaptive skills.

Recognition and Assessment of the Post-Ictal Child

A. The post-ictal state is an often ambiguous and arbitrary period between the clinical termination of a seizure and the individual's return to baseline.
   1. The duration and manifestations of this period of time vary considerably between individuals with epilepsy.
   2. Similarly, the physiologic, motor, linguistic, cognitive, and behavioral features are remarkably heterogeneous.

3. The obscure onset of a state is more typical of a dialeptic seizure, during which there is sudden loss of awareness, responsiveness, motor activity, and subtle automatisms. Examples of dialeptic seizures are absence, atypical absence, and focal impaired awareness events. The beginning of a post-ictal period, therefore, is straightforward with generalized tonic or tonic–clonic episodes.

B. From a patient care point of view, knowing the end of a post-ictal state has practical and patient safety implications. Certainly, knowledge about, and identifying, the end of this state permits the nurse to feel comfortable about moving on to his/her next responsibility, either clinical or with regard to documentation.

C. Typically, eye closure denotes the end of a seizure, and in fact, the presence of eye closure ictally is strongly sensitive and specific for the events' likelihood of being a paroxysmal nonepileptic attack.

D. As the patient becomes hemodynamically stable, the nurse can now focus upon the diagnostically and clinically observed important ictal semiology and post-ictal deficits.

1. The physical features and post-ictal deficits inform localization and may or may not support the epileptologists' hypothesis in the context of a presurgical evaluation. The astute nurse can be of inestimable value to the epileptologist as her/his eyes and ears supplement or can be superior to the ictal correlates seen on video as it is not uncommon for the child to be off camera or blocked from camera view by a family member or caregiver. Ictal speech arrest with rapid return of baseline linguistic functions suggests a nondominant hemispheric localization.
2. A Todd's paresis localizes the seizure onset zone to the contralateral hemisphere. Individuals with left temporal lobe epilepsy have more prominent post-ictal memory deficits, while right temporal lobe epilepsy associates with visual memory impairments.

E. The most common post-ictal symptoms and signs are confusion, headache, migraine paresis, wandering, ictal nose rub automatisms, coughing, dysmemory, amnesia, anxiety, panic, dysphoria/depression, agitation, combativeness, and psychosis.

F. Post-ictal headaches occur in children and adults, with migraine and headaches slightly more common in children. Post-ictal aggression is a rarely observed feature, occurring in approximately 0.5%. Post-ictal psychosis was noted in 4% of subjects.

G. The duration of post-ictal symptoms and signs is remarkably heterogeneous and difficult to quantify. Paresis, wandering, and automatisms tend to last less than 48 h.

H. Fatigue and depression have been reported to last from 10 min to approximately 12 days.

I. Post-ictal unresponsiveness has the highest mean-weighted proportion relative to the occurrence with pooled meta-analysis of higher quality studies.

J. In addition to the more dramatic or obvious post-ictal symptoms, exhaustion, frustration, shame, embarrassment, psychomotor slowing, and memory loss, more extreme mental symptoms include delirium and psychosis.
K. Physical symptoms to be aware of include sphincter incontinence, thirst, nausea, presyncope, myalgias, and frank joint pain. Always consider dislocations and fractures as possible causes of "paresis" or reduced range of motion of shoulders as they can accompany violent convulsive events in those at risk for pathological fractures.

Assessment in the Unconscious Child

An unconscious patient introduces limitations in the breadth and scope of the nursing neurological assessment. Any assessment elements that require cooperation and active participation are no longer available. The following guidance assumes mental status has been assessed and there is no eye opening or verbal response, even with stimulation. This could be due to either acute neurological condition or purposeful sedation with or without the use of paralytics. In this case, the nurse must resort to more primitive elements of the neurological assessment.

A. Cranial Nerves
    1. Pupillary Response—Pupillary response should be assessed in an unconscious child in the same manner as in an awake child. It is not uncommon for this to be one of the few assessment findings available in either severely neurologically impaired patients or those heavily sedated. Pinpoint pupils are a common finding in heavily sedated patients. Pupillometry can be a helpful tool in these circumstances.
    2. Cough or Gag—When pupillary assessment is not available (nonreactive or pinpoint), assessing gag and/or cough is an acceptable alternative to understand the brain stem function. Cough in an intubated patient can be assessed when suctioning. In a nonintubated patient, gag can be assessed by stroking the posterior of the oropharynx with a tongue depressor, suction catheter, etc.
B. Motor Function
    1. Movement—Unresponsive patients require more effort to stimulate movement. Assess for spontaneous, purposeful, or abnormal movement. Start by utilizing the same techniques for assessing responsiveness—verbal, light touch, and then noxious stimulus. Using a normal speaking voice or light touch, assess for spontaneous and/or purposeful movement. If neither are present, apply noxious stimuli and assess for withdrawal or localization. Noxious stimuli can be applied centrally or peripherally. Central stimuli include orbital notch pressure or trapezius pinch. Peripheral stimulation includes nail bed pressure. Response only to peripheral stimulation indicates spinal reflexes, not cerebral function. Assess both upper and lower motor functions, as well as right and left.

2. Localization—It is the act of reaching across the midline toward the central noxious stimuli on the opposite side. This is a positive finding and indicates intact sensation and cortical functioning [11].
3. Withdrawal—While applying peripheral stimulation (nail bed pressure), assess for reflexive movement, which does not cross midline, away from the stimulus. This reflects an intact thalamus with cortical impairment [11].
4. Nonpurposeful Movement—This includes withdrawal, muscle contractions, abnormal flexion (decorticate posturing), and abnormal flexion (decerebrate posturing) [11].

C. Vital Signs—In an unconscious patient with a limited exam, monitoring and interpreting vital signs in the context of neurological insult become even more critical. Often, these patients are intubated, so the nurse must heavily rely upon heart rate and blood pressure for both early and late signs of neurological decompensation. Blood pressure has a direct relationship to cerebral perfusion, as described below. Sustained bradycardia should be treated as an ominous sign and treated as such.

D. Intracranial Pressure (ICP)—When available, either with an implanted intracranial pressure monitor or a transduced external ventricular drain, understanding the intracranial pressure and correlating it to the neurological exam and vital signs can be the most valuable tool in understanding your patient's overall neurological status. Increased intracranial pressure can result in secondary neurological insult.

Due to ethical constraints, "normal" ICP in children has not been rigorously studied or defined; thus, pediatric norms are most often extrapolated from adult data, which shares lack of clear definition [12]. One study did find ICP to be inversely correlated to age, decreasing by 0.69 mmHg by a decade [13]. This would imply that the pediatric patient population can tolerate incrementally higher ICP than adults. Note that ICP can be very dependent on body position and activity and must be considered.

The managing provider team should define the ICP threshold specific to the patient, considering their age and pathological process. ICP and mean arterial pressure (MAP) must be considered together to understand the impact on the overall health of brain tissue. MAP must overcome ICP to allow for even minimal brain perfusion. This is measured as cerebral perfusion pressure (CPP). MAP minus ICP equals CCP (MAP−ICP = CPP).

References

1. DiBrito SR, Cerullo M, Goldstein SD, Ziegfeld S, Stewart D, Nasr IW. Reliability of Glasgow Coma Score in pediatric trauma patients. J Pediatr Surg. 2018;53(9):1789–94.
2. Caruana M, Hackenbruch SN, Grech V, Farrugia R. Inconsistency in the application of Glasgow Coma Scale in pediatric patients. Med Princ Pract. 2024;33(1):41–6.
3. Wijdicks EF, Bamlet WR, Maramattom BV, Manno EM, McClelland RL. Validation of a new coma scale: the FOUR score. Ann Neurol. 2005;58(4):585–93.

4. Czaikowski BL, Liang H, Stewart CT. A pediatric FOUR score coma scale: interrater reliability and predictive validity. J Neurosci Nurs. 2014;46(2):79–87.
5. Kirschen MP, Smith KA, Snyder M, et al. Serial Neurologic Assessment in Pediatrics (SNAP): a new tool for bedside neurologic assessment of critically ill children. Pediatr Crit Care Med. 2021;22(5):483–95.
6. Olson DM, Stutzman S, Saju C, Wilson M, Zhao W, Aiyagari V. Interrater reliability of pupillary assessments. Neurocrit care. 2016;24:251–7.
7. Martin TJ. Horner syndrome: a clinical review. ACS Chem Neurosci. 2018;9(2):177–86.
8. Dinallo S, Waseem M. Cushing reflex. StatPearls [Internet]. StatPearls Publishing; 2023.
9. Scharf RJ, Scharf GJ, Stroustrup A. Developmental milestones. Pediatr Rev. 2016;37(1):25–38.
10. Hair EC, Jager J, Garrett SB. Helping teens develop healthy social skills and relationships: what the research shows about navigating adolescence. 2002.
11. Hill M, Moreda M, Navarro J, Mulkey M. Assessing patients with altered level of consciousness. Crit Care Nurs. 2023;43(4):58–65.
12. Norager NH, Olsen MH, Pedersen SH, Riedel CS, Czosnyka M, Juhler M. Reference values for intracranial pressure and lumbar cerebrospinal fluid pressure: a systematic review. Fluids Barriers CNS. 2021;18:1–10.
13. Chambers I, Stobbart L, Jones P, et al. Age-related differences in intracranial pressure and cerebral perfusion pressure in the first 6 hours of monitoring after children's head injury: association with outcome. Child's Nerv Syst. 2005;21:195–9.
14. Chambers IR, Jones PA, Lo TM, et al. Critical thresholds of intracranial pressure and cerebral perfusion pressure related to age in paediatric head injury. J Neurol Neurosurg Psychiatry. 2006;77(2):234–40.

Suggested Reading

Cartwright C, Battick K, et al. Neurological assessment of the hospitalized child. 2023

Petersen MC, Kube DA, Whitaker TM, Graff JC, Palmer FB. Prevalence of developmental and behavioral disorders in a pediatric hospital. Pediatrics. 2009;123(3):e490–5. https://doi.org/10.1542/peds.2008-2750.

Horridge K. SINDA: standardized infant neuro developmental assessment an instrument for early detection of neurodevelopmental disorders Edited by Mijna Hadders-Algra Uta Tacke Joachim Pietz Heike Philippi. London: Mac Keith Press, 2022 £45.00 (Paperback), pp 200 ISBN: 9781911612612. Dev Med Child Neurol. 2022;64:924–5. https://doi.org/10.1111/dmcn.15179

DeMyer's The Neurologic Examination: A Programmed Text, 7e Eds. José Biller, et al. McGraw-Hill Education 2016

Shimony N, Jallo G. Pediatric neurosurgery board review: a comprehensive guide. 1st ed. Springer; 2023. https://doi.org/10.1007/978-3-031-23687-7.

Transport of the Critically Ill Neurologic Patient

Ladonna K. Bingham, Julie Bacon, and Christine Muller

Description

A critically ill neurologic patient may require movement to imaging, the ICU, operating room, or another hospital for a higher level of care. Transport of a critically ill patient is a high-risk event with the potential for adverse or unexpected events. Patient decompensation, herniation, cardiopulmonary arrest, loss of life-sustaining devices, extubation, equipment issues, and delay in medications and care are all documented adverse events during the transport of the critically ill. Prior to moving the patient, proper preparation should be made to have the needed personnel, medications, and equipment. Careful planning, ensuring qualified and trained personnel, and functioning equipment can minimize the risk of transport [1].

Intrahospital Transport

For transport within the hospital, an assessment of the patient should take place prior to transport. Patients with seizures, increased intracranial pressure, changes in mental status, agitation, concern for intracranial hemorrhage or herniation, apnea,

L. K. Bingham
Pediatric Critical Care Medicine, Critical Care Transport, Center for Simulation and Innovation Johns Hopkins All Children's Hospital Saint Petersburg, St. Petersburg, FL, USA
e-mail: lbingha2@jhmi.edu

J. Bacon
Chief Flight Nurse Lifeline Johns Hopkins All Children's Hospital Saint Petersburg, St. Petersburg, FL, USA
e-mail: julie.bacon@jhmi.edu

C. Muller (✉)
Hough Family Institute for Brain Protection Sciences Johns Hopkins All Children's Hospital Saint Petersburg, St. Petersburg, FL, USA
e-mail: cmuller5@jhmi.edu

K. Battick et al. (eds.), *Nursing Guide for Pediatric Neuroscience Patients*,
https://doi.org/10.1007/978-3-032-22664-8_2

changes in breathing patterns, intubation, desaturations, bradycardia, tachycardia, hypotension, hypertension, arrhythmias, or poor perfusion should be considered high-risk, and appropriate personnel and equipment should be available before transport. Prior studies have shown a change in vital signs in as many as 70% of critically ill pediatric patients during transport and equipment-related problems in 10% of intrahospital transports [2, 3]. Several factors have been reported to decrease morbidity and mortality associated with transport, including optimizing patient status prior to transport, staff training on safe transport practices, familiarity with the transport equipment, prechecking the equipment, and having experienced clinicians accompany the patient on transport [4–6].

Intrahospital transport can be divided into three phases: the pre-transport or planning stage, the transport, and the post-transport phase. The pre-transport phase should include good communication between the physicians and nurses in both the sending and receiving areas. The team caring for the patient should decide who needs to be present for safe transfer of the patient. For critically ill patients, two trained staff should move the patient. If the patient is intubated or at risk of decompensation, a respiratory therapist or someone who can manage the airway should be present. If the patient is at risk of herniation, instability, arrest, or need for intubation, a provider should travel with the patient.

Preparing the patient:

1. In patients with high ICP (intracranial pressure), the head should be kept midline with the chin in a neutral position and the head of the bed elevated to 30 degrees whenever possible [7].
2. If there is concern for spinal injury, a proper sized collar should be used, and the cervical spine should be held during transfers and repositioning.
3. If there is concern for acute mental status changes or decompensation, GCS less than 8, or increased ICP with pCO2 above 40, the patient should be intubated. The goal pCO2 for patients with increased ICP is in the mid-30s.
4. The patient's vital signs should be assessed for stability prior to moving.
5. Seizures are common in patients with head injuries and should be treated immediately.
6. All lines and tubes should be properly secured to prevent dislodgement, which is a frequent adverse event during transport. The ETT (endotracheal tube), central line, EVD (external ventricular drain), ICP monitor cords, and tubing should be carefully placed so that there is no tension on them during transport.
7. Any medications that may be needed should be available, and all drips should have ample medication available for transport.
8. A transport checklist such as the one below can be utilized to prepare for a safe transport.

Pre-transport intrahospital checklist for transfers between the EC, OR, ICU, and/or radiology should include the following:

1. Nursing report given to the receiving unit?
2. Oxygen (full tank) placed on bed?
3. Bag valve mask with proper size mask connected, even if the patient is intubated?
4. Working portable suction on bed?
5. Patient connected to monitor/defibrillator/ETCO2/pulse ox?
6. EVD-clamped before moving the patient or bed? Remember to keep the system upright.
7. ICP should be monitoring the pressures during transport.
8. Emergency medications:
   (a) Seizure/sedation—benzodiazepine
   (b) Intracranial hypertension—mannitol or 3% hypertonic saline
   (c) Cardiac decompensation—epinephrine
   (d) Consider paralytic if intubated
9. Any drips should have at least three times more medication than needed for transport.
10. NS or LR connected with tubing for bolus and/or flushing medications?
11. All tubes and lines well secured, especially ETT, arterial line, EVD, and central line?
12. Blankets/warming pad available for patients at risk of hypothermia (especially infants).
13. Patient should be calm and cooperative or appropriately sedated and restrained.
14. Equipment should be properly working with ample battery available.
15. Before moving, assess the patient and their vital signs. Do you have necessary personnel (RN, RT, MD if unstable)? Generally, a critical patient should have at least two trained personnel for transport.
16. If the patient is intubated, an RT should be present and holding the secured tube during any repositioning or transfers of patient between beds. ETT position should be confirmed before and after transport. Know the goal ETCO2, which should be in the 30s with increased ICP.
17. Keep the head midline during transport. Someone should hold c-spine during repositioning and transfers if there is concern for spinal injury.
18. Additional blood products and push–pull setups if patient requires or has required a massive transfusion.
19. Enteral nutrition, if being given, should be off during transport.
20. Before you move–is the receiving area ready for the patient?

During the transport phase, the patient should have the following measures:

1. Continuous monitoring which includes mental status, pulse oximetry, heart rate, telemetry, and frequent blood pressure checks.
2. Continuous ETCO2 monitoring is considered the standard of care if the patient is intubated. The goal for ETCO2 and pCO2 with increased ICP is lower 30s.
3. If the patient has an EVD, it should be clamped prior to moving the patient or repositioning in bed.

4. Intracranial pressure can also be monitored if an ICP monitor has been placed. Generally, an ICP of greater than 20 mmHg is considered high, and a physician should be aware of the elevated ICP. Therapies to try and bring down the ICP include the following:
   (a) Positioning the head midline to improve venous drainage. Check to make sure the monitor is zeroed.
   (b) Elevating the head of the bed to 30 degrees.
   (c) Giving additional sedation.
   (d) If these measures do not work, mannitol or 3% hypertonic saline can be used to help reduce cerebral edema.
   (e) Pentobarbital and paralysis can also be trialed.
5. Patients with critical illness or increased ICP need an appropriate blood pressure for cerebral perfusion, so a goal MAP should be selected prior to transport. Epinephrine or norepinephrine can be used to maintain the MAP.
6. The c-spine should be stabilized during transport with a cervical collar.
7. Cushing's triad is the combination of bradycardia, hypertension, and change in respiration and is a sign of increased ICP and impending brain herniation. A physician should be aware of these vital sign changes and ICP treated immediately [5].

In the post-transport phase:

1. Monitoring of the heart rate, saturation, blood pressure, ICP, and ETCO2 should continue.
2. Patient placed in bed with head midline and bed elevated 30 degrees, if concern for ICP.
3. If the EVD was clamped for transport, it should be unclamped and leveled.
4. The ICP monitor will need to be zeroed.
5. Mental status and pupils should be checked.
6. Nursing should verify medications and drips.
7. IV lines will need to be untangled and checked that they are not kinked or clamped.
8. The endotracheal tube depth should be checked and good bilateral breath sounds and appropriate ETCO2 confirmed.
9. Other tubes such as the NG, Replogle, Salem Sump, or chest tubes should be reattached to suction or appropriate drainage containers [8].

Sample: Pre-transport Checklist for Transports Within the Hospital

Equipment and materials	Yes	No	N/A
Monitor/defibrillator			
Bag-valve-mask			
Sufficient oxygen			
IV tubing (extra for MRI)			
Discontinue feeds			

Equipment and materials	Yes	No	N/A
Pumps charged and working			
Portable suction			
Lines and tubes secure			
Clamp EVD before moving			
Medications:			
Sufficient IV medication			
Sufficient sedation			
Sufficient inotropes			
Mannitol or 3% hypertonic saline			
Emergency seizure med			
Paralytic			
Additional meds			
CT scan with contrast?	Yes	No	N/A
Large bore IV			
Enteral contrast given			
Renal protection given			
Monitor:			
ICP monitoring			
Telemetry, sat, bp			
Alarms on and audible			
Continuous ETCO2			
Arterial line			
Head midline			
Transport ventilator:			
On/working			
O2 on/enough in tank			
ETT depth			
RN, RT, MD available			
Receiving unit ready			
Blood products needed			

Sample: Reminders During Intrahospital Transport

Monitor:
Frequent vital signs (q5–15 min)
Telemetry
Intercranial pressure
Oxygen saturations
Continuous ETCO2
Equipment:
Unclamp EVD if able in radiology?
Notify provider for:
Change in mental status or pupils
Increase in ICP or ICP >20
Desaturation, apnea or respiratory distress
Changes in telemetry
Bradycardia
Hypo- or hypertension
Seizures

Sample: Post-transport Checklist for Transports Within the Hospital

Equipment:
Move back to unit monitor
Elevate head of bed 30 degrees
Check ICP
Level EVD and Unclamp
Place back on ventilator with humidity
Verify ETT depth
Continuous ETCO2 monitoring
Ensure appropriate vital signs
Untangle IV tubing
Check medications and pumps
Place NG to suction
Physical exam:
Check pupils and mental status, head midline
Bilateral breath sounds
Perfusion
Notify provider for:
Change in mental status or pupils
Increase in ICP or ICP >20
Desaturation, apnea or change in breath sounds
Changes in telemetry
Bradycardia or tachycardia
Hypo- or hypertension
Seizures

Interhospital Transport

Some patients require transport to another hospital for imaging, surgery, or specialty pediatric care. Critically ill patients are at high risk of morbidity or mortality during transport. All monitoring and care should continue during interhospital transport. In general, the level of care should not decrease during transport. Transport should be performed by a minimum of two personnel with transport training, usually one person as an RN, with the second being an RT, RN, or paramedic. There is lower morbidity and mortality when a specialized pediatric critical care team is utilized, and the patient receives the same level of monitoring and care that is available in the ICU. There will be times and locations when such a team is not available, so each institution should have alternative plans in place and be aware of resources available to them such as local adult critical care teams and EMS. There are minimum standards for the transport of critically ill children, and any service performing these transports should at least meet these guidelines [1]. This includes continuous monitoring of telemetry, heart rate, and pulse oximetry using equipment appropriately sized for pediatrics. Frequent blood pressure monitoring and assessment of pupils and mental status should be performed. Transport personnel should be able to treat the possible emergencies for that patient such as intubation for apnea or respiratory failure, identification and treatment of seizures, management of arrhythmias and blood pressure, treatment of ICP, and cardiopulmonary arrest.

When a new team assumes care of the patient, there should be a physician-to-physician conversation with the receiving physician accepting the patient. During this conversation, the referring physician should ask for advice if needed and the receiving physician should offer medical advice for stabilizing and treating the patient. Unnecessary lab and radiologic studies should be avoided prior to transfer. Also, during this conversation, a mode of transport should be selected and agreed upon. Traditionally, the referring physician chooses the team and mode of transport, but many pediatric centers with subspecialty services offer pediatric critical care transport teams and utilize a mode of transport matrix. The literature does not support a scoop-and-run approach to interfacility transport. Studies show increased mortality and loss of life-sustaining equipment when transferred by a general helicopter team instead of a pediatric critical care team, "which brings the ICU to the patient". Most pediatric patients, including trauma cases, do not go emergently to the operating room except for a few surgical emergencies such as a large epidural hematoma or mass with midline shift, acute symptomatic hydrocephalus, spinal fracture with associated neurological injury, and penetrating injury with unstable vital signs. Such patients would suffer irreversible harm if there is a delay in neurosurgical intervention; hence, the fastest mode of transport should be used. This may be one-way ground transport, EMS, or helicopter. The referring hospitals should be aware that there is often a delay when using EMS because new 911 calls take priority over patients already in a hospital. Likewise, helicopter providers will often not specify if there will be delays due to simultaneous calls. When scheduling the transport, the time of arrival for the transport team should be established. If there are delays in getting a local team or helicopter to bedside, the pediatric critical care transport team from the receiving hospital should be used. A specialized pediatric critical care team should be used for patients who require close neurological monitoring or ICU level care but are not in need of immediate surgical intervention. Environmental stressors such as vibration, movement, and temperature changes can cause significant changes to heart rate, blood pressure, and ICP during transport. For transports greater than 200 miles, a fixed wing aircraft may need to be utilized. This usually takes longer to coordinate, and the transport team should be well-trained in flight physiology and the effects it will have on the patient. If there is a pneumothorax, it should be decompressed prior to fixed wing flight. The stomach should also be decompressed and cuffs on tubes such as the ETT and foley fluid-filled prior to takeoff.

The referring hospital should place an IV and begin stabilizing the patient while waiting for the transport team. Missed diagnosis and missed treatments worsen outcomes. Oxygenation, ventilation, and perfusion should be treated prior to and during transport. Medical emergencies such as pneumothorax and hemorrhage should also be treated. Studies show improved mental status and survival when critically ill and trauma patients are resuscitated early [9]. A nurse-to-nurse communication should also occur prior to the patient leaving the referring institution. A consent or EMTALA form should be signed by the family; if the family is not available in a life-threatening emergency, this should be documented in the medical record with reasons for transfer [1].

A checklist such as the EMSC Pediatric Transport Checklist [10] or the one below should be utilized.

Interfacility Preparation Checklist

Called receiving hospital, name of accepting physician ______________________
Special equipment/DME for patient including extra trachs, ventilator parts or feeding tubes
Any continuous meds or fluids with 3 times more in bag than needed for transport
Patient NPO or any enteral feeds stopped
Lines and tubes secured
Chart copied including vitals, physical exam, MAR, labs
Copy of X-rays and imaging studies or pushed to cloud
All forms including Backer Act or DNR form
Consent or EMTALA form signed by family
Sign out given to receiving nurse

A resuscitated patient with appropriate oxygenation, ventilation, heart rate, and blood pressure will handle transport with the fewest emergencies and have the best chance of full recovery without brain or organ injury. To smooth the transition and facilitate timely transport, it is helpful to the transport team if the following actions have been taken. These items should not delay the call to the receiving hospital or the patient leaving with the transport team but are things that can be done to improve patient care while waiting for the transport team to arrive.

1. A combative patient is unsafe for transport. So, if needed, the patient should be on sedation with 3 times more medication than needed for transport in a syringe/bag.
2. Seizure prophylaxis done (if applicable), and seizures treated.
3. In bed with head midline and head of bed elevated to 30 degrees, if ICP elevated.
4. Appropriately sized neck collar in place. Appropriately secured to backboard, if spinal injury.
5. Patient intubated, if necessary, on a ventilator with appropriate settings and continuous waveform capnography and blood gas performed.
6. Chest X-ray to verify ETT position.
7. Chest tube placed if needed.
8. IV or IO access obtained.
9. Blood pressure in appropriate range for age/size. If requiring vasoactives, the syringe or bag should have 3 times more medication than needed for the transport available.
10. Normal saline, lactated Ringers or maintenance IVFs running.
11. Labs printed and available.
12. Salem sump or Replogle in place.
13. Chart copied and already at bedside.
14. It is helpful to give the family realistic expectations for transport and outcomes. Most teams do not allow family in the back of the ambulance but allow a

caregiver to ride up front. Not all teams allow a parent to fly, so ask what the policy is for family to ride along.

15. If there is a significant chance that the patient may die during transport or while the receiving hospital tries to get them emergently to the operating room, the family should be aware that this is a concern.

For the Interhospital Transport Team

Transport should not lower the level of care. Any team transporting a pediatric neurologically critically ill patient should be trained and competent to manage the patient and possible emergencies related to their illness. They should also have training on the transport environment and risks of transport. During transport, the patient should have the following:

1. All tubes and lines well secured, especially ETT, arterial line, EVD, and central line.
2. Continuous monitoring which includes mental status, pulse oximetry, heart rate, telemetry, and frequent blood pressure checks.
3. Frequent neuro checks and assessments of pupils. Change in pupils can be a marker of increasing intracranial pressure, herniation, or seizure.
4. Seizures should be treated; benzodiazepines can be used as first-line treatment.
5. Patient should be calm and cooperative or appropriately sedated and restrained.
6. If the patient has an EVD, it should be clamped prior to moving the patient or repositioning in bed.
7. Intracranial pressure can also be monitored if an ICP monitor has been placed. Generally, an ICP of greater than 20 mmHg is considered high. Therapies to try and bring down the ICP include the following:
   (a) Positioning the head midline to improve venous drainage. Check to make sure the monitor is zeroed.
   (b) Elevating the head of the bed 30 degrees.
   (c) Giving additional sedation.
   (d) If these measures do not work, mannitol or 3% hypertonic saline can be used to help reduce cerebral edema.
8. Patients with critical illness or increased ICP need an appropriate blood pressure for cerebral perfusion, so a goal MAP should be selected prior to transport. Epinephrine or norepinephrine can be used to maintain the MAP.
9. If needed, the c-spine should be stabilized during transport with a cervical collar and backboard.
8. Cushing's triad is the combination of bradycardia, hypertension, and change in respiration and is a sign of increased ICP and impending brain herniation. Elevated ICP should be treated immediately [7].

9. Continuous ETCO2 monitoring is considered the standard of care if the patient is intubated. The goal for ETCO2 and pCO2 with increased ICP is 35 but could be lowered to 30 if there are signs of impending brain herniation.
10. ETCO2 can also be used to monitor patients with decreased mental status.
11. Blankets or warming pads are used for patients at risk of hypothermia (especially infants).

References

1. Warren J, Fromm RE Jr, Orr RA, Rotello LC, Horst HM, American College of Critical Care Medicine. Guidelines for the inter- and intrahospital transport of critically ill patients. Crit Care Med. 2004;32(1):256–62. https://doi.org/10.1097/01.CCM.0000104917.39204.0A. PMID: 14707589
2. Wallen E, Venkataraman ST, Grosso MJ, Kiene K, Orr RA. Intrahospital transport of critically ill pediatric patients. Crit Care Med. 1995;23(9):1588–95. https://doi.org/10.1097/00003246-199509000-00020. PMID: 7664562
3. Papson JP, Russell KL, Taylor DM. Unexpected events during the intrahospital transport of critically ill patients. Acad Emerg Med. 2007;14(6):574–7. https://doi.org/10.1197/j.aem.2007.02.034. PMID: 17535981
4. Haydar B, Baetzel A, Elliott A, MacEachern M, Kamal A, Christensen R. Adverse events during intrahospital transport of critically ill children: a systematic review. Anesth Analg. 2020;131(4):1135–45. https://doi.org/10.1213/ANE.0000000000004585. PMID: 32925334
5. Harish MM, Siddiqui SS, Prabu NR, Chaudhari HK, Divatia JV, Kulkarni AP. Benefits of and untoward events during intrahospital transport of pediatric intensive care unit patients. Indian J Crit Care Med. 2017;21(1):46–8. https://doi.org/10.4103/0972-5229.198326. PMID: 28197051; PMCID: PMC5278590
6. Venn AM, Sotomayor CA, Godambe SA, Vazifedan T, Jennings AD, Qureshi FA, Mullan PC. Implementation of an intrahospital transport checklist for emergency department admissions to intensive care. Pediatr Qual Saf. 2021;6(4):e426. https://doi.org/10.1097/pq9.0000000000000426. PMID: 34235354; PMCID: PMC8225371
7. Pinto VL, Tadi P, Adeyinka A. Increased intracranial pressure. [Updated 2023 Jul 31]. In: StatPearls [Internet]. Treasure Island: StatPearls Publishing; 2025. Available from: https://www.ncbi.nlm.nih.gov/books/NBK482119/.
8. Brunsveld-Reinders AH, Arbous MS, Kuiper SG, de Jonge E. A comprehensive method to develop a checklist to increase safety of intra-hospital transport of critically ill patients. Crit Care. 2015;19(1):214. https://doi.org/10.1186/s13054-015-0938-1. PMID: 25947327; PMCID: PMC4438434
9. Little WK. Golden hour or golden opportunity: early management of pediatric trauma. Clin Pediatr Emerg Med. 2010;11(1):4–9., ISSN 1522-8401,. https://doi.org/10.1016/j.cpem.2009.12.005.
10. EMSC Pediatric Transport Checklist. https://media.emscimprovement.center/documents/Provider_Check_List_V8_1.pdf

Intracranial Pressure Monitoring in Pediatric Neurosurgery: Nursing Management and Care

Guirish Solanki, Katie Herbert, Tracey Rowberry, Amy Drew, and Fardad Afshari

Abbreviations

BTF	Brain Trauma Foundation
BP	Blood pressure
CCRN	Critical Care Registered Nurse
CFAM	Cerebral Function Analyzer Monitor
CNS	Central nervous system
CNRN	Certified Neuroscience Registered Nurse
CPP	Cerebral perfusion pressure
CSF	Cerebrospinal fluid
CT	Computed tomography
EEG	Electroencephalogram
EVD	External ventricular drain
GCS	Glasgow Coma Score
ICU	Intensive care unit
ICP	Intracranial pressure
kPa	Kilopascals

G. Solanki (✉) · K. Herbert · F. Afshari
Department of Neurosurgery, Birmingham Women's and Children's Hospital, Birmingham, West Midlands, UK
e-mail: guirish.solanki@nhs.net; katie.herbert@nhs.net; fardad.afshari@nhs.net

T. Rowberry
Neurocritical Care Lead & Paediatric Critical Care, Birmingham Women's and Children's Hospital, Birmingham, West Midlands, UK
e-mail: tracey.rowberry@nhs.net

A. Drew
Department of Craniofacial Surgery, Birmingham Women's and Children's Hospital, Birmingham, West Midlands, UK
e-mail: amy.drew@nhs.net

K. Battick et al. (eds.), *Nursing Guide for Pediatric Neuroscience Patients*,
https://doi.org/10.1007/978-3-032-22664-8_3

mmHg	Millimeters of mercury
MRI	Magnetic resonance imaging
NIRS	Near-infrared spectroscopy
NICE	National Institute for Health and Care Excellence
NPi	Neurological Pupil Index
ONSD	Optic nerve sheath diameter
$PaCO_2$	Partial pressure of carbon dioxide
PICU	Pediatric intensive care unit
SIGN	Scottish Intercollegiate Guidelines Network
SOP	Standard operating protocol
TBI	Traumatic brain injury
TCD	Transcranial Doppler
WHO	World Health Organization

Nursing Care and Protocols for ICP Monitoring

Effective nursing management of ICP monitors is vital to ensure accurate readings and patient safety. This includes the proper setup and calibration of devices, vigilant monitoring, maintenance of system integrity, troubleshooting false or absent readings, and thorough documentation. Nursing care must also encompass measures to prevent secondary increases in ICP and respond to monitor alarms appropriately. In the following sections, we detail nursing protocols for each monitoring method.

General Nursing Considerations

Core nursing principles for neurologically compromised pediatric patients include maintaining sedation and analgesia to prevent agitation, optimizing nutrition, maintaining a good bowel regime, avoiding fever, and positioning the head in a neutral midline position with the bed elevated ~30° to aid venous drainage, and minimizing environmental stressors. Positioning alterations may occur due to cervical spine stability in some traumatic brain injuries. Pain is managed aggressively as per NICE guidelines, and care activities are clustered where possible to allow rest while avoiding simultaneous stimuli that could raise ICP. In PICU, procedural sedation can be used prior to painful interventions. Airway management is crucial, with suctioning performed only as needed and with pre-oxygenation to prevent hypoxia or hypercarbia. Hourly neurologic assessments (e.g., consciousness using the Glasgow Coma Score, pupil reactivity, limb movement) are documented alongside ICP values. In PICU, cerebral perfusion pressure (CPP) values may also be calculated and documented. Any discrepancies between clinical signs and ICP readings should prompt troubleshooting or further investigation as per local observation and monitoring policies. Interdisciplinary communication is essential for addressing sustained ICP elevations or concerning trends.

Classification of ICP Monitoring Methods

Invasive Techniques

Invasive methods directly measure pressure inside the skull, providing the most accurate ICP readings:

- *External Ventricular Drain (EVD)*
  Catheter placed in lateral ventricle; allows accurate ICP measurement and therapeutic cerebrospinal fluid (CSF) drainage. Considered most accurate due to bedside calibration capability but does not offer a continuous monitoring capability due to the need for CSF drainage.
- *Intraparenchymal Monitors*
  Small transducers (fiber-optic or strain-gauge) placed directly into brain tissue (usually frontal lobe); provide continuous ICP readings without CSF drainage capability. Highly accurate, but may experience baseline drift over time.
- *Subdural/Epidural Sensors*
  Less invasive (no penetration of brain tissue), placed in subdural or epidural spaces; less commonly used due to reduced accuracy and calibration issues, usually inserted intraoperatively for post-surgical monitoring.
- *Lumbar CSF Pressure*
  Performed in cases of suspected or known idiopathic intracranial hypertension or pseudotumor cerebri to assess the baseline CSF pressure or for regular monitoring and therapeutic drainage to lower CSF pressure.
- *Lumbar CSF Drains*
  Indirect ICP monitoring through spinal CSF drainage; *mainly therapeutic* rather than precise ICP measurement. Must be carefully managed to prevent complications.
- *Telemetric ICP Monitors*
  Implantable wireless sensors transmit ICP data transcutaneously; emerging technology mainly for long-term monitoring, not yet common in pediatric settings.

Each invasive method has distinct indications. Generally, EVDs are preferred if ventricles are accessible due to combined monitoring and therapeutic capabilities outside of the PICU. Intraparenchymal monitors are alternatives for small ventricles or bilateral comparisons, preferential in PICU due to continuous multimodal monitoring capabilities. Risks of invasive monitoring (infection, hemorrhage) are low but require careful techniques.

Noninvasive Techniques

Noninvasive methods estimate ICP without skull penetration, avoiding risks but offering lower accuracy, used mostly as supplementary tools:

- *Clinical Examination*
  Frequent neurological assessments for signs of raised ICP (e.g., fontanelle bulging in infants, headache, and altered mental status in older children). Quantitative pupillometry objectively tracks pupil reactivity changes related to ICP.
- *Optic Nerve Sheath Diameter (ONSD) Ultrasound*
  Ultrasound measurement through the eyelid; enlarged ONSD suggests raised ICP. Quick bedside method, useful for trend monitoring rather than precise ICP values.
- *Transcranial Doppler (TCD) Ultrasonography*
  Measures cerebral blood flow velocities; changes in pulsatility indicate ICP shifts indirectly. Requires skill and provides trends rather than exact ICP values.
- *Neuroimaging (CT/MRI)*
  Detects signs of raised ICP (midline shift, edema) but not reliable for excluding elevated ICP alone; clinical assessment still necessary.
- *Near-Infrared Spectroscopy (NIRS)*
  Continuous, noninvasive monitoring of cerebral oxygenation (rSO_2); indirectly suggests ICP increases but influenced by other factors, providing trends rather than absolute values.
- *Tympanic Membrane Displacement*
  Experimental, nonroutine technique assessing ICP indirectly via ear pressure response; not commonly used clinically.
- *CSF Outflow Analysis*
  Experimental methods estimating intracranial compliance; specialized use, semi-invasive, not routinely practiced.

Overall, noninvasive methods are supportive tools rather than replacements, indicating potential ICP changes and guiding decisions for invasive monitoring.

Nursing Management of External Ventricular Drains (EVDs)

- *Setup and Calibration*: Accurate EVD setup involves aligning the transducer's zero-reference point with the foramen of Monro (typically at the tragus level). The system is leveled and zeroed to atmospheric pressure at least once per shift or after interruptions. The drainage system height is adjusted with head-of-bed changes to maintain alignment. Drainage pressure levels are set as per provider orders, with protocols varying between intermittent or continuous drainage methods. Accurate ICP readings require momentarily closing the drain during measurement which poses risk if not reopened to drain in those reliant on CSF drainage to reduce ICP.
- *Monitoring and Maintenance*: Nurses perform hourly checks of ICP values, CSF volume drained, and CSF characteristics (e.g., clarity, color). The system is inspected hourly for kinks, air bubbles, or clots. Dressing integrity at the insertion site is monitored for dryness and signs of CSF leakage. Overdrainage

precautions include clamping the drain during patient repositioning and re-leveling it afterward.

- *ICP Waveform Assessment*: Nurses assess waveform morphology (e.g., P1–P2–P3 peaks) to identify rising ICP or technical issues like dampened waveforms. Troubleshooting includes checking for occlusions, air bubbles, or transducer misalignment.
- *Troubleshooting and Avoiding Misreading*: If readings are inconsistent with clinical signs, nurses systematically inspect the catheter, tubing, and transducer connections. Flushing is avoided unless ordered due to infection risks; lowering the drainage chamber briefly can confirm patency. Equipment issues are resolved step-by-step while keeping the neurosurgeons and the intensivists informed.
- *CSF Drainage and Temporary Clamping*: Nurses follow specific orders and local protocols for opening or closing drains based on ICP thresholds. Overdrainage risks are mitigated by maintaining prescribed chamber levels and clamping during repositioning. All suspicions of a blocked EVD are urgently escalated to the neurosurgical team after local troubleshooting (local guidance should be followed).
- *Infection Prevention*: Infection control includes keeping dressings sterile and dry, using strict aseptic techniques during system access, and minimizing manipulation. Fever prompts CSF sampling for infection evaluation.

Documentation Detailed records include hourly ICP values, CSF volume drained, waveform observations, neurological assessments including pupillary shape, size, symmetry, and reactivity along with the GCS (if nonsedated or anesthetized), interventions (e.g., drain adjustments), alarm settings, and troubleshooting steps. This ensures continuity of care and provides a medicolegal record of monitoring accuracy.

Nursing Management for ICP Monitoring

- *Setup and Calibration*: Intraparenchymal ICP monitors, such as fiber-optic or microchip probes, are pre-calibrated by the manufacturer, neurosurgeon, or PICU nurses before insertion. Unlike EVDs, they do not require bedside zeroing post-insertion, except for specific devices like pneumatic strain gauges that allow recalibration. It is therefore vital that calibration is performed prior to insertion. In PICU, ICP may integrate with other multimodal monitoring systems that will need calibrating as per local guidance each shift. Nurses assist with setup, procedural support, documentation, and ensuring proper cable connections and confirming initial readings for accuracy. Alarm settings for minimum and maximum allowed pressures and detailed intervention instructions are set in the monitoring systems and recorded. Device-specific calibration procedures should be followed as per manufacturer and hospital guidelines.
- *Securing and Site Care*: These probes are anchored to the skull via bolts or sutures, with cables secured to prevent accidental displacement. The insertion

site is covered with a sterile dressing, which is inspected daily for infection signs like redness or swelling. Dressing changes follow hospital protocols, maintaining strict aseptic techniques.

- *Monitoring and Troubleshooting*: Continuous ICP monitoring requires nurses to set alarm limits (e.g., 20 mmHg) and watch for baseline drift over time. Discrepancies between clinical signs and monitor readings may indicate drift or malfunction. Nurses troubleshoot by checking connections, replacing cables if needed, and ensuring cables remain dry and intact. Dislodged monitors require immediate sterile coverage and neurosurgical notification.
- *Use and Limitations*: Intraparenchymal monitors provide localized pressure readings, which may vary due to intracranial gradients in cases of focal lesions. Bilateral monitors may be used in rare cases, requiring clear labeling and diligent monitoring of each side for therapeutic decisions.
- *Documentation*: Nurses document hourly ICP and/or CPP values, neurological assessments, site conditions, and any technical issues or interventions. Detailed records ensure continuity of care and provide a medicolegal record of monitoring accuracy and patient safety.

Nursing Considerations for Noninvasive ICP Monitoring

Though less technically demanding than invasive methods, noninvasive ICP monitoring requires nurses to ensure accurate data collection, proper techniques, and thoughtful integration of findings into patient care.

- *Neurologic Assessments*
  Frequent neurological observations (consciousness, pupils, limb movement) are essential as per local guidance Subtle changes like increased sleepiness, delayed responses, or motor deficits should raise concern. In infants, assess fontanelle (bulging when calm/upright = possible raised ICP) and measure head circumference daily if ordered, using a consistent technique.
- *Pupillometry*
  Use the same device and method each time. Document the pupil size and Neurological Pupil Index (NPi); values <3 or a drop >0.7 from baseline or a difference in NPi of >0.7 between the left and right pupil suggest concern and require escalation to a clinician.
- *Optic Nerve Sheath Ultrasound (ONSD)*
  Nurses support the procedure by positioning the child (midline, eyes closed), assisting if needed, and recording results. Enlarged sheath (>5–6 mm depending on age) may indicate raised ICP.
- *Transcranial Doppler (TCD)*
  Coordinate timing, position the child appropriately, and document vitals. Note ventilatory status, as $PaCO_2$ affects pulsatility index. Report any findings suggesting poor cerebral compliance and document reported mean flow velocity (MFV) and pulsatility index (PI).

- *Near-Infrared Spectroscopy (NIRS)*
  Ensure good sensor contact and troubleshoot signal issues. Escalate concerns of low rSO_2 (<50–60%), sudden drops (>20%), or a difference of 10–20% between the left and right hemispheres and cross-check with vitals and exam.
- *Data Integration*
  Nurses synthesize trends across tools (e.g., rising ONSD, high TCD PI, drowsiness) to identify potential ICP elevation early—even before a monitor is placed. Early communication of clinical concern is vital.

Summary

Noninvasive monitoring relies on the nurse's clinical judgment, proper technique, and pattern recognition. Accurate documentation of all assessments (neurological exams, pupillometry, ONSD, etc.) builds a clear picture of evolving intracranial status and guides escalation of care when needed.

Patient Care in the PICU Versus Ward Settings

PICU Care In the PICU, children with ICP monitors receive intensive care with a high nurse-to-patient ratio (1:1 or 1:2), enabling continuous monitoring and rapid interventions. Patients are often intubated and sedated, especially in severe cases like traumatic brain injury (GCS ≤8). Nurses manage ICP spikes by adjusting ventilator settings under provider guidance, administering hyperosmolar therapy, or initiating tiered protocols for ICP thresholds. Advanced equipment, such as arterial and central venous lines, allows real-time calculation of cerebral perfusion pressure (CPP) and precise management with vasoactive infusions. The environment is tightly controlled to reduce stimuli that could exacerbate ICP, with measures like pre-oxygenation before suctioning and spacing care activities. Continuous end-tidal CO_2 monitoring supports temporary hyperventilation strategies. Neurosurgeons and intensivists are readily available for emergencies, ensuring immediate escalation when needed.

Ward Care On the ward, the nurse-to-patient ratio is lower (1:3 or 1:4), and care focuses on stabilized patients transitioning out of critical care. Continuous ICP monitoring may be replaced by intermittent readings, with nurses relying more on clinical observations to detect changes. Patients are often more mobile, requiring strict safety measures such as bed alarms, sitter supervision for younger children, and securing EVD tubing to prevent dislodgment. Nurses ensure proper leveling of EVDs and sterile handling while educating families about safety precautions, such as avoiding head repositioning or interfering with the drain. Family involvement is crucial for monitoring and preventing complications.

Monitoring Frequency Differences In the PICU, vital signs and ICP are continuously monitored and recorded hourly or more frequently during crises. On the ward, documentation may occur less often (e.g., CSF output every 2–4 h), focusing on clinical signs like headache or vomiting to detect elevated ICP. Nurses escalate care to the PICU if neurologic status worsens or ICP trends upward.

Resource Availability The PICU is equipped for immediate interventions like mannitol administration or intubation during ICP surges. On the ward, such resources require calling a Rapid Response team, emphasizing that active ICP management issues should remain in the PICU until fully stabilized.

Communication and Handover Transitioning patients from PICU to ward requires thorough handover to ensure continuity of care. The PICU nurse educates ward staff on device management protocols and signs of complications. Competency training for ward nurses is essential for managing devices like EVDs safely. Neurosurgery NPs or ICU outreach teams often support ward staff in managing complex cases.

Family Education Parents are educated about the function of ICP monitors or drains, safety measures, and how to respond to alarms or changes in the child's condition. Their presence can help soothe the child and reduce agitation-related ICP spikes while ensuring they do not interfere with medical equipment.

In summary, PICU care offers intensive surveillance and immediate intervention for unstable ICP patients, while ward care supports stabilized cases with less frequent monitoring but requires vigilance in detecting clinical changes and ensuring safety protocols are followed. Both settings demand meticulous observation and prompt action to safeguard patient outcomes.

Complications of ICP Monitoring and Their Prevention

ICP monitoring, while essential, carries risks. Nurses play a critical role in preventing, detecting, and responding to complications such as *infection, hemorrhage, catheter obstruction, device malfunction, over drainage*, and *accidental dislodgment*.

Infection (Ventriculitis/Meningitis)

Occurs in up to 10% of pediatric EVD cases. Caused by microbial entry during insertion or handling.

Prevention:
- Strict aseptic technique
- Minimize system access
- Antimicrobial catheters or single-dose prophylactic antibiotics if protocol allows
  Signs: Fever, altered mental status, cloudy/bloody CSF
  Action: Obtain CSF cultures, anticipate device replacement, assess daily for EVD removal

Hemorrhage

Low but serious risk (~1–2%) during insertion or from chronic over-drainage.

Prevention:
- Check and correct coagulation labs pre-procedure.
- Avoid excessive drainage or lowering chamber below ordered level.
- Monitor for neurological changes or bulging fontanelle.
  Action: Suspected bleeding may require imaging and drainage adjustments.

Catheter Obstruction

Often caused by clots or debris; results in false ICP readings and reduced drainage.

Prevention:
- Monitor for flat waveform or absent CSF despite high ICP.
- Maintain proper positioning and avoid stagnant blood in tubing.
  Action: Gentle flushing only per protocol; notify neurosurgery if blockage persists.

Monitor Malfunction/Measurement Drift

Sensor drift can lead to inaccurate ICP values.

Prevention:
- Correlate readings with the clinical condition.
- Perform periodic checks if zeroing is available.
  Action: Report inconsistencies; rely on clinical assessment while troubleshooting.

Over-Drainage or Pressure Fluctuations

Excessive CSF loss can cause headaches, slit ventricles, or subdural bleeds.

Prevention:

- Follow prescribed drain levels; clamp before repositioning.
- Reopen slowly after clamping to avoid sudden pressure changes.
- Verify transducer level regularly (too low = falsely high ICP, too high = falsely low).

Dislodgment or Misuse

Children may dislodge EVDs, causing CSF leakage or loss of monitoring.

Prevention:

- Secure catheter and tubing.
- Use supervision or soft restraints if needed.
- Educate cooperative children.
  Action: Cover site with sterile pad, keep child flat, alert neurosurgery, save system for culture if needed.

Summary

Nurses are the first line of defense. Prevention of complications require the following:

- Aseptic handling
- Careful leveling and calibration
- Device and patient assessment
- Prompt documentation and escalation

Early signs (e.g., waveform changes, subtle lab abnormalities) often appear in nursing observations. Meticulous care and detailed documentation help prevent and manage complications effectively.

Discussion

Modern intracranial pressure (ICP) management in pediatric patients relies on protocols from organizations like the Brain Trauma Foundation (BTF), NICE, and WHO. Nurses are pivotal in implementing these evidence-based interventions, balancing technical expertise with clinical and holistic care.

Indications for ICP Monitoring

- *Severe TBI*: BTF recommends ICP monitoring for children with GCS ≤8 and abnormal CT findings (Level III recommendation).
- *Other Conditions*: Considered in cases of CNS infections, stroke, or hydrocephalus with signs of elevated ICP.
- *Guidelines*: NICE emphasizes imaging/monitoring over clinical signs alone to exclude high ICP.

ICP and CPP Thresholds

- *Critical Levels*: Maintain ICP <20 mmHg; CPP ≥40 mmHg (adjusted by age: 40–50 mmHg for young children, closer to adult targets [50–60 mmHg] in adolescents).
- *Nursing Role*: Titrate interventions (analgesia, sedation, CSF drainage, vasopressors, PCO2, temperature, and seizure management) to stabilize CPP, ensuring adequate cerebral perfusion.

Tiered Therapy Approach

1. *First-Tier Interventions*
   - *Ventilation*: Target $PaCO_2$ 35–40 mmHg (4.5–5.0 kPa); brief hyperventilation ($PaCO_2$ 30–35 = 3.9–4.6 kPa) for herniation and secretion clearance. The conversion is: mmHg × 0.133322 = kPa. Maintain adequate oxygenation.
   - *Sedation/Analgesia*: Use opioids, benzodiazepines; neuromuscular blockade if refractory.
   - *Positioning*: Head elevation (30°), midline position.
   - *CSF Drainage*: EVD utilization as per guidance.
   - *Hyperosmolar Therapy*: Hypertonic saline (preferred) over mannitol due to safety profile; 0.9% sodium chloride as IV maintenance or feed as indicated. Aim for sodium around 145–150 mmol/L
   - *BP Support*: Fluids/vasopressors to maintain CPP. Noradrenaline preferred for vasoconstriction; maintain normal electrolyte levels.
   - *Temperature/Seizure Control*: Maintain normothermia, avoid hyperthermia; prophylactic anticonvulsants (e.g., levetiracetam), seizure surveillance (CFAM, EEG) as indicated.
2. *Second-Tier Interventions*
   - *Hyperventilation* (Mild hyperventilation: CO_2 4.0–4.5 kPa, moderate: 3.6–4.0 kPa, severe: ≤3.5 kPa)
   - *Titrated hypothermia for seizure control if indicated*
   - *Barbiturate Coma*: For refractory ICP, with hemodynamic and CFAM/EEG monitoring
   - *Decompressive Craniectomy*: Considered if medical management fails
   - *Advanced Monitoring*: Brain tissue oxygen probes in select cases

Global and Resource-Limited Settings

- WHO prioritizes preventing hypoxia/hypotension, head elevation, and accessible therapies (e.g., mannitol).

Research Evidence

- *ICP Monitoring*: Mixed outcomes in pediatric studies; benefits linked to protocolized care rather than monitoring alone.
- *Interventions*: Hypertonic saline favored; hypothermia and corticosteroids not routinely recommended.
- *Nursing Impact*: Meticulous care reduces complications (e.g., infection, DVT) and improves outcomes.

Training and Competencies

- *Education*: Formal training on devices (EVD, ICP catheters, CFAM/EEG monitoring, pupillometry), simulations for emergencies
- *Certifications*: CCRN/CNRN/PICU Specialist Course encouraged; annual competency assessments
- *Soft Skills*: Family communication, psychosocial support, ethical decision-making

Conclusion

Intracranial pressure (ICP) monitoring in pediatric neurosurgery is a vital yet intricate aspect of care, requiring advanced technology and skilled nursing. Nurses play a pivotal role in ensuring accurate data through proper management of invasive and noninvasive monitors, meticulous calibration, hourly checks, and timely interventions. Holistic care, including patient comfort, minimal stimulation, and family involvement, is equally critical.

Nurses act as first responders to high ICP alarms, stabilizing patients through interventions like elevating the head of the bed or draining CSF. They prevent complications with aseptic techniques and vigilant observation while integrating evidence-based guidelines into individualized care plans. Their expertise extends to educating families, coordinating multidisciplinary teams, and contributing to quality improvement initiatives such as EVD care bundles or research on new monitoring methods.

With ongoing training and experience, pediatric neurosurgical nurses adapt to evolving technologies and practices, aiming to protect the developing brain. Their blend of technical skill, evidence-based knowledge, and compassionate care ensures ICP monitoring improves outcomes and enhances the safety of pediatric neurosurgical care.

The information in this chapter is drawn from current guidelines and literature, among other sources. These provide an evidence-based foundation for the practices described. Nurses should remain updated as guidelines are periodically revised and new evidence emerges in this rapidly developing field.

Further Reading

Brain Trauma Foundation's 2019 Pediatric Severe TBI Guidelines. https://braintrauma.org/coma/guidelines/pediatric#:~:text=To%20Improve%20Overall%20Outcomes

NICE head injury management recommendations. nice.org.uk

AANN nursing practice guidelines for ICP monitoring. Care of the Patient Undergoing Intracranial Pressure Monitoring/External Ventricular Drainage or Lumbar Drainage. AANN Clinical Practice Guideline Serie. https://www.bmc.org/sites/default/files/Patient_Care/Specialty_Care/Stroke_and_Cerebrovascular_Center/Medical_Professionals/Protocols/AANN%20Guideline%20caring%20for%20ICP%20Monitor%20External%20Vent%20Drain%20or%20Lumbar%20Drainage.pdf

Recent research findings on ICP monitoring efficacy. pmc.ncbi.nlm.nih.gov, frontiersin.org

Haydel MJ, Weisbrod LJ, Saeed W. Pediatric head trauma. [Updated 2024 Feb 16]. In: StatPearls [Internet]. Treasure Island: StatPearls Publishing; 2025. Available from: https://www.ncbi.nlm.nih.gov/books/NBK537029/.

Pedersen SH, Lilja-Cyron A, Astrand R, Juhler M. Monitoring and measurement of intracranial pressure in pediatric head trauma. Front Neurol. 2020;10:1376. https://doi.org/10.3389/fneur.2019.01376.

Raboel PH, Bartek J Jr, Andresen M, Bellander BM, Romner B. Intracranial pressure monitoring: invasive versus non-invasive methods – a review. Crit Care Res Pract. 2012;2012:950393. https://doi.org/10.1155/2012/950393. Epub 2012 Jun 8. PMID: 22720148; PMCID: PMC3376474

Kochanek PM, Tasker RC, Carney N, Totten AM, Adelson PD, Selden NR, Davis-O'Reilly C, Hart EL, Bell MJ, Bratton SL, Grant GA, Kissoon N, Reuter-Rice KE. CPNP- guidelines for the management of pediatric severe traumatic brain injury. 3rd ed. Update of the Brain Trauma Foundation Guidelines.

Neuroimaging Basics

Amanda Johnson and Asim Choudhri

Definition

Imaging of the neuroaxis is imperative for the diagnosis and treatment of most neurological diseases. The type of image obtained is decided based on the information to be gathered for the patient, the ability to obtain the image, and acuity of the patient. In addition, each type of image has risks and benefits that should be reviewed prior to obtaining.

1. Ultrasound (Fig. 1)
    (a) Head
        (i) Anterior fontanelle must be open [1].
            1. Images are better with larger fontanelles.
            2. Ultrasound waves do not pass easily through bone.
        (ii) Visualize the brain cortex and cerebral spinal fluid spaces (CSF).
        (iii) Early evaluation for macrocephaly.
            1. Concern for ventriculomegaly
            2. Intraventricular hemorrhage
            3. Mass or lesion

A. Johnson (✉)
Department of Neurologic Surgery, The University of Chicago Medicine and Biological Sciences, Chicago, IL, USA
e-mail: Amanda.Johnson@bsd.uchicago.edu

A. Choudhri
Department of Pediatric Neuroradiology, LeBonheur Children's Hospital, Memphis, TN, USA
e-mail: achoudhri@uthsc.edu

K. Battick et al. (eds.), *Nursing Guide for Pediatric Neuroscience Patients*,
https://doi.org/10.1007/978-3-032-22664-8_4

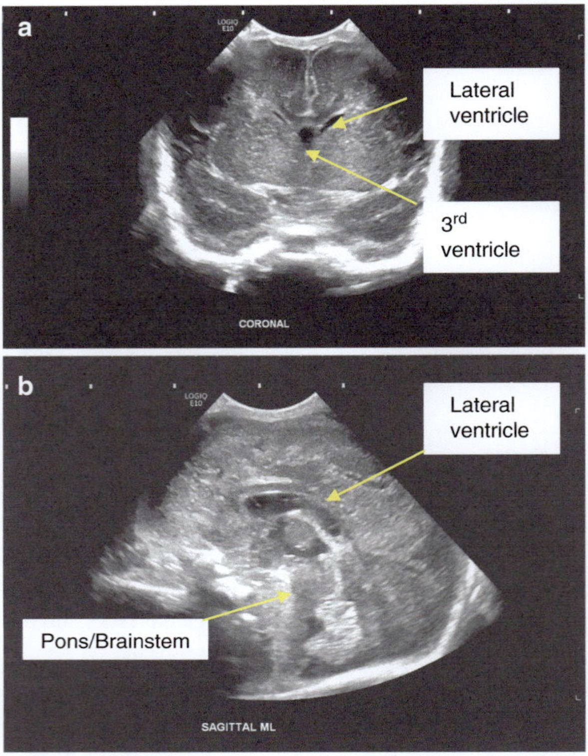

Fig. 1 Normal cranial ultrasound: (**a**) coronal view of lateral and third ventricle; (**b**) sagittal view of lateral ventricle, pons/brainstem, and cerebellum

(b) Spinal (Fig. 2)
  (i) Infants with concern for complex sacral dimple or other cutaneous findings [2].
    1. Larger sacral dimple
    2. Multiple dimples
    3. Deep or indurated dimple
    4. Hemangioma
  (ii) Visualize the end of the spinal cord and potential decreased motion of cord.
  (iii) Early evaluation for tethered spinal cord.
    1. Can have false positives
    2. Should not be the only image to diagnose tethered cord syndrome

(c) Benefits
  (i) No radiation
  (ii) No sedation
  (iii) Quick to complete
    1. Less than 10 min
  (iv) Low cost to patient
  (v) No need for intravenous access

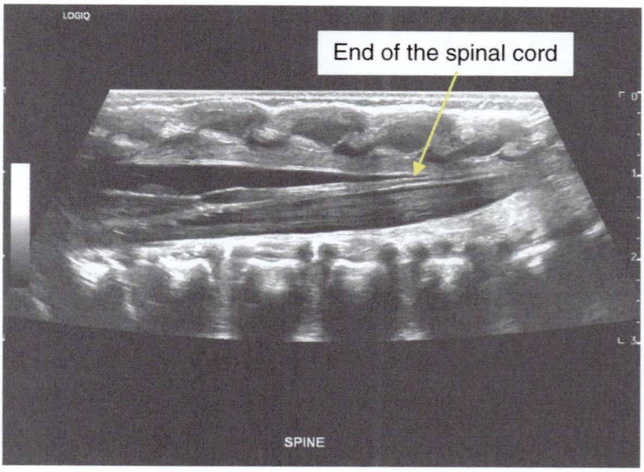

Fig. 2 Spinal ultrasound with normal lying conus

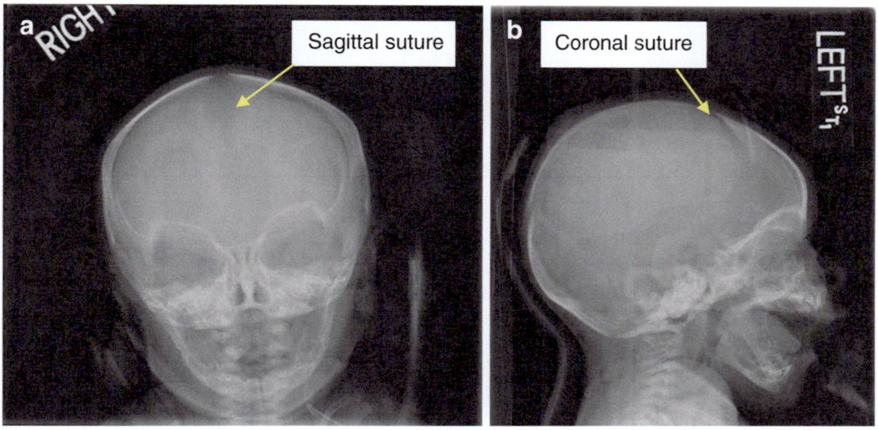

Fig. 3 Infant skull plain film radiograph: (**a**) anteroposterior (AP) view revealing patent sagittal suture; (**b**) lateral view revealing patent coronal suture

- (d) Risks
  - (i) Low-quality image
  - (ii) Potential to miss disease process

2. Plain film radiograph, cranial and spinal (Figs. 3 and 4)
   - (a) Assess bony abnormalities
     - (i) Skull or spinal fracture
     - (ii) Craniosynostosis
     - (iii) Spinal dysraphism
     - (iv) Medical devices

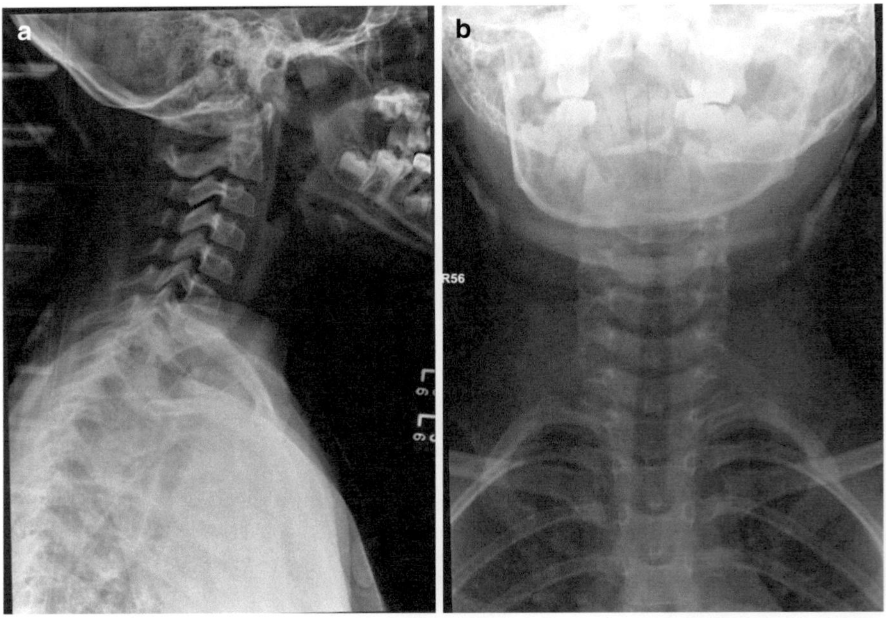

Fig. 4 (**a**) Lateral cervical spine radiograph to assess alignment; (**b**) AP cervical spine radiograph

1. Ventriculoperitoneal, ventriculopleural, ventriculoatrial shunts
2. Vagal nerve stimulators
3. Baclofen pumps

(v) Assess spinal alignment
1. Scoliosis
2. Traumatic injury

(b) Benefits
(i) Quick to obtain
1. Less than 10 min

(ii) No sedation
(iii) Low cost to the patient
(iv) No need for intravenous access

(c) Risks
(i) Radiation exposure
(ii) If concern, might need further imaging evaluation

3. Computed topography (CT) scan of head and spine are radiograph "slices" of images in cross section to produce multiple plain images (Fig. 5).
(a) The "slices" of images are axial, sagittal, coronal, and 3D reconstruction. The "slices" of the image can be of different thicknesses and are stacked on each other to produce a picture based on the tissue density. The thicker the "slice," the larger the gap in the overall image. The thinner the "slice," the smaller the gap in the overall image [3].

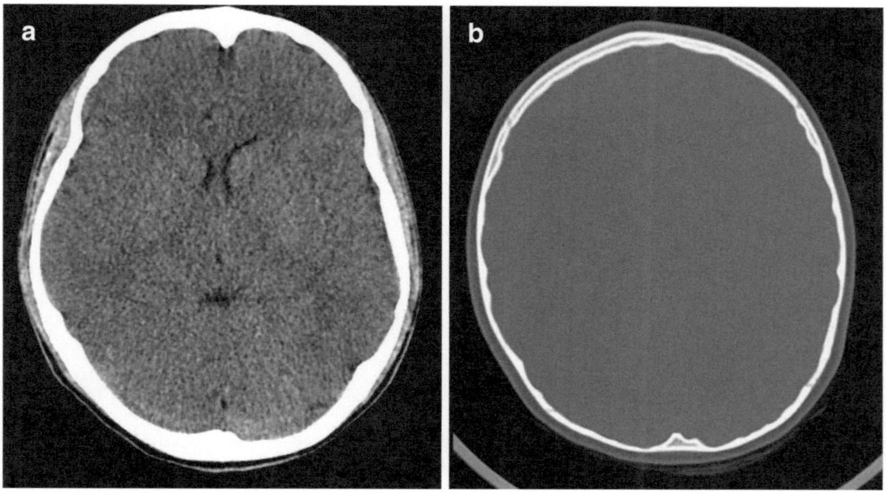

Fig. 5 (**a**) Axial image of head CT scan revealing no intracranial process; (**b**) axial image of head CT with bone windows

(i) Fluid is black.
(ii) Tissue is gray.
(iii) Bone/calcium is white.

(b) Head imaging
  (i) Able to be completed at any age
  (ii) Assess bone
    1. Fracture
    2. Craniosynostosis
  (iii) Assess brain cortex and ventricular size
    1. Hemorrhage
    2. Tumor
    3. Infection
    4. Ventriculomegaly

(c) Spine imaging (Fig. 6)
  (i) Assess bone
    1. Fracture
    2. Alignment
  (ii) Not ideal for direct view of the spinal cord

(d) Benefits [4]
  (i) Quick to complete
    1. Most images are less than 2 min
  (ii) Better quality image than a plain radiograph or ultrasound

(e) Risks
  (i) Radiation exposure [4–6].
    1. Multiple CT scans over a lifetime can increase risk for cancer.

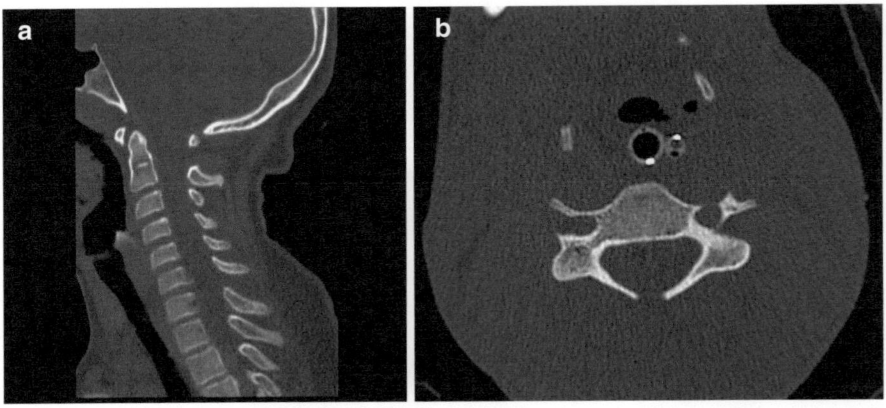

Fig. 6 (**a**) Sagittal image of cervical spine CT scan bone window revealing normal alignment. (**b**) Axial image of cervical spine CT scan

2. Low-dose radiation imaging is available.
3. Remove orbits from imaging to help decrease glaucoma rate.

(ii) Depending on the image and age of patient, sedation might be needed.
(iii) Higher cost to patient.
(iv) Might need intravenous access if contrast images are obtained.

4. Magnetic Resonance Image (MRI) (Fig. 7) of the brain and spine are obtained using different radiofrequency pulses and gradients to create a particular sequence and can be obtained at any age. There are multiple types of MRI images, including vascular imaging (arteries [MRA] and veins [MRV]), functional, and spectroscopy [7].
   (a) Each sequence has a different focus
      (i) T1-weighted images
         1. Best for looking at the anatomy.
         2. Fluid will be dark, gray matter will be gray, white matter will be light gray, fat will be bright white, and inflammation will be dark.
         3. Axial, coronal, and sagittal views.
      (ii) T2-weighted images
         1. Best for fluid density.
         2. Fluid will be white, gray matter will be light gray, white matter will be dark gray, and inflammation will be bright white.
         3. Axial, coronal, and sagittal views.
      (iii) Fluid-attenuated inversion recovery (FLAIR) sequence
         1. Best for evaluating subtle changes not visible on T1, leptomeningeal enhancement, and subarachnoid hemorrhage
         2. Axial and sagittal views
      (iv) Diffusion-weighted
         1. Best for evaluating edema, ischemic process, tumor, or infection
         2. Evaluating the ease of water moving within the cells
         3. Axial view

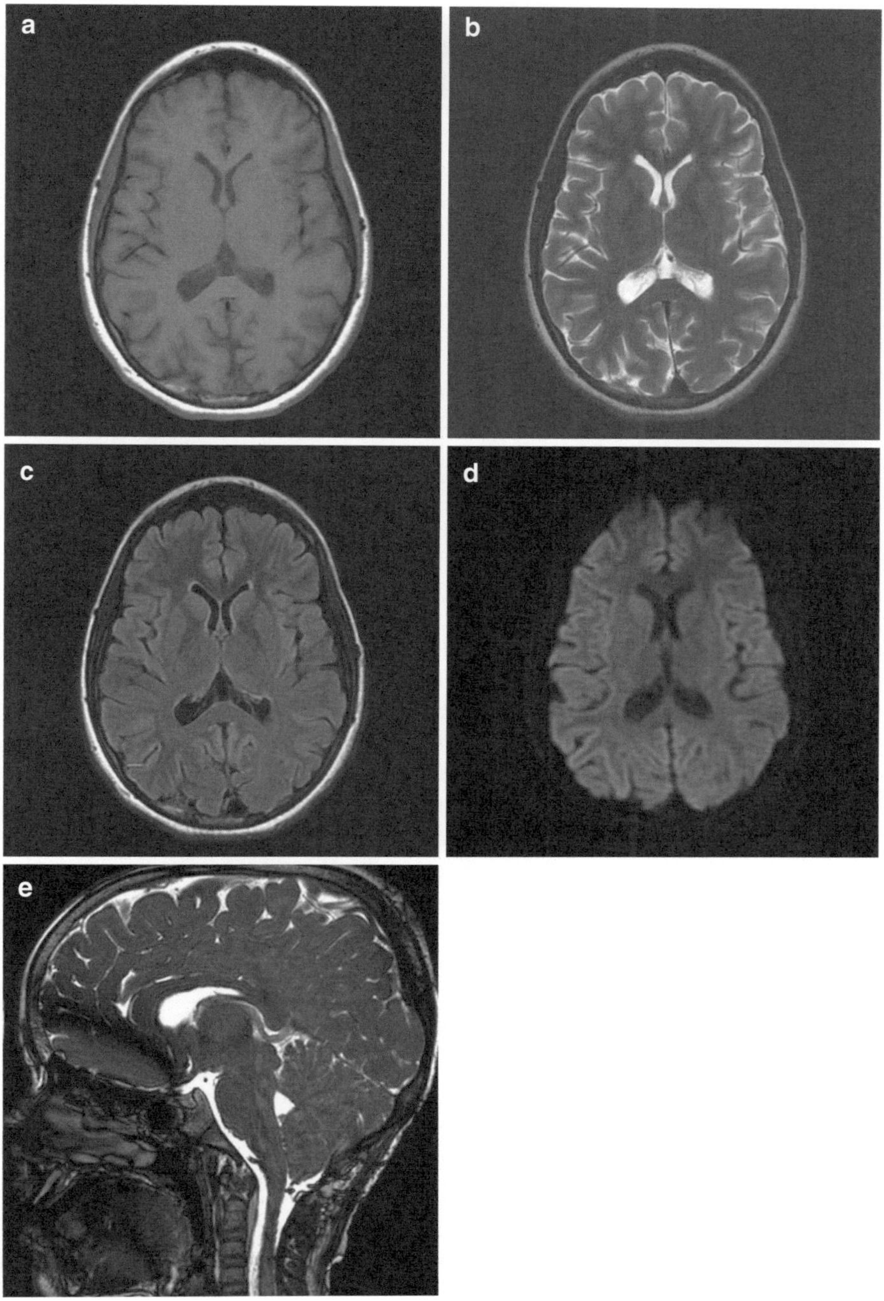

Fig. 7 (**a**) T1-weighted axial image. (**b**) T2-weighted axial image. (**c**) FLAIR axial image. (**d**) Diffusion-weighted axial image. (**e**) Flow sequence sagittal image

(v) Flow-sensitive
1. Best to evaluate the flow of CSF
2. Sagittal view
(b) Brain imaging
(i) Assess the brain cortex.
1. Hemorrhage
2. Tumor
3. Infection
4. Diffuse axonal injury
(ii) Assess ventricles.
1. Size
2. Obstruction of flow
(c) Spine imaging
(i) Assess spinal cord and spaces surrounding the cord.
(ii) Assess ligaments and muscles.
(iii) Assess the discs.
(iv) Not ideal to assess bony disease.
(d) Benefits
(i) No radiation
(ii) Best-quality image
(e) Risks
(i) Takes time to complete image.
1. Brain without contrast is about 20 min.
2. Spine without contrast is about 40 min.
3. Shorter sequencing is becoming available.
(ii) High expense to the patient.
(iii) Likely will need sedation depending on the age of the patient.
1. If sedation needed, intravenous access will be needed.
(iv) Consider if there is metal in the patient, i.e., braces, VP shunt valves.
1. This can obscure the image.

Noncontrast Versus Contrast Imaging (Fig. 8)

There are considerations when deciding if the image should be completed without or with contrast. Contrast should be considered if there is concern for infection, neoplasm, vascular problem, or demyelinating disease [8]. If the child presents with nonspecific symptoms, imaging almost always starts as a noncontrast study. If contrast images are needed, it is best to obtain both noncontrast and contrast imaging to be able to compare the noncontrast to contrast images.

1. Contrast for CT scans
   (a) Iodine-based contrast is used.
2. Contrast for MRI scans
   (a) Gadolinium-based contrast is used.

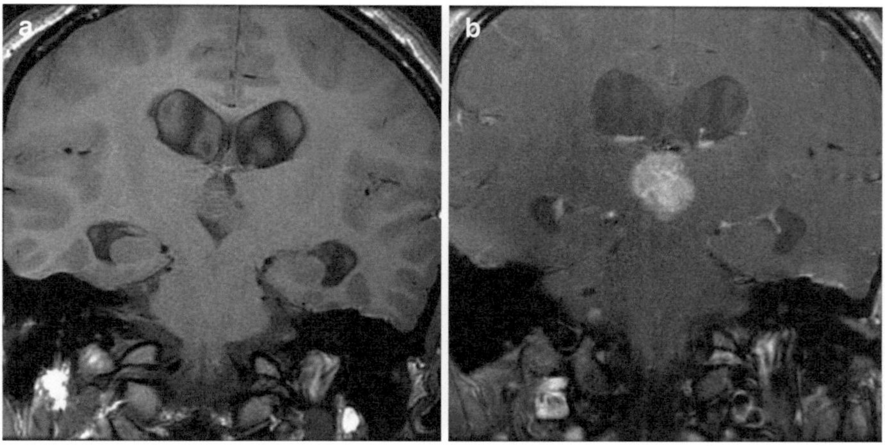

Fig. 8 (**a**) Noncontrast coronal T1 image with enlarged ventricles. (**b**) Contrast coronal T1 image revealing heterogeneous enhancing lesion in the region to the tectum/pineal gland causing obstructive hydrocephalus

3. Risks of contrasts
   (a) Invasive to child
      (i) Requires intravenous access
   (b) Potential allergic reaction
      (i) Most common with iodine-based contrast
   (c) Consider renal function
      (i) Contrast is metabolized through the kidneys.
   (d) Consider if the child is pregnant
   (e) Concern for longer retention of gadolinium circulating in the body

How to Review an Image and a Radiologist Report

When reviewing CT and MRI scans, begin with the same sequences each time the images are reviewed. All images are mirrored. The right side is on the left side of the image, and the left side is on the right side of the image. Start with axial imaging and then review sagittal and coronal imaging. If reviewing a CT scan, review both the brain and bone images to evaluate for intracranial process on the brain imaging and a bony process on the bone images. When reviewing MRI scans, look at the T1 and T2 sequences first and then move to the FLAIR and DWI sequences.

Radiologist Report

1. Read both sections of the radiologist report.
   (a) The findings
      (i) Detailed description of each area of the image.
         1. Review brain parenchyma.

2. Review ventricles and other CSF spaces.
3. Review vasculature.
4. Review bone (most often on CT).
(ii) Report specific section of scan to review for abnormal finding.
(iii) Report specific measurements of abnormal findings.
(b) Impression
(i) Summary of the findings

Abnormalities on Imaging

Interpreting the common abnormal findings on imaging can be valuable to understand the next steps in the care for the patient. Some abnormal findings will require neurosurgical intervention to prevent permanent neurological deficits or even death. There might be additional imaging required based on the type of study to reveal abnormal findings.

Definitions of Abnormal Findings

1. Intraventricular hemorrhage (IVH) (Fig. 9)
   (a) Hemorrhage within the ventricle
   (b) Caused by
      (i) Prematurity
      (ii) Significant trauma
      (iii) Vascular malformation
2. Ventriculomegaly/Hydrocephalus (Fig. 10)
   (a) Enlarged ventricle system
   (b) Caused by
      (i) Idiopathy
      (ii) Tumors
      (iii) Obstruction
      (iv) Hemorrhage

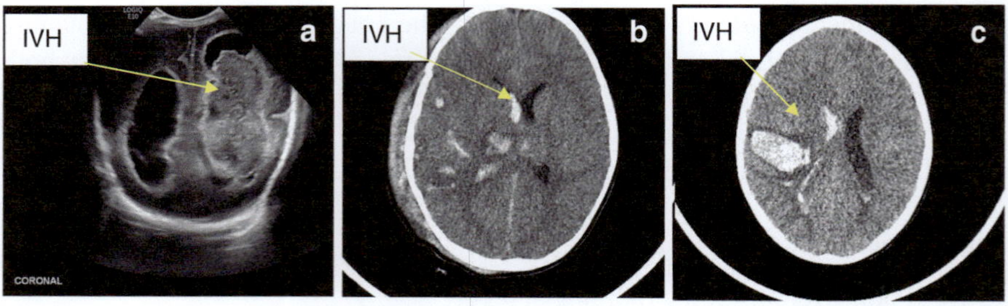

Fig. 9 (**a**) Head ultrasound coronal image revealing hyperdensity of the ventricle, which is blood, from prematurity. (**b**) Non-infused head CT axial image with hemorrhage in the right lateral ventricle after significant trauma. (**c**) Non-infused head CT with hemorrhage in the right ventricle from AVM rupture

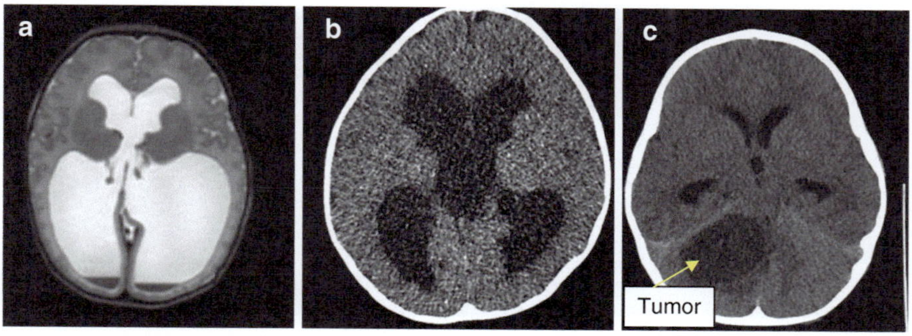

Fig. 10 (**a**) MRI T2 axial image revealing idiopathic ventriculomegaly in a newborn. (**b**) Non-infused head CT axial image revealing enlarged lateral and third ventricles related to obstruction of the aqueduct. (**c**) Non-infused head CT axial image revealing large posterior fossa tumor causing ventriculomegaly

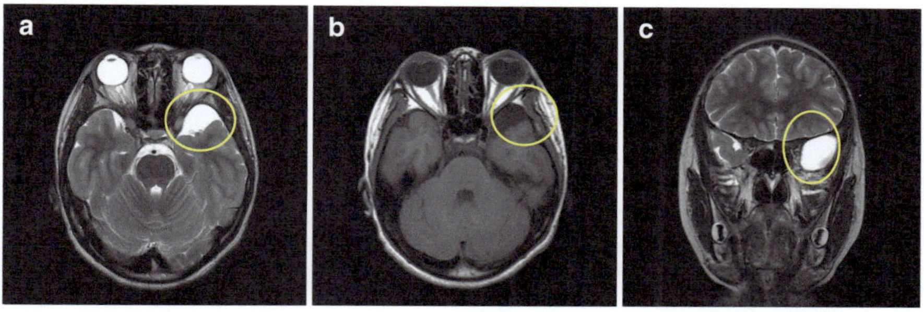

Fig. 11 All sequences revealing left temporal arachnoid cyst. (**a**) MRI T2 axial sequence. (**b**) MRI T2 axial sequence. (**c**) MRI T2 coronal sequence

3. Arachnoid cyst (Fig. 11)
   (a) Fluid-filled space within the brain parenchyma
   (b) Often incidental finding
4. Epidural collection (Fig. 12)
   (a) Hemorrhage or empyema within the potential epidural space
   (b) Does not cross the suture lines
   (c) Can be either arterial or venous
   (d) Caused by
      (i) Trauma
      (ii) Infection
5. Subdural collection (Fig. 13)
   (a) Hemorrhage, CSF, or empyema within the potential subdural space
   (b) Can cross the suture lines
   (c) Disruption of bridging veins
   (d) Caused by

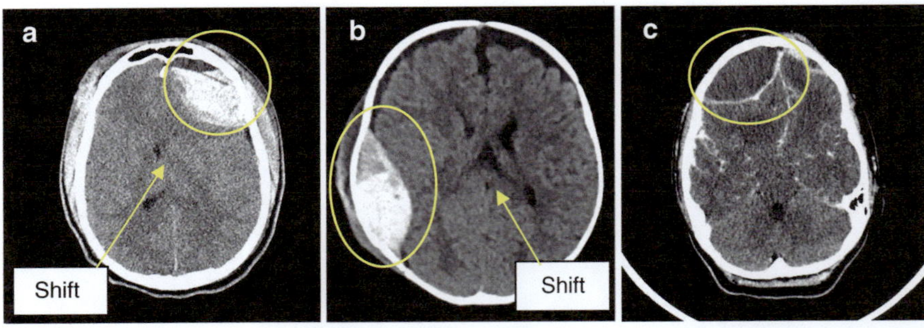

Fig. 12 (**a**) Head CT axial image with left frontal epidural with midline shift. (**b**) Head CT axial image with right parietal epidural with midline shift. (**c**) Infused head CT axial image with right frontal epidural abscess

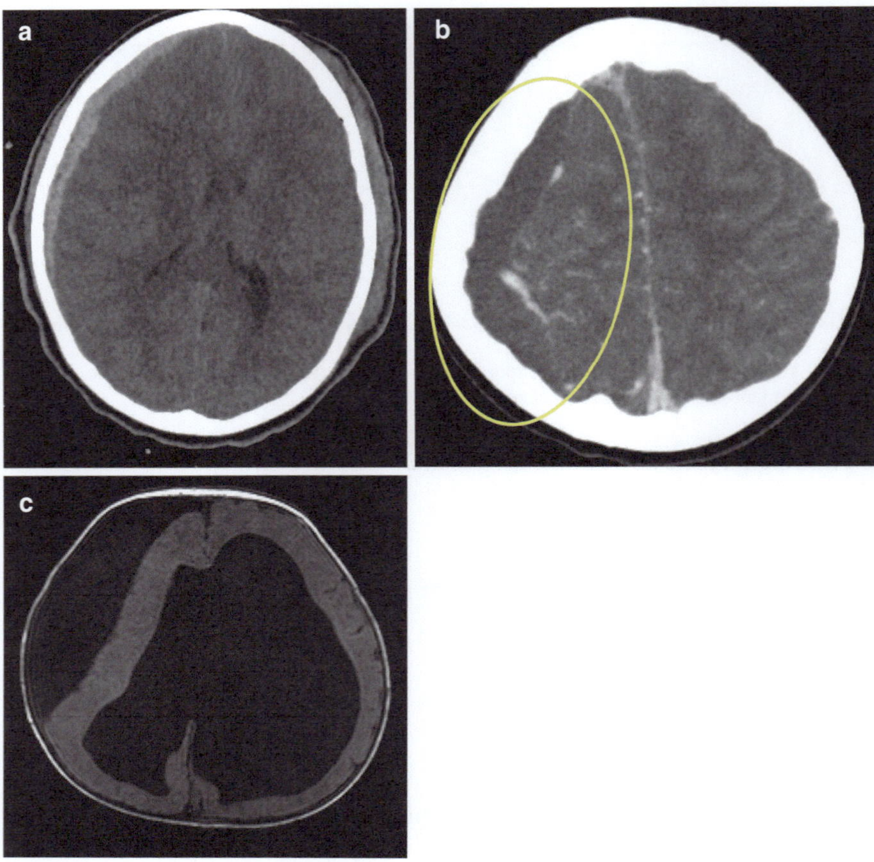

Fig. 13 (**a**) Non-infused head CT revealing right-side subdural hematoma from trauma. (**b**) Infused head CT revealing right-side subdural empyema from sinusitis. (**c**) Non-infused MRI revealing right-side subdural CSF fluid collection after shunt placement

        (i) Trauma
        (ii) Infection
        (iii) Acute decrease in size of ventricles from shunt or external ventricular drain
6. Mid-line shift (Fig. 14)
    (a) Shift of one hemisphere toward another
    (b) Caused by
        (i) Hemorrhage
        (ii) Tumor
        (iii) Infection
7. Uncal herniation (Fig. 15)
    (a) Part of the temporal lobe descends through the tentorium.
    (b) Compresses cranial nerve III (oculomotor).
    (c) Caused by
        (i) Increased intracranial pressure
8. Tonsillar herniation (Fig. 16)
    (a) Cerebellar tonsils descend through the foramen magnum
    (b) Compresses brainstem and pons
        (i) Can cause brain death
    (c) Caused by
        (i) Increased intracranial pressure
        (ii) Tumor
        (iii) Chiari malformation

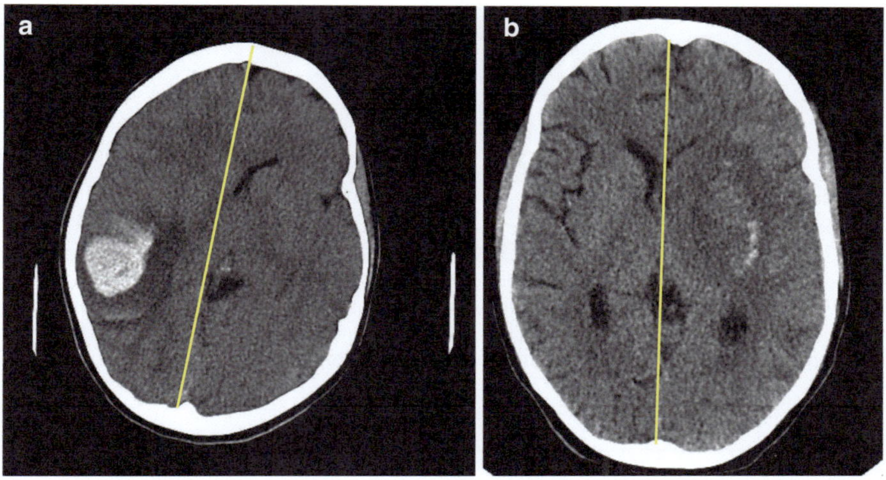

Fig. 14 (**a**) Non-infused head CT with midline shift to the left from large right intracranial hemorrhage with effacement of the right lateral ventricle. (**b**) Non-infused head CT with midline shift to the right from left middle cerebral artery stroke

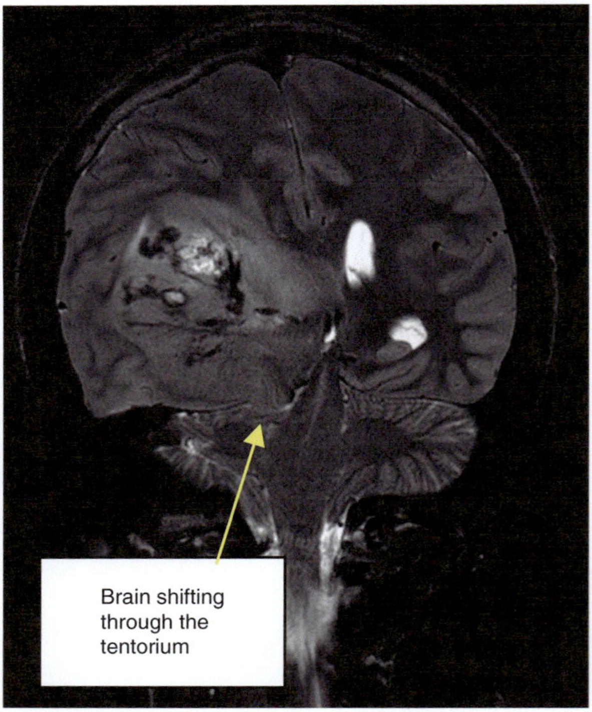

Fig. 15 MRI T2 coronal sequence revealing large right parietal mass causing uncal herniation

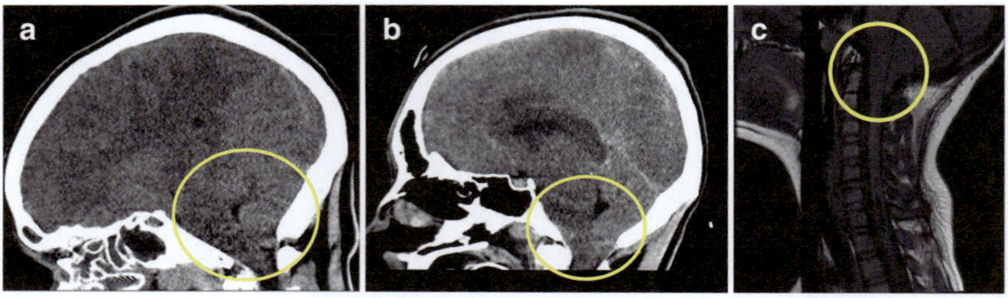

Fig. 16 (**a**) Non-infused head CT revealing tonsillar herniation from significant hypoxic injury. (**b**) Non-infused head CT revealing tonsillar herniation from significant trauma. (**c**) MRI cervical spine sagittal T2 sequence revealing tonsillar decent from Chiari malformation

Nursing Care and Treatment

Coordination of imaging with radiology is imperative to ensure images are completed in a timely fashion. Certain images, particularly MRI scans, might need to involve either anesthesia, intensive care service, or sedation service, which adds another component to coordination. Protocols for transporting patients to radiology will be institution-dependent; however, safety of the patient is the priority. Communication between radiology, providers, and caregivers will be often led by nursing to ensure everyone is informed.

What to Expect for Each Image

1. Head or spinal ultrasound
   (a) Can be completed at the bedside or in radiology department.
   (b) Patient does not need a nothing-by-mouth order (NPO).
   (c) Patient does not need intravenous access.
   (d) Caregivers can stay with the child while the image is completed.
2. Plain film radiographs
   (a) If patient is of childbearing age, pregnancy test should be completed prior to imaging.
   (b) Can be completed at the bedside or in the radiology department.
      (i) Some images must be completed in radiology department.
         1. Upright plain films of the spine
   (c) Patient does not need a NPO.
   (d) Patient does not need intravenous access
   (e) Caregivers will need to step away from the patient while the image is being taken.
      (i) Some institutions allow caregivers to wear lead to stay with patient while imaging is being done.
3. CT scan
   (a) If patient is of childbearing age, pregnancy test should be completed, if possible.
   (b) If obtaining contrast imaging, renal function might need to be evaluated prior to image completion.
   (c) Consider if patient has electroencephalogram (EEG) leads in place; they need to be CT-compatible or they will cause distortion of the image, making it hard to interpret.
   (d) Patient will need to be transported to the radiology department.
      (i) Patient will need to be transferred to CT scan table.
      (ii) If patient has intravenous medications to be infused, ensure there is ample length of tubing to transfer from bed to CT scan table.
      (iii) If patient is intubated, respiratory therapy personnel will need to accompany the patient to radiology department. Whether ventilator accompanies the patient to the CT scan is institution-dependent.
   (e) For CT imaging of head and spine, the patient does not need a NPO; however, if anesthesia or sedation is needed for the image to be completed, NPO status will be needed.
   (f) Intravenous access will be needed for contrast-infused imaging or if anesthesia or sedation is needed.

(i) Intravenous access type and gage will be institution-dependent for contrast images. Check with radiology prior to transporting patient to the radiology department.

(g) Caregivers will need to step away from the patient while the image is being taken because of the radiation exposure.
   (i) Some institutions will allow caregivers to wear lead to stay with the patient.

(h) Noncontrast imaging will be completed first and then contrast imaging will be completed.
   (i) The CT technologist will give contrast either by hand push or by machine injection depending on the size and location of intravenous access.
   (ii) Imaging will be completed immediately after the contrast has been delivered.

(i) Ventriculograms or cisternograms
   (i) CT imaging with contrast injected directly into the CSF space to evaluate for obstruction to CSF pathway.
      1. Provider with privileges from neurosurgical service or radiology will sterile-prepare contrast.
      2. Contrast is then slowly injected either into a shunt, external ventricular drain, or via lumbar puncture.
         (a) If injected into external ventricular drain, drain will be clamped for a certain length of time to allow contrast to stay within the ventricular system.
      3. Time between injection and the image being obtained will be provider-dependent.

4. MRI scans
   (a) If obtaining contrast imaging, renal function might need to be evaluated prior to image completion.
   (b) Consider if patient has electroencephalogram (EEG) leads in place; they need to be MRI-compatible or removed prior to transport.
   (c) Prior to having patient transported, a screening form regarding potential metal in the body will need to be completed.
      (i) If patient has any metal in the body, it will need to be evaluated for safety while in MRI scan.
         1. Baclofen pumps
            (a) Will need to be slowed or stopped
         2. Vagal nerve stimulators
            (a) Will need to be stopped
         3. VP shunt valves
            (a) If programmable, might need to be reprogrammed
         4. Aneurysm clips or coils
         5. Retained foreign body
            (a) Bullet
         6. Endotracheal tube or trach with metal

   (ii) Clothing with snaps or clasps will need to be removed.
   (iii) Piercings will need to be removed.
- (d) Patient will need to be transported to the radiology department.
   - (i) Patient will need to be transferred to MRI table without any metal.
     1. Metal electrocardiogram (EKG) leads will need to be replaced with MRI-compatible MRI leads.
   - (ii) If patient has intravenous medications infusing, ensure there is ample length of tubing because the intravenous pumps will have to remain outside of the room.
   - (iii) If patient is intubated, a special MRI-compatible ventilator will be needed.
- (e) For MRI imaging of head and spine, the patient does not need to a NPO; however, if anesthesia or sedation is needed for the image to be completed, NPO status will be needed.
- (f) Intravenous access will be needed for contrast-infused imaging or if anesthesia or sedation is needed.
   - (i) Intravenous access type and gage will be institution-dependent for contrast images. Check with radiology prior to transporting patient to the radiology department.
- (g) Caregivers will need to step away from the patient while the image is being taken.
   - (i) There might be option for music or a movie while the patient is having imaging completed to help with distraction.
- (h) Noncontrast imaging will be completed first; then, contrast imaging will be completed.
   - (i) The MRI technologist will give contrast either by hand push or by machine injection depending on the size and location of intravenous access.
   - (ii) Imaging will be completed immediately after the contrast has been delivered.
- (i) Nursing considerations
   - (i) MRI scans can take a long time to complete depending on the images prescribed. If patient is required to be monitored by a nurse during the scan, nurse staffing ratios will need to account for a nurse to be off the unit.

What to Teach Patients and Caregivers About Imaging

The nurse should prepare the patient and caregiver for the type of image to be completed. The child life department should be requested, if available in the institution, to help with education to the patient. The child life department often has pictures of the different machines that will take the pictures and what the different radiology rooms look like to help prepare. The child life department can also help with distraction techniques during the image process.

1. Key points for each image
   (a) Head or spinal ultrasound
      (i) Takes only minutes to complete.
      (ii) The technologist will have to use a gel on the head or back to be able to get the image. The gel is usually warmed.
   (b) Plain radiographs
      (i) Takes only minutes to complete.
      (ii) Sometimes, the patient will have to turn to their side and have multiple imaging taken.
      (iii) Lead will be used to protect certain areas of the body from the radiation.
   (c) CT scan
      (i) The patient will be on a hard table to have the image completed and strapped in with a safety strap.
      (ii) The table will move in and out of a doughnut-shaped tube while the images are being taken.
      (iii) The patient will need to stay still while the images are being taken.
      (iv) The images take about 30–60 s to complete.
   (d) MRI scan
      (i) The patient will have to have all metals removed prior to the image. If the patient has braces, this might interfere with the image of the brain.
      (ii) A screening form will need to be completed prior to the image.
      (iii) The patient will be on a hard table to have the image completed and strapped in with a safety strap.
      (iv) The table will move in and out of a doughnut-shaped tube while the images are being taken. There will be a cage placed over the face for brain imaging.
      (v) Ear plugs will be provided because the machine makes loud noises while each sequence is obtained. Music or movies might be available to help with distraction from the loud noise.
      (vi) The patient will need to stay still while the images are being taken.
      (vii) Most sequences will take 2–5 min to complete. The number of sequences will be dependent on the imaging that was prescribed. An MRI brain without contrast takes about 20 min to complete.
      (viii) Caregivers will have to wait in either the patient's room or waiting room while the images are being completed.

References

1. Gupta P, Sodhi K, Saxena A, Khandelwal N, Singhi P. Neonatal cranial sonography: a concise review for clinicians. J Pediatr Neurosci. 2016;11(1):7–13. https://doi.org/10.4103/1817-1745.181261.
2. Choi S, Yoon H, Hwang J, Suh C, Jung A, Cho Y, Lee J. Incidence of occult spinal dysraphism among infants with cutaneous stigmata and proportion managed with neurosurgery. JAMA Netw Open. 2020;3(7):e207221. https://doi.org/10.1001/jamanetworkopen.2020.7221.

3. Kayhanian S, Young A, Rory P, Donnelly J, Scoffing D, Garnett M, Fernandes H, et al. Radiological correlate of raised intracranial pressure in children: a review. Front Pediatr. 2018;6:32. https://doi.org/10.3389/fped.2018.00032.
4. Burstein B, Upton J, Terra H, Neuman M. Use of CT for head trauma:2007-1015. Pediatrics. 2018;142(4):e20180814.
5. Barreto I, Tuna I, Rajderkar D, Ching J, Governale L. Pediatric craniosynostosis computed tomography: an institutional experience in reducing radiation dose while maintaining diagnostic image quality. Pediatr Radiol. 2022;52:85–96. https://doi.org/10.1007/s00247-021-05205-6.
6. Cappellari A, Bruschi G, Beretta G, Molisso M, Bertolozzi G. How can specialist advice influence the neuroimaging practice for childhood headache in emergency department. Children. 2023;10(12):1837. https://doi.org/10.3390/children10121837.
7. Vossough A. Newer MRI techniques in pediatric neuroimaging. Semin Roentgenol. 2023;58(1):131–44.
8. Azhari A, Truzzi A, Neoh M, Balagtas J, Tan H, Goh P, et al. A decade of infant neuroimaging research: what have we learned and where are we going? Infant Behav Dev. 2020;58:101389. https://doi.org/10.1016/j.infbeh.2019.101389.

Hydrocephalus

Paula Zakrzewski and Ulrich-W Thomale

Description

Hydrocephalus is an imbalance between cerebral spinal fluid (CSF) production and absorption. This results in spinal fluid accumulation which finally increases the intracranial pressure inside the head. In infants, when the fontanelle is still open or the calvarium is thin, the condition will result in disproportionate growth of the head (macrocephaly). In older children, when the skull bone is more rigid, increased intracranial pressure is more likely to develop. Pathophysiologically, there are distinct factors involved in the development of hydrocephalus. In a simplified understanding, six relevant factors have been shown to be most relevant:

1. Overproduction of CSF
2. Malabsorption of CSF
3. Obstruction of major CSF pathways (between the ventricles and the external CSF spaces)
4. Obstruction of minor CSF pathways (within the brain tissue)
5. Impaired pulsatility
6. Venous congestion

In this context, hydrocephalus is not a disease by itself but a result based on an underlying pathological origin. Factor No. 3 leads to a noncommunicating

P. Zakrzewski (✉)
Hough Family Institute for Brain Protection Sciences, Johns Hopkins All Children's Hospital, St. Petersburg, FL, USA
e-mail: pzakrze1@jhmi.edu

U.-W. Thomale
Department of Pediatric Neurosurgery, Charite Universitaetsmedizin, Berlin, Germany
e-mail: uthomale@charite.de

K. Battick et al. (eds.), *Nursing Guide for Pediatric Neuroscience Patients*,
https://doi.org/10.1007/978-3-032-22664-8_5

hydrocephalus, while all other factors are related to communicating type of hydrocephalus. Typical diseases which are linked to hydrocephalus are:

- Intraventricular hemorrhage
- Severe CSF infection
- Brain tumors
- Brain trauma
- Congenital malformation of the brain
- Others

Among congenital malformations, relevant syndromes with considerable risk for developing hydrocephalus are:

- Myelomeningocele (spina bifida)
- Encephalocele
- Arachnoid cysts
- Aqueductal stenosis
- Dandy Walker malformations
- Syndromal craniosynostosis
- Others

Most of the diseases need interdisciplinary care, and hydrocephalus may only be one of the clinical problems relevant for the patient.

Signs and Symptoms

The signs and symptoms of hydrocephalus depend on the age of the patient and the anatomy of the skull and also on the acuteness or chronicity of the pathophysiology of slowed or impaired CSF flow. Table 1 gives a good overview of the relation of symptoms toward age and various stages of acuity.

In shunted patients, overdrainage (negative intracranial pressure) symptoms may be misinterpreted with increased intracranial pressure, which are remarkably similar. The best way to distinguish underdrainage from overdrainage is to correlate the symptoms with body position and activity.

Underdrainage: Symptoms are more severe in lying position but may be similar in standing position.

Overdrainage: Symptoms are more severe in standing position and after activity. Symptoms will improve after lying flat and with continuous fluid intake.

Infection:

In shunted patients, symptoms for shunt infection are necessary to distinguish:

- Reddish, inflammation or swelling along the shunt
- Wound healing problems (reddish wound, exudate, purulent drainage)
- Neck stiffness (nuchal rigidity)

Table 1 Scheme for clinical symptoms related to various stages of hydrocephalus according to age and acuity

<table>
<tr><th></th><th>Infancy</th><th>Children</th><th>Adolescence</th></tr>
<tr><td>Acute</td><td colspan="3">Impaired consciousness
Vomiting
Bradycardia
Loss of consciousness
Arterial hypertension</td></tr>
<tr><td rowspan="3">Subacute</td><td>Sunset phenomenon</td><td colspan="2" rowspan="3">Headache
Nausea
Papilledema
Lethargy
Visual decline
Strabism/double vision</td></tr>
<tr><td>Irritability</td></tr>
<tr><td>Impaired food intake</td></tr>
<tr><td rowspan="3">Chronic</td><td>Macrocephaly</td><td colspan="2">Motor and cognitive developmental delay/decline</td></tr>
<tr><td>Tense and bulging fontanelle</td><td></td><td>Gait disturbances</td></tr>
<tr><td>Gaping sutures</td><td></td><td>Incontinence</td></tr>
</table>

- Fever
- General: stomach ache, nausea, lethargy

When no local signs but only general signs are present, other sources of infection must be excluded before invasive tests for the shunts are performed.

In principle, a shunt infection is very much unlikely if the previous shunt surgery was more than 6–9 months prior and no sepsis occurred in between.

Physical Examination

Most often, patients will have a normal neurological exam. Patients with examination findings can be categorized into the following groups:

1. Consciousness and orientation
   (a) Pediatric Glasgow Coma scale
   (b) Orientation to time, location, and situation
2. Headache characterization
   (a) More severe in the morning (in lying position)
   (b) More severe during the day or after activity (in the standing position)
3. Cranial nerve signs
   (a) Vision/visual field
   (b) Bulb position/ disconjugate gaze
   (c) Nystagmus
4. Motor signs

(a) Gait instability
(b) Impaired coordination

5. Head anatomy

(a) Head circumference—(corrected) age-related percentile measure (relation to body size percentile)
(b) Fontanelle status / suture status
(c) Head shape (any bulging structures)

6. Hemodynamic

(a) Heart rate
(b) Blood pressure

7. In shunted patients

(a) Exclude CSF collection or wound problems.
(b) Exclude swelling or infectious signs along the shunt.
(c) Get information about the shunt type (VA/VP/SDP).
(d) Where is the ventricular catheter placed?
(e) Get information about the valve type (fixed pressure valve; adjustable valve) and pressure setting.
(f) When was the last surgery on the shunt performed?

Labs and Diagnostics

Labs

1. There are no lab studies in primary hydrocephalus diagnosis.
2. In shunted patients with suspected infection, blood samples with leukocytosis and C-reactive protein (CRP) level should be taken.
3. CSF samples should be taken only if other sources of infection are excluded and the CRP is higher than 7 mg/L.

Imaging (if available, always compare to previous images): See Fig. 1

1. Ultrasonography

   - In open fontanelle, it is the imaging of choice. Look for ventricular width (ventricular indices, relation of internal to external CSF spaces), Doppler flow (resistance index, end-diastolic flow).

2. Computer Tomography: Evaluation of ventricular width of each ventricle and external CSF spaces. Due to radiation exposure, it might be exclusively used in urgent cases, and MRI is preferred on a routine basis.

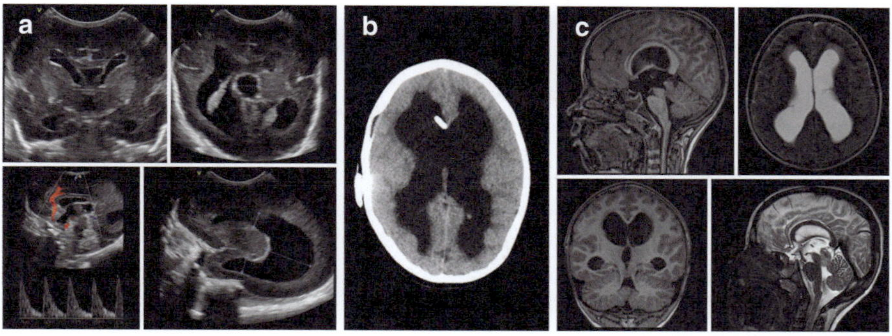

Fig. 1 (**a**) Ultrasound of infant. (**b**) Head CT. (**c**) Brain MRI, each with hydrocephalus conditions

3. MR imaging: Imaging of choice in closed fontanelles. Limited or quick sequence brain MRI imaging may be considered, especially in noncompliant children.
   (a) T1/T2 sequences: Ventricular width, width of external CSF spaces
   (b) T1/T2 sequences: Disproportion of internal and external CSF spaces
   (c) T1/T2 sequences: Exclusion of mass effects disturbing CSF flow
4. MRI Flow Studies: Impairment of any CSF flow dynamics; after ETV: flow void at 3rd ventricular floor?
   - In shunted patients: Check for adjustable valves (MRI stable for setting changes?).
   - In shunted patients: Correct ventricular catheter position.

Additional Imaging for shunted patients

1. X-Ray of the shunt: Evaluates for disconnections, displacement of shunt components, type of valve, valve setting, and peritoneal catheter length
2. Ultrasonography of the abdomen: Evaluates for free fluid and pseudocyst
3. Ophthalmology: Evaluates for papilledema, optic coherence tomography (OCT)

Treatment

Medications

1. There are no medications to treat a hydrocephalus.
2. For symptom relief, medications are beneficial to reduce headaches or pain and usually consist of acetaminophen or ibuprofen, and to reduce nausea, usually zofran is used.

3. In patients with idiopathic intracranial hypertension (IIH; formerly pseudotumor cerebri), acetazolamide can reduce the intracranial pressure by improving the intracranial compliance.

Surgery

- Surgery is to relieve intracranial pressure and to balance the CSF dynamics. In general, four different surgical options exist to treat hydrocephalus:
- Treat exclusively the primary cause.
- Apply temporary treatment options.
- Endoscopic techniques.
- Implantation of a CSF-diverting shunt system.

1. Treat the primary cause:
   (a) In arachnoid cysts causing hydrocephalus: perform cyst fenestration
   (b) In tumors causing hydrocephalus: perform craniotomy for tumor removal
2. Temporary treatment options are applied if time is needed before the definite treatment can be achieved (see 1) or in premature babies if a shunt system cannot yet be implanted.
   (a) Ventricular access device (VAD): Closed system and minimal invasive procedure. Placed usually in the frontal horn, it consists of a ventricular catheter connected with a reservoir, placed subcutaneously. The reservoir can be punctured repeatedly to get CSF samples and remove CSF volume Usually applied in premature babies with intraventricular hemorrhage (IVH). Disadvantage: ICP control is not continuous.
   (b) Ventricular subgalleal shunt (VSGS): Closed system like VAD with side opening and subgaleal pocket as CSF collection to enhance the CSF resorption extracranially. Needs less punctures compared to VAD. Usually applied in premature babies with IVH. Disadvantages: May have higher risk for overdrainage, CSF leak, and infection.
   (c) External ventricular drainage (EVD): Open system to remove the CSF to an external collection system. Catheter is usually placed in the frontal horn (but also posterior horn) with relatively long subcutaneous tunneling. ICP measurement and volume monitoring can be carried out. Usually applied in premature babies (less common), in patients with CSF infection, before tumor removal, or patients with impaired consciousness. Drainage level is regulated by the height of the reservoir placed relative to the external auditory canal. Disadvantage: May cause under or overdrainage, if drainage level is not properly controlled. Might be more prone to infections as being an open system.
3. Neuroendoscopy is a camera-aided minimal invasive surgical technique to either clean the ventricles or to re-establish CSF flow if CSF communication between different compartments is impaired.

(a) Neuroendoscopic lavage (NEL): Method to clean the ventricles (usually supratentorial only) forms polluted CSF, hematoma, or infectious debris. In cases of IVH, neuroendoscopy might be applied as an alternative or in combination with other temporizing measures in premature babies to reduce the amount of blood in the ventricles and reduce the shunt dependency as well as secondary shunt complications. In ventriculitis, it is applied to clean the ventricles more efficiently from germs and inflammatory material to reduce multiloculated hydrocephalus, shunt reinfection, or other shunt complications. Multidisciplinary expertise is warranted and more relevant in patients with high amounts of intraventricular debris.

(b) Endoscopic ventriculozisternostomy (ETV): It is an alternative to a shunt system implantation and is indicated in patients with noncommunicating hydrocephalus with major CSF pathway obstruction, usually at the level of the Sylvian aqueduct or the outlets of the fourth ventricles. Typically, a pressure gradient is seen at the level of the third ventricle (membranes are bulged outward) and the origin of the obstruction as a mass or a membrane. During the intervention, a frontal burr hole is applied to insert the endoscope through the lethal in the third ventricle and to open the membrane at the floor of the third ventricle under endoscopic view in order to achieve a free flow from the third ventricle (internal CSF space) into the prepontine cistern (external CSF space) as CSF flow bypass. Disadvantage: This will not work in all patients with obstruction, especially infants younger than 6 months of age and patients with other causes of CSF dynamic pathology, and may not treat hydrocephalus sufficiently (resulting in compensated intracranial pressure).

(c) Choroid plexus coagulation (CPC): The choroid plexus is mainly located in the lateral ventricles (lesser amounts in the 3rd and 4th ventricles) and is responsible for CSF production. The obliteration of the choroid plexus by endoscopic coagulation can reduce CSF production and thereby re-establish a balance between CSF production and CSF absorption. It is often combined with ETV. The aim is to avoid shunt dependency in hydrocephalus patients. Disadvantage: It will not work in all patients, especially in whom other factors of hydrocephalus development are still dominant, and may not treat hydrocephalus sufficiently (resulting in compensated intracranial pressure) and remains to be controversial.

(d) Endoscopic cyst fenestration (ECF): This is indicated in arachnoid cysts with hydrocephalus and multiloculated hydrocephalus. In arachnoid cysts (especially suprasellar arachnoid cysts) which are related to hydrocephalus, the ECF can connect the CSF in the cyst with normal CSF spaces and can re-establish CSF flow. It may not work in infants if other factors for hydrocephalus development play a key role but should always be tried as the first choice. In multiloculated or multicystic hydrocephalus (often a consequence of intraventricular inflammation or ventriculitis), endoscopy needs often be combined with shunt implantation. The aim is to connect all isolated CSF-producing compartments by fenestration and to simplify the shunt system. Neuronavigation is essential in these patients since regular anatomy is often severely disturbed. During the active inflammation process, multiple repeated interventions might become necessary.

(e) Endoscopic stenting (EST): The combination of fenestration and placing a stent by endoscopic means to sustainably keep CSF communication patent at the respective opening may be applied in isolated ventricles and in multiloculated hydrocephalus. The first applies typically for isolated 4th ventricle by placing an aqueduct stent. It might be helpful especially during infancy if fenestrations at any location may re-occlude more likely. Precise planning of the entry point and neuronavigation is essential.

4. CSF-diverting shunt implantation is indicated in continuous hydrocephalus dynamics in communicating type of hydrocephalus and if no primary choice exists or is feasible to re-establish regular CSF flow in noncommunicating hydrocephalus.

   (a) Ventriculoperitoneal Shunt (VPS): Most frequent type of shunt implantation. A ventricular catheter is placed in the frontal or occipital horn (recommended under any kind of guidance) connected to a subcutaneous tubing in which a reservoir and a valve are included. The reservoir can be a burr hole reservoir or an inline reservoir and enables the possibility of CSF sample collection and pumping tests. The latter might check on proximal and distal flow patency (the latter depending on the reservoir and valve used). The valve is supposed to regulate adequate CSF drainage. The peritoneal catheter is placed after subcutaneous tunneling of the proximal shunt system usually via a paraumbilcal incision in microsurgical technique. Another option is laparoscopic guided implantation. A sufficient length (at least 35 cm) of intraperitoneal catheter placement is recommended to compensate for further growth of the patient.
   (b) Ventriculoarterial shunt (VAS): It is usually the first alternative to VPS if impaired resorption capacity is present in the peritoneal cavity (e.g., after enterocolitis or peritonitis). The distal catheter is then placed in the Seldinger technique under ultrasonic and X-ray guidance via a small neck incision just above the jugular vein. Microsurgical placement with dissection of the respective vessels is also feasible. The catheter length should be sufficient to place the catheter tip in the cardiac atrium.
   (c) Ventricular pleural shunt (VPlS): Another alternative if both the above options do not apply. An intercostal incision will enable access to the pleural cavity. Underdrainage and/or breathing impairment might be possible restrictions for the patients.
   (d) Lumboperitoneal shunt (LPS): It is another option if the ventricles are very small and CSF needs to be sustainably drained. A lumbar catheter is placed at the level of L4/5, and a sufficient catheter length is placed in the spinal canal. A subcutaneous catheter is connected to it and is equipped with a valence system before placing it via a paraumbilical incision into the peritoneal cavity. This shunt system is usually contraindicated in active small children because of a higher incidence of secondary Chiari malformation with

long-term devastating consequences. The LPS, however, might be an alternative in IIH patients during adolescence with small ventricles and after repeated proximal catheter occlusions.

(e) Consideration of valves used for shunt systems: There are multiple valve systems on the market, and in general, clinical studies were not able to distinguish the quality of different shunt valves. In general, there are fixed pressure valves on the market (low pressure, medium pressure, high pressure) and adjustable valves (which might be or might not be resistant to external magnetic forces, e.g., MRI, in terms of their adjustment setting). In addition, valves might incorporate overdrainage-compensating units (anti-siphon devices or gravitational devices), which should compensate for the different height levels of connected compartments (head and peritoneum) in the standing position of the patient. Advantages of fixed pressure valves are that they are simple, relatively cheap, and easy to implant. Adjustable valves have the opportunity to adjust the draining level and possibly treat the patient without necessarily performing another surgery. Overdrainage-compensating units are considered to be more physiological in CSF drainage ability and are applied with the goal of avoiding long-term problems of CSF overdrainage. In more modern treatments of hydrocephalus, adjustable valves in combination with overdrainage compensation units are indicated in pediatric hydrocephalus patients.

5. Preoperative needs

   (a) Temporizing measures: Imaging—Ultrasound images in prematurity, preoperative blood samples—normal electrolytes, complete blood counts, hemostasis, infectious workup, and neonatal stability, confirming the possibility to undergo surgery.
   (b) Endoscopy: Navigated MRI preferable; thin sliced T2 showing the membranes to be targeted.
   (c) Shunt: Imaging (for hydrocephalus and if applicable shunt), blood test as described above (a).

6. Intraoperative needs: All procedures should include strict anti-infectious protocol (Hydrocephalus Clinical Research Network protocol), especially if implants are used.

   (a) Temporizing measures: Intraoperative ultrasound, implants, instrumentation.
   (b) Endoscopy: Endoscopy instrumentation set—need to be checked for function. Neuronavigation system or any other guidance if applicable.
   (c) Shunt: Shunt instrument sets. Implants—appropriate valve, for tubing systems, antibiotic impregnation of the catheters or intraoperative use of vancomycin bath (500 mg/250 mL saline) to fill the shunt for additional prophylaxis. Valve type and setting (and overdrainage protection unit) must be checked or carefully selected. Double gloving, minimal handling of implants during surgery, limit traffic in the OR, consider using re-disinfective

measures during surgery with antiseptic wound and mucous membrane disinfectant on wounds and implants.

Nursing Care and Treatment

Management of external ventricular, subdural, and lumbar drains.

What Is Most Critical?

1. External neurosurgical drains are named after the location where the proximal catheter of the drain is located.
   (a) Ventricular (EVD)
   (b) Subdural (SDD)
   (c) Lumbar (LD)
2. These are gravity-based systems, and it is extremely important to make sure the patient and family are aware that any position changes can affect the drainage of CSF from the brain or spine. Incorrect positions can cause over- or underdrainage of CSF, which can lead to symptoms or complications for the patients. This can contribute to prolonged hospitalization.
3. Due to risk of serious harm, it is strongly recommended to provide adequate training to staff caring for patients with an EVD. This could include annual education, hands on skills with an EVD not hooked to a patient, and easily accessible tools/instructions on EVD management and troubleshooting.

Immediate Postoperative Care

1. The drain exit site may or may not have an occlusive dressing over it. Institutional policy should be followed for the management of the drain, incision, and wound care per surgical team orders.
2. The drain orders are specific to each individual patient and will include:
   (a) Level system 0 cmH_2O or 0 mmHg to the external auditory meatus (EAM) or tragus of the ear for EVD or SDD. Level system 0 cmH_2O or 0 mmHg at the lumbar exit site for LD.
   (b) Drainage height, usually measured in cmH_2O or mmHg.
   (c) Clamped vs unclamped.
   (d) CSF labs include protein, glucose, cell count, culture, and can be collected per institutional policy.

Daily Management of the Drain

1. Level the EVD/SDD/LD per manufacturer instructions. These systems can include a string level or laser level. Ensure to level zero reference point in line with the patient's EAM/tragus; see picture below.

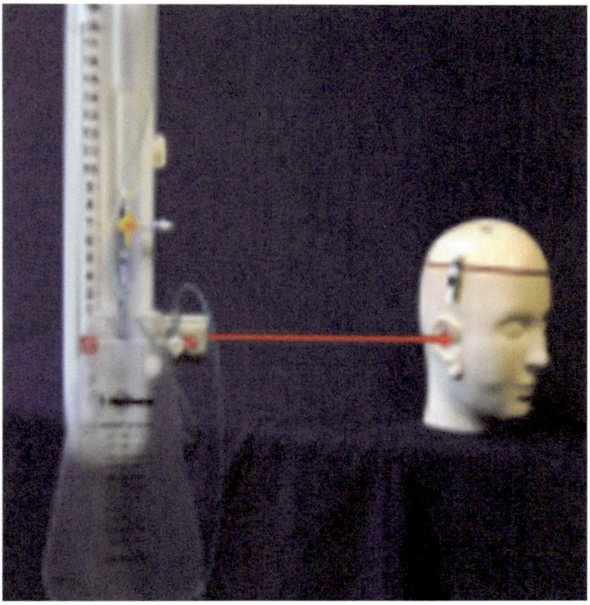

2. Confirm that the chamber is at the prescribed drainage height as shown below.

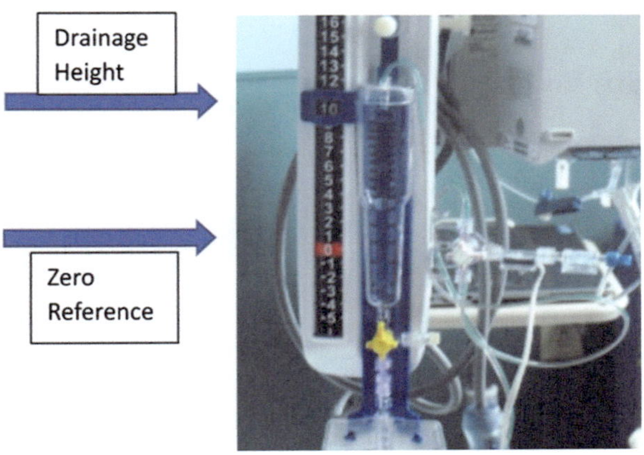

3. Make sure all stopcocks are open to the patient and open to the chamber.
4. Confirm fluctuance of CSF within the tubing or dripping in the chamber.

Important Tips

1. Clamp drain with any and all position changes, transporting, suctioning, turning, or sitting up.
2. Patients can remain clamped as long as they remain asymptomatic or per provider orders for therapy, imaging, etc.
3. For infants or nonverbal patients with an unclamped EVD, it is important that their family members or care providers are educated not to move the patient without the assistance of nursing staff.
4. Notify providers:

   (a) If CSF is no longer fluctuating in the tubing
   (b) Any leakage from the incision or drain exit site
   (c) Any signs of infection at the incision or drain exit site
   (d) Acute bloody CSF drainage

Lumbar Drain

1. Review orders to determine if CSF drainage is by gravity or demand.
2. If by gravity, refer to EVD instructions.
3. If by demand, RN must visually watch the lumbar drainage while the drain is open at all times as overdrainage can cause brain herniation and can be fatal. Drain the prescribed demand amount, i.e., open, drain 10 mL every hour and clamp.
4. Follow institutional policy as some hospitals require two RNs to be present for on-demand drainage.
5. Notify the provider with any drainage at the catheter exit site.

How to Obtain CSF Labs from an EVD

1. Obtain sample as per institutional policy.
2. Obtain supplies:

   (a) 3 mL syringe
   (b) Mask and gloves
   (c) Blue end cap
   (d) Scrub site or approved institutional cleaning product

3. Perform hand hygiene. Apply a mask and gloves.
4. There must be at least 2 mL of CSF in the chamber to obtain the specimen.
5. If the patient is ordered to be clamped and there is no CSF in the chamber, simply open the drain, allow 4 mL to drain into the chamber, and re-clamp.
6. To draw CSF from the chamber, clamp EVD stopcocks as shown below.

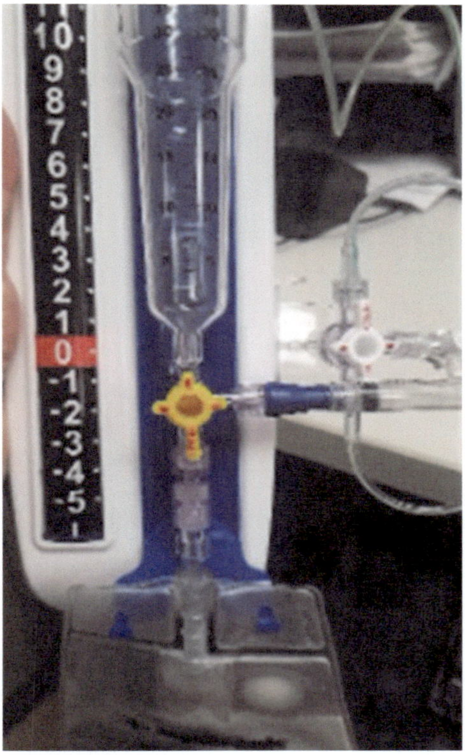

7. Scrub EVD port closest to the chamber with the institution-approved antiseptic cleaning agent for 15 seconds and allow it to dry.
8. Attach 3 mL syringe onto the needle-free connector and obtain 2–3 mL.
9. Place a blue end cap on the syringe.
10. Return the EVD system as ordered, clamped vs unclamped. Verify patient ID with the lab label per policy. Place the label on the syringe and send it to lab services per policy.

Nursing Care and Treatment

Postoperative management of shunts is surgeon-specific and thus may vary on a case-by-case basis.

What Is the Most Critical?

1. Shunts can malfunction at any time, even immediately postop if the ventricular catheter is inserted in a poor position.
2. Level of consciousness:

(a) Any changes in consciousness indicate the potential for life-threatening complications. Notify a provider immediately.
(b) If the postoperative neurological exam differs from the preoperative exam in any way, notify a provider immediately.

Immediate Postoperative Care

1. Pain control
   (a) Schedule acetaminophen and ibuprofen.
   (b) Some recommend IV Toradol postoperative day (POD) 1 for 24 h, unless there is concern for bleeding during the surgery.
   (c) Minimize narcotics.
      (i) Usually not needed for pain control and will often cause constipation, nausea, or emesis.
      (ii) Use with caution as it can mimic shunt malfunction symptoms.
2. Nausea control
   (a) Nausea and vomiting can occur due to anesthesia.
   (b) Control with anti-emetics.
3. Neck mobility/chest pain
   (a) For any patient with a new distal tube inserted, the tunneling of the tubing can cause pain along the tubing tract site, including the neck.
   (b) This is a normal finding. Some infants or developmentally delayed patients may not want to move their neck.
   (c) Nonsteroid anti-inflammatory medications are helpful in treating the pain for these patients.

What to Watch for

1. Incision
   (a) Some surgeons may place a dressing; others will not. If one is placed, it will often be removed over the course of 1–3 days.
   (b) CSF: Monitor and notify for any clear fluid from the wound. Also notify for any swelling or fluid collection around the shunt valve or tubing. This can indicate a shunt malfunction or increased intracranial pressure causing the CSF to leak around the shunt components.
   (c) Purulence: Monitor and notify for any purulent or yellow discharge from the wound, excessive redness, warmth, or pain at the incision that might indicate an infection.
   (d) Dehiscence: Monitor and notify for any openings of the incision.

2. Headaches

   (a) Postoperative and incisional headaches are expected.
   (b) If out of proportion to what is expected, this may indicate the development of intracranial pressure, especially if coupled with nausea, emesis, or a change in the level of consciousness. Notify a provider immediately with changes or concerns.
   (c) Positional headaches, especially those worse when sitting up or standing, may indicate a low-pressure headache. Some patients can take some time to become acclimated to a new shunt valve or shunt setting. Encourage patients to make position changes slowly.

Wound Care

1. Keep the incisions clean and dry.

   (a) Do not submerge incisions under water, i.e., swimming, until cleared by the neurosurgical team.
   (b) Frequency and initiation of wound care is surgeon-specific and can include:

      (i) For incision closure with absorbable or nylon sutures or staples: Can be washed as soon as postoperative day #1. Use soap and water with a clean washcloth or sponge, and dry thoroughly.
      (ii) Skin glue, i.e., Dermabond: Can be cleaned as soon as postoperative day #1 or as late as 7 days postoperatively. Use soap and water with a clean washcloth or sponge, and dry thoroughly.

2. Continue to monitor for redness and drainage.

Discharge Teaching

Parents should teach back/return demonstrate the following:

1. Signs and symptoms of shunt malfunction which can include:

   (a) Headache
   (b) Nausea and vomiting
   (c) Lethargy
   (d) Irritability
   (e) Bulging fontanelles for infants

2. Wound care:

   (a) Wash the incision per surgeon preference.
   (b) Assess for redness, drainage, or dehiscence.
   (c) Incisions can be closed with glue, absorbable, or nylon sutures.

    (i) Glue: As the skin heals, the glue will flake off. Do not pull the glue as it can tear the skin.
    (ii) Absorbable sutures can take up to 90 days to fully dissolve.
    (iii) Nylon sutures: Patient should return for postoperative wound check for suture removal 10–14 days after surgery.

  (d) Do not submerge incisions under water until cleared by the neurosurgical team.
  (e) Do not allow the patient to scratch or itch the incision as this can cause the incision to break open or become infected.

3. Pain Control

  (a) Acetaminophen and ibuprofen scheduled around the clock may be helpful for the first 1–2 days after discharge from the hospital and then transitioned to every 6 h as needed.
  (b) Narcotics may be prescribed as needed and given for breakthrough pain.

4. Activity

  (a) May resume prior therapies, i.e., physical, occupational, after shunt revision.
  (b) Recommend no contact sports, physical education class, or sweat-inducing activities until postoperative wound evaluation.
  (c) Contact your neurosurgical provider via office phone number or electronic medical record for the following concerns:

    (i) Fever
    (ii) Drainage, redness, swelling, warmth. or significant pain from the incision site
    (iii) Pain uncontrolled by recommended OTC or prescribed medications
    (iv) Changes in neurological examination

5. Follow-up appointment

  (a) Schedule a follow-up appointment date and time prior to discharge.

Diagnosis Support

Hydrocephalus is often a lifetime disease, for which patients and families can benefit from support groups, educational resources, and general navigation of living with hydrocephalus. There are a few options, one being the Hydrocephalus Association which offers a wide array of support, including a phone application to track treatment history, tools to transition from pediatric to adult care, and many other support services.

Suggested Reading

1. American Association of Neuroscience Nurses. Evidence-based clinical review: intracranial monitoring, brain tissue oxygen monitoring, bispectral monitoring [Webinar]. American Association of Neuroscience Nurses; 2023. https://apps.aann.org/store/product-details?productId=749992881.
2. Holleman J, Johnson A, Zakrzewski P. Hydrocephalus and intracranial shunt disorders. In: Bolick BN, Reuter-Rice K, Madden MA, Severin PN, editors. Pediatric acute care: a guide for interprofessional practice. 2nd ed. Elsevier; 2020. p. 840–2.
3. Jallo GI, Kothbauer KF, Epstein FJ, editors. Handbook of pediatric neurosurgery. Thieme Medical Publishers; 2018.
4. Hydrocephalus Association | We're here to support you. https://www.hydroassoc.org/.

Craniosynostosis

Pamela Gehrich and Eric M. Jackson

Introduction

Craniosynostosis, initially described by Virchow in 1851, is a pathological condition resulting from the early closure of one or more skull sutures [1]. The condition can be classified as either primary or secondary, occurring in approximately 1 in 2000–2500 live births worldwide [2]. Primary craniosynostosis is often attributed to unclear causes in the literature, while secondary is attributed to diseases and disorders and comes with other health issues. Depending on the number of sutures involved, a variety of complications may impact the child's neurodevelopmental status, and outcomes can vary. Craniosynostosis can present as an isolated suture closure or as part of a syndrome. See Table 1. There are many syndromes described in the literature, with the most common being Apert, Crouzon, Pfeiffer, and Muenke. See Table 2, Figs. 1, 2, and 3.

P. Gehrich (✉)
Clinical Education & Research, Johns Hopkins All Children's Hospital, Saint Petersburg, FL, USA
e-mail: pgehric1@jhmi.edu

E. M. Jackson
Neurosurgery, Johns Hopkins and Johns Hopkins School of Medicine, Baltimore, MD, USA
e-mail: ejackson@jhmi.edu

K. Battick et al. (eds.), *Nursing Guide for Pediatric Neuroscience Patients*,
https://doi.org/10.1007/978-3-032-22664-8_6

Table 1 Single-suture craniosynostosis [1, 9]

Categories of craniosynostosis	Sutures affected	Prevalence	Features
Scaphocephaly or dolichocephaly 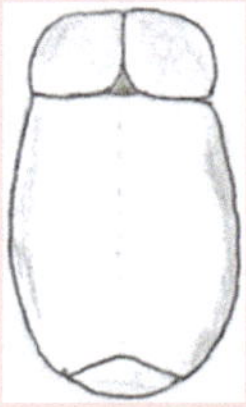	Sagittal	40–60%	Hull-shaped skull; premature sagittal suture fusion resulting in cranial elongation of anteroposterior axis.
Anterior plagiocephaly 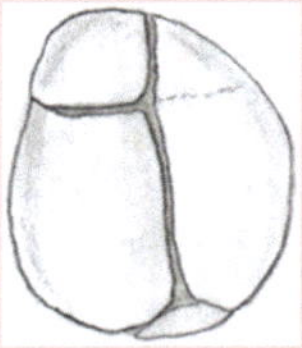	Unicoronal	11–20%	Flattening of forehead with eyebrow elevation and ear displacement of the affected side. Chin and nose deviate to the unaffected side. Also described as twisting of skull.
Synostotic trigonocephaly 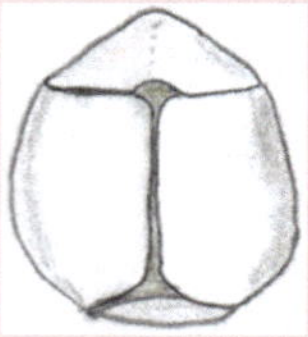	Metopic	10–30%	Temporal narrowing on both sides creating a triangle-shaped or pointed forehead and wide, flat back due to premature metopic closure.
Posterior plagiocephaly, typical lambdoid suture synostosis 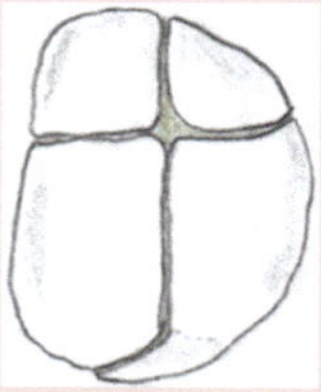	Lambdoid	2–5%	Temporal narrowing on both sides due to premature closing of unilateral lambdoid suture. Forehead bulges forward on the opposite sides of the defect, while the same side appears flattened, giving a trapezoid shape. The ear on the affected side is low-set.
Multiple sutures	Combination	3–7%	Cranial shape dependent on sutures affected.

Illustration by: A. Scott Gehrich

Table 2 Syndromic craniosynostosis [1, 10]

Syndrome-related craniosynostosis	Sutures affected	Common features
Apert syndrome	Coronal, combination	Tall cranium, cone-like, with flattened and elongated forehead. Bilateral temporal widening with flattened occiput. Cleft palates and syndactyl are seen as well.
Crouzon	Bicoronal, combination	Cranial shortening with wide and flattened/large forehead.
Pfeiffer	Combination	Tall cranium, elongated/large forehead.
Muenke	Coronal sutures	Tall cranium, elongated/large forehead with shortened skull.

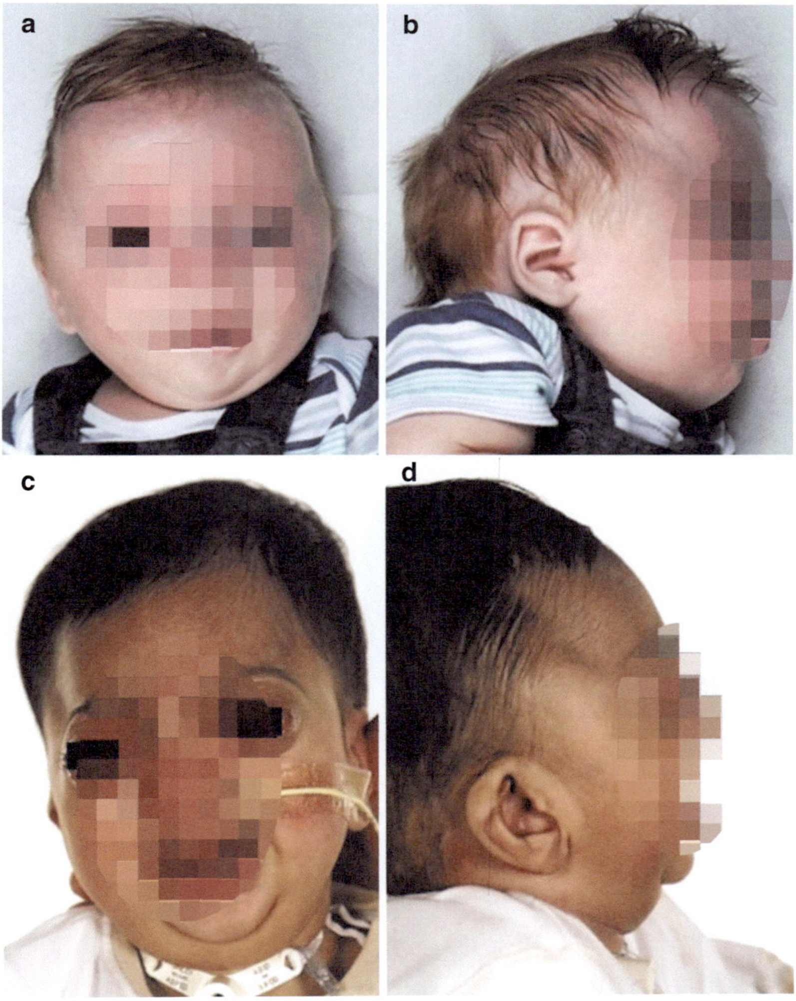

Fig. 1 Crouzon syndrome. (**a**) Anterior view; (**b**) lateral view; (**c**) severe case—anterior view; (**d**) lateral view. (Adapted from Mavridis et al. [15, p. 153])

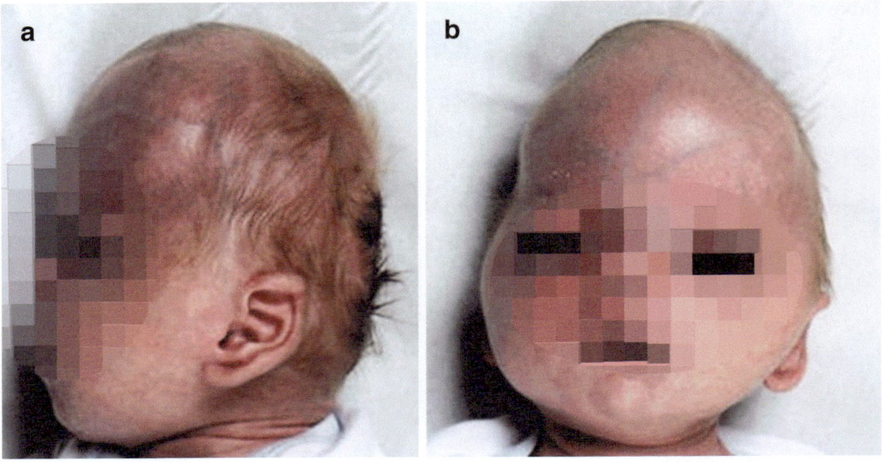

Fig. 2 Pfeiffer syndrome. (**a**) Lateral facial view; (**b**) anterior facial view. (Adapted from Mavridis et al. [15, p. 154])

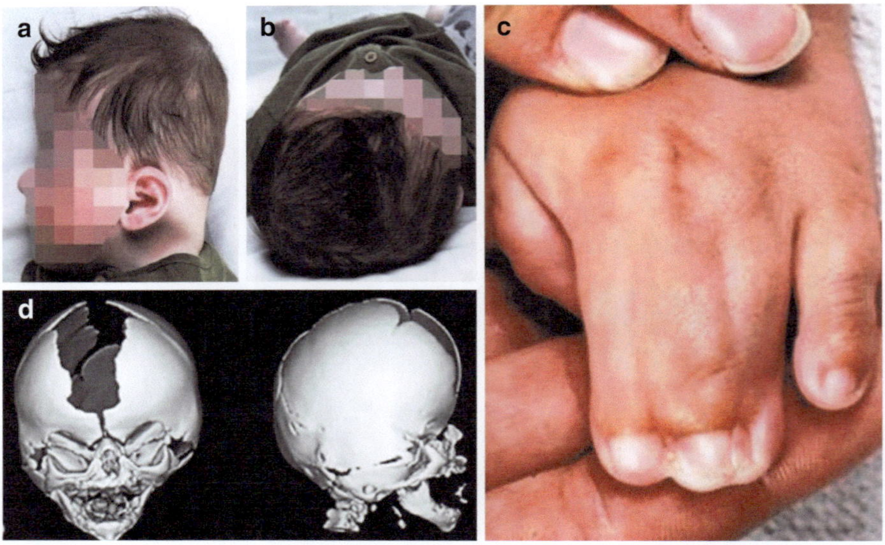

Fig. 3 Apert syndrome: (**a**) Lateral view; (**b**) superior view; (**c**) hand digits' syndactyly; (**d**) 3D CT reconstruction of skull (anterior and lateral views). (Adapted from Mavridis et al. [15, p. 151])

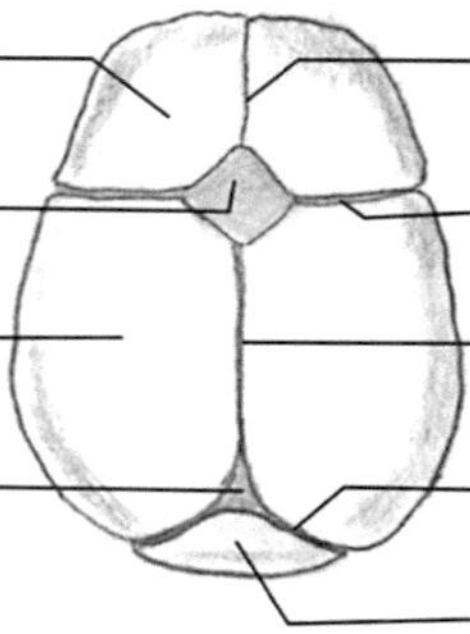

Fig. 4 Diagram showing the superior newborn skull with sutures and fontanelles. (Illustration by: A. Scott Gehrich)

Cranial Anatomy

Newborn infants have skulls made of bony plates separated by sutures. Cranial sutures serve to ease the baby's passage through the birth canal and later enable the brain to expand and grow with its volume quadrupling during the first 2 years of life. The major sutures are as follows: the metopic, coronal (2), sagittal, and lambdoid (2) sutures. Additional sutures that contribute to calvarial development are considered minor: the frontonasal, temporosquamosal, and frontosphenoidal sutures [3]. The sutures that meet the skull to form the anterior fontanelle include the following: the sagittal, metopic, and coronal sutures, palpable just behind the forehead at the midline. The posterior fontanelle is formed by the intersection of the sagittal and lambdoid sutures [3]. See Fig. 4.

There is a pattern to the closures of both sutures and fontanelles. The median closure of the anterior fontanelle is about 13.8 months, with the closure ranging from about 3 to 25 months [4, 5]. The posterior fontanelle closure is normal from 2 months to 1 year. The anterolateral fontanelle closes around 3 months of age, while the posterolateral fontanelle closes at 1 year. The metopic suture is typically closed before 1 year, while the remaining sutures remain open to accommodate craniofacial growth into adulthood [3–5].

Pathological Process

In craniosynostosis, early fusion limits skull growth in a direction perpendicular to the affected suture. As the brain grows, the compensatory skull growth occurs parallel to the affected suture, resulting in deformity [3]. Sagittal synostosis is the most common of all craniosynostosis not associated with a syndrome [7, 8, 14]. See Table 1 and Fig. 5.

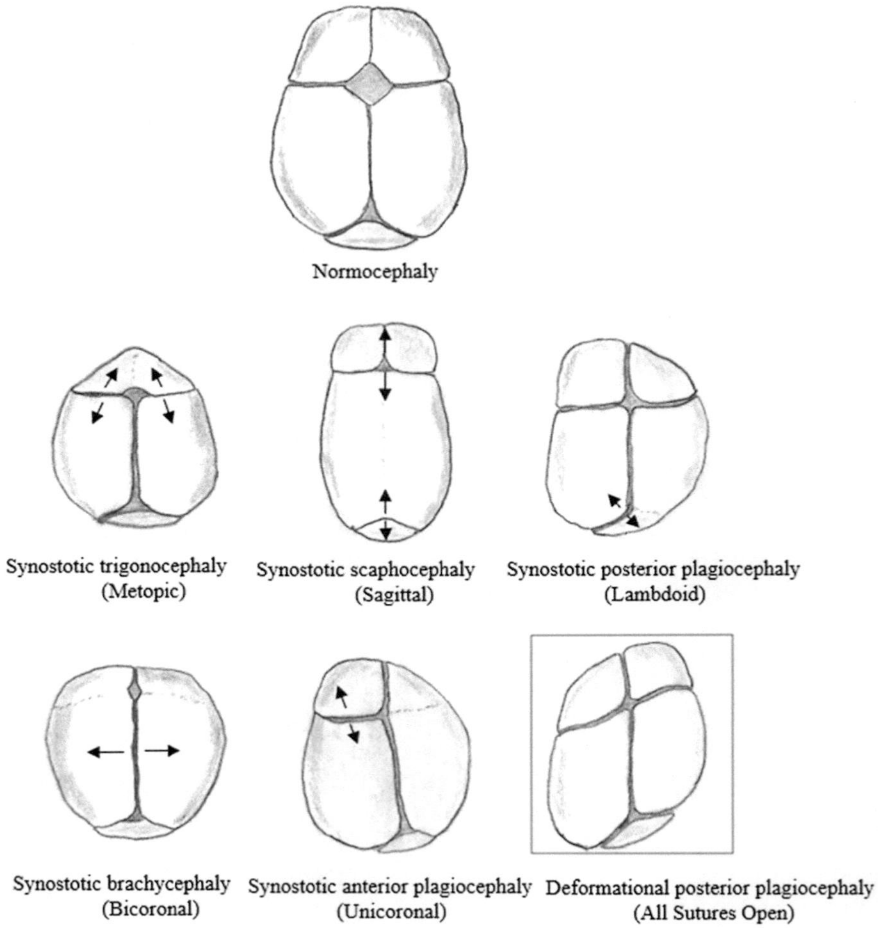

Fig. 5 Diagram depicts skull deformities associated with suture synostosis. (Illustration by: A. Scott Gehrich)

Diagnosis Definition for Nonsyndromic Craniosynostosis

1. Nonsyndromic is the most common type of craniosynostosis.
   (a) Can be identified at birth.
   (b) Molding may occur at birth, normalizing by 3 months.
   (c) Deformities worsen as brain grows.
   (d) Early recognition helps to allow for earlier interventions with less invasive surgical options.

Diagnosis Definition for Syndromic Craniosynostosis [10]

1. Syndromic craniosynostosis comprises 15% of all cases.
   (a) Physical exam and radiographic studies identify structural abnormalities.
   (b) Parents should be referred to a multidisciplinary team including a geneticist.
      (i) There are up to 180 syndromes linked to defects.
      (ii) Varying presentation of symptoms occurs, including cranial, face, and limb deformities.
   (c) Treatment includes medical and surgical management.

   Figures below are examples of syndromes indicated in Table 2.

Signs and Symptoms/Complications

Craniosynostosis is often identified at birth but may be more noticeable in the first few months of life as the baby's skull develops. Identification is dependent on severity and suture involvement.

1. Signs and symptoms of craniosynostosis include the following:
   (a) Mis-shaped skull
   (b) Raised and hard ridge along affected sutures
   (c) Facial asymmetry
   (d) Slow skull growth
   (e) Increased head circumference
   (f) Increased intracranial hypertension (bulging fontanelle; papilledema; projectile vomiting; increased irritability; high-pitch cry, headaches)
   (g) Cranial nerve involvement (vision, hearing, speech issues)
   (h) Visible scalp veins
   (i) Poor feeding
   (j) Poor weight gain
   (k) Developmental delays
   (l) Cognitive impairment
   (m) Coordination issues
   (n) Self-esteem and social isolation related to abnormal appearance

Diagnosis

The most common way to diagnose craniofacial deformities is by physical examination. It is important to obtain a full history when completing a physical examination for diagnosis. Physical/neurological examination includes the assessment of suture fusion and identification of congenital abnormalities and/or dysmorphic features. In addition to abnormal skull shape, the identification of signs and symptoms of elevated ICP should be investigated. Vision, feeding, growth, and developmental issues should be reviewed. Family history questions should include the discussion of utero exposure to teratogenic drugs, maternal smoking, nutritional factors, uterine restraint, fetal position, and pregnancy complications.

The gold standard for radiological studies used in identifying craniosynostosis is a low-dose 3D CT scan due to its accuracy compared to X-rays or ultrasound of skull. Magnetic resonance imaging (MRI) tends to be used for syndromic cases. For surgical planning, a 3D CT scan of the skull is standard to objectify the abnormality [14].

Genetic testing is offered to all patients when craniosynostosis is suspected.

Patient Management

It is common for patients who suffer from craniosynostosis to be managed by a pediatric multidisciplinary team.

1. Craniofacial team members may include the following:
   (a) Craniofacial surgery
   (b) Genetics
   (c) Neurology
   (d) Neurosurgery
   (e) Pediatrician
   (f) Radiology
   (g) Audiology
   (h) Ophthalmology
   (i) Orthodontics
   (j) Anesthesiology
   (k) Critical care
   (l) Nursing
   (m) Psychology
   (n) Social work
   (o) Case management

Differential Diagnosis: Positional Plagiocephaly

There are a variety of conditions that may cause positional plagiocephaly, including congenital muscular torticollis and positional deformities [3]. It is important to identify and differentiate the causes for plagiocephaly in order to provide the best treatment for conditions. Posterior plagiocephaly caused by craniosynostosis can be confused with deformational (positional) plagiocephaly [3]. An assortment of forces may cause positional plagiocephaly such as birth canal, mattress, car seat, swing, stroller, or any hard surfaces for a prolonged period of time.

Congenital torticollis occurs when the sternocleidomastoid muscle becomes fibrotic or shortened and causes lateral tilt of head, impacting passive cervical range of motion, causing the neck to stiffen. This positioning may result in facial hemihypoplasia or plagiocephaly [11].

Management and Treatment

Positional Plagiocephaly Prevention

Since the American Academy of Pediatrics launched its "Back to Sleep Campaign" in 1992 related to SIDS prevention, there has been a significant increase in positional plagiocephaly cases [12].

1. Ways to reduce the incidence of positional plagiocephaly includes the following:
   (a) Supervised tummy time (strengthens neck, shoulder, and arm muscles).
   (b) Frequent repositioning in crib (do not lay down in same spot/change direction).
   (c) Change crib location so infant does not look in one dominant area (example, toward door).
   (d) Avoid too much time in car seats, bouncers, carriers, or on hard surfaces.
   (e) Change or rotate positions of infant when holding, carrying, or feeding.

Treatment for positional plagiocephaly if above techniques fail may include cranio-orthotic device or band therapy. Helmet therapy applies gentle pressure to affected area where growth is not desired; leaving space on the side where growth is preferred can help with reshaping the head [9]. Length and time of treatment are dependent on age at presentation. See Fig. 6.

1. Treatment options include the following:
   (a) Families should consult a provider prior to utilizing helmets since products are custom-made and fitted.
   (b) The optimal age range for treatments is typically between 6 and 12 months.

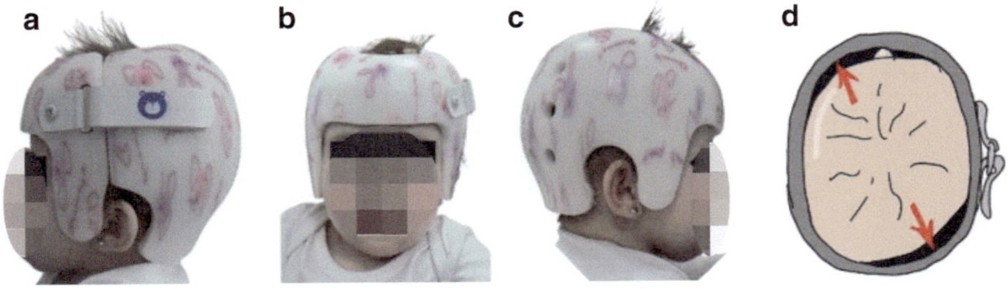

Fig. 6 Cranio-orthotic therapy. (**a–c**) Lateral and frontal views; (**d**) principle of orthotic therapy. (From Chrenko et al. [16])

(c) Helmets/bands are worn at all times except for bathing/cleaning.
(d) Scalp should be monitored for redness and breakdown to prevent issues.

Congenital Torticollis

For congenital torticollis, physical therapy with exercises to stretch the muscles of neck may be warranted. Occasionally, cases seen later in childhood may require a surgical intervention to correct skull deformity. See Fig. 7.

Surgical Approach

Surgical intervention for craniosynostosis is indicated to reduce the risk of increased ICP and manage the head shape. There are two main types of surgeries for craniosynostosis, "minimally invasive" or endoscopic-assisted and traditional open cranial vault remodeling. See Table 3.

1. Strip craniectomy plus helmet is a common primary approach for young children who have single suture involvement.
2. Another approach for sagittal synostosis involves strip craniectomy with spring placement rather than helmet therapy.

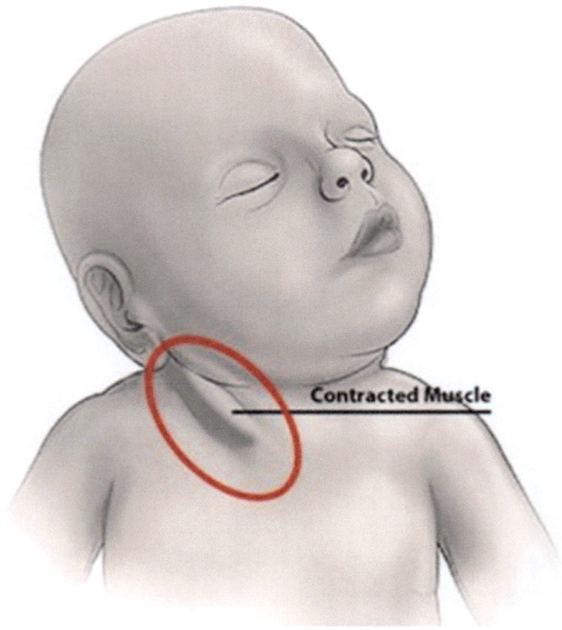

Fig. 7 Contracted muscle seen in congential toricollis. (Adapted from Maqsood [17, p. 147])

Table 3 Surgical interventions [6, 13, 14]

Suture affected	Surgical approach/ treatment option(s)	Typical age of patient	Length of surgical procedure	Nursing considerations
Sagittal	Open vault remodeling	6–12 months	4–5 h	LOS 4–5 days High rate of transfusion Surgical drain No helmet required postop
	Endoscopic	2–3 months	1–2 h	LOS typically 1 day Minimal EBL Helmet or springs postop required
Coronal/ metopic	Open vault remodeling or fronto-orbital advancement	6–12 months	4–5 h	LOS 4–5 days High rate of transfusion Surgical drain No helmet required postop
	Endoscopic	2–3 months	1–2 h	LOS typically 1 day Minimal EBL Helmet postop required
Lambdoid (very rare)	Open vault remodeling	6–12 months	4–5 h	LOS 4–5 days High rate of transfusion Surgical drain No helmet required postop
	Endoscopic	2–3 months	1–2 h	LOS typically 1 day Minimal EBL Helmet postop required

3. Fronto-orbital advancement/remodeling may be utilized for correcting coronal, metopic, or multi-suture synostosis.
4. Cranial vault remodeling and reconstruction allow for reshaping of bones in a single surgery.
5. Posterior vault distraction is a surgical intervention used to gradually stretch the bone and skin while expanding the back of skull, providing intracranial space. The family is taught how to turn distractors, allowing for gradual expansion of bone and tissue.

Any patient who undergoes a surgical intervention for craniosynostosis is at risk for a variety of complications. Risks are associated as in all surgical procedures.

1. Surgical complications include the following:
   (a) General anesthesia
   (b) Bleeding/ blood loss
   (c) Infection
   (d) Scarring
   (e) Injury to neurovascular structures
   (f) Neurologic abnormalities
      (i) Blindness
      (ii) Weakness
      (iii) Seizures
   (g) Cerebral edema
   (h) Coma/death (very rare)

Postoperative Care

Postoperative care for a patient after cranial surgery is important to reduce the risk of complications. The bedside nurse is responsible for monitoring the patient and identifying any abnormal findings to report to providers. The level of monitoring and care may vary based on the acuity of patient's condition. The patient will be admitted to either the pediatric intensive care unit or general surgical/neurosurgical unit.

General care includes the following:

1. Monitoring the level of consciousness (LOC)
   (a) Notify a provider immediately of any changes.
   (b) Any neurological changes such as severe headaches, seizures, decreased LOC, vision changes, difficulty speaking, new numbness, weakness, or change in mental status should be reported immediately.
2. Vitals signs
   (a) Temperature, heart rate, blood pressure, pulse oximetry.
   (b) Notify a provider if vitals are outside of ordered parameters.
   (c) Fevers are common after open procedures; follow orders for notification.
3. Monitor surgical site for any of the following:
   (a) Swelling (expected, and eyes may swell closed; notify a provider for severe swelling).
   (b) Bleeding (notify a provider for excessive bleeding or bruising, monitoring for signs of anemia).
   (c) Signs of infection, redness, drainage.
   (d) Signs of CSF leakage.
4. Nausea prevention
   (a) Administering anti-emetics
5. Pain control
   (a) Scheduled acetaminophen and NSAIDS depending on age.
   (b) Use of narcotics is limited due to potential change in LOC.

6. Activity/mobility
   (a) It is important for the patient to be out of bed as ordered.
   (b) Elevation of head is important to reduce swelling. Patients should not lay on one side but alternate to avoid unilateral swelling.
7. Diet
   (a) It may take up to 48 h postop for the patient to return to a normal feeding schedule.
8. Surgical site care/wound care
   (a) Keep incision clean and dry.
   (b) May wash with mild soap and water after 48 h.
      (i) Pat dry with towel.
      (ii) Do not scrub incision or soak it in water.
   (c) If dressing is in place, keep it covered until the provider instructs removal.
   (d) Drain may be present to avoid accumulation of fluid under skin, usually removed 1–2 days after surgery.

Discharge Teaching

1. Complications to contact Neurosurgery/Plastic Surgery office.
   (a) Fever
   (b) Drainage, redness, swelling, warmth, or significant pain from the wound
   (c) Pain uncontrolled by prescribed medications
   (d) Changes in neurological examination/level of consciousness
2. Describe any activity restrictions and medication regimen (if any) for home.
3. Pain medications include acetaminophen and ibuprofen. Medication should be taken as directed and family instructed not to give any medication not prescribed. Report any uncontrolled pain to provider.
4. Nonpharmacological interventions that may assist in providing comfort include the following:
   (a) Cold packs.
   (b) Positioning.
   (c) Soft music.
   (d) Calming environment.
   (e) Comfortable environment.
      (i) Reduce noise and lights.
   (f) Clean area to reduce the risk of infections.

Conclusion

Craniosynostosis can be overwhelming for parents and caregivers when diagnosed. It is important to diagnose early and provide interventions to limit complications. The role of nurses caring for these patients include providing postoperative care, pain management, and identifying any abnormal postoperative complications.

References

1. Girgin Fİ, Abdullayev R, Sakar M, Dağçınar A, Ozturk MN. Comparison of syndromic and non-syndromic craniosynostosis cases followed in a tertiary pediatric intensive care unit: a case control study. Child's Nerv Syst. 2024;41(1):12.
2. Betances EM, Mendez MD, Das JM. Craniosynostosis [Internet]. PubMed. Treasure Island: StatPearls Publishing; 2020. Available from: https://www.ncbi.nlm.nih.gov/books/NBK544366/.
3. UpToDate [Internet]. Uptodate.com. 2025 [cited 2025 Feb 27]. Available from: https://www.uptodate.com/contents/overview-of-craniosynostosis?csi=2e10057d-126d-4c6d-9d0d-824800733dc3&source=contentShare.
4. Vu HL, Panchal J, Parker EE, Levine NS, Francel P. The timing of physiologic closure of the metopic suture: a review of 159 patients using reconstructed 3D CT scans of the craniofacial region. J Craniofac Surg. 2001;12(6):527–32.
5. Kiesler J, Ricer R. The abnormal fontanel. Am Family Phys [Internet]. 2003;67(12):2547–52. Available from: https://www.aafp.org/pubs/afp/issues/2003/0615/p2547.html.
6. Sullivan LE, Li R, Tong VS, Jagasia P, Bonfield CM, Golinko MS, et al. Craniosynostosis: current evaluation and management. Ann Plastic Surg [Internet]. 2024;93(6S Suppl 3):S144–9. Available from: https://pubmed.ncbi.nlm.nih.gov/39527402/.
7. Sandoval JI, De Jesus O. Scaphocephaly [Internet]. PubMed. Treasure Island: StatPearls Publishing; 2022. Available from: https://www.ncbi.nlm.nih.gov/books/NBK567753/.
8. Welcome to Zscaler Directory Authentication [Internet]. Lww.com. 2025 [cited 2025 Feb 28]. Available from: https://journals.lww.com/annalsplasticsurgery/fulltext/2024/12003/craniosynostosis__current_evaluation_and.3.aspx.
9. Conrady CD, Patel BC, Sharma S. Apert syndrome [Internet]. Nih.gov. StatPearls Publishing; 2020. Available from: https://www.ncbi.nlm.nih.gov/books/NBK518993/.
10. Gundrathi J, Cunha B, Mendez MD. Congenital torticollis [Internet]. PubMed. Treasure Island: StatPearls Publishing; 2021. Available from: https://www.ncbi.nlm.nih.gov/books/NBK549778/.
11. Positional Plagiocephaly [Internet]. AANS. 2024. Available from: https://www.aans.org/patients/conditions-treatments/positional-plagiocephaly/.
12. Bonanthaya K, Panneerselvam E, Manuel S, Kumar VV, Rai A, editors. Oral and maxillofacial surgery for the clinician. Singapore: Springer Singapore; 2021.
13. Alexiou G, Velasquez R, Colasanti D, Kozyrev S, Baluszek S, Muhammad J, et al. Pediatric neurosurgery for clinicians. Springer eBooks. Springer Nature; 2022.
14. Craniosynostosis imaging: practice essentials, radiography, computed tomography. eMedicine [Internet]. 2023. Available from: https://emedicine.medscape.com/article/407856-overview?form=fpf.
15. Mavridis IN, Wimalachandra WSB, Rodrigues D. Craniofacial syndromes. Pediatr Neurosurg Clin. 2022:147–61.
16. Chrenko R, Plž A, Nedomová B, Kuniaková D. Diagnostic and treatment possibilities in the management of positional plagiocephaly. Wien Med Wochenschr (1946) [Internet]. 2024. https://doi.org/10.1007/s10354-02401056-6. Available from: https://pubmed.ncbi.nlm.nih.gov/39436546/.
17. Maqsood A. Congenital muscular torticollis. Springer eBooks; 2022. p. 145–53.

Chiari Malformation

Kentlee Battick and S. Hassan A. Akbari

Description

A chiari malformation type I (CM1) refers to the descent of the cerebellar tonsils below the level of the hole at the bottom of the skull (foramen magnum) that allows the brain to send the spinal cord to a person's extremities (Fig. 1). Typically, a CM1 is defined as having 5 mm or more of tonsillar descent below the foramen magnum. Less than 5 mm is termed tonsillar ectopia, is usually considered a normal variant, is usually asymptomatic, and usually does not require treatment. A CM1 can occur for secondary reasons such as hydrocephalus, spinal tethering, or tumors; these are treated by treating the underlying condition. However, CM1 is most often idiopathic, with no known reason. There are several theories on why idiopathic cases occur, ranging from abnormal development to a small posterior fossa (most posterior part of the cranium) [1].

Cerebrospinal fluid (CSF) usually flows through the ventricular system of the brain and drains into the spinal canal as well as into a thin channel of fluid in the spinal cord itself, termed the central canal. Usually, this is not visible on MRI, but CM1, for reasons that are still unclear, can cause abnormal amounts of fluid in the

Supplementary Information The online version contains supplementary material available at https://doi.org/10.1007/978-3-032-22664-8_7.

K. Battick (✉)
Hough Family Institute for Brain Protection Sciences Johns Hopkins All Children's Hospital, St Petersburg, FL, USA
e-mail: kbattic2@jhmi.edu

S. H. A. Akbari
Johns Hopkins University, Hough Family Institute for Brain Protection Sciences, Johns Hopkins All Children's Hospital, St. Petersburg, FL, USA
e-mail: sakbari3@jhmi.edu

K. Battick et al. (eds.), *Nursing Guide for Pediatric Neuroscience Patients*,
https://doi.org/10.1007/978-3-032-22664-8_7

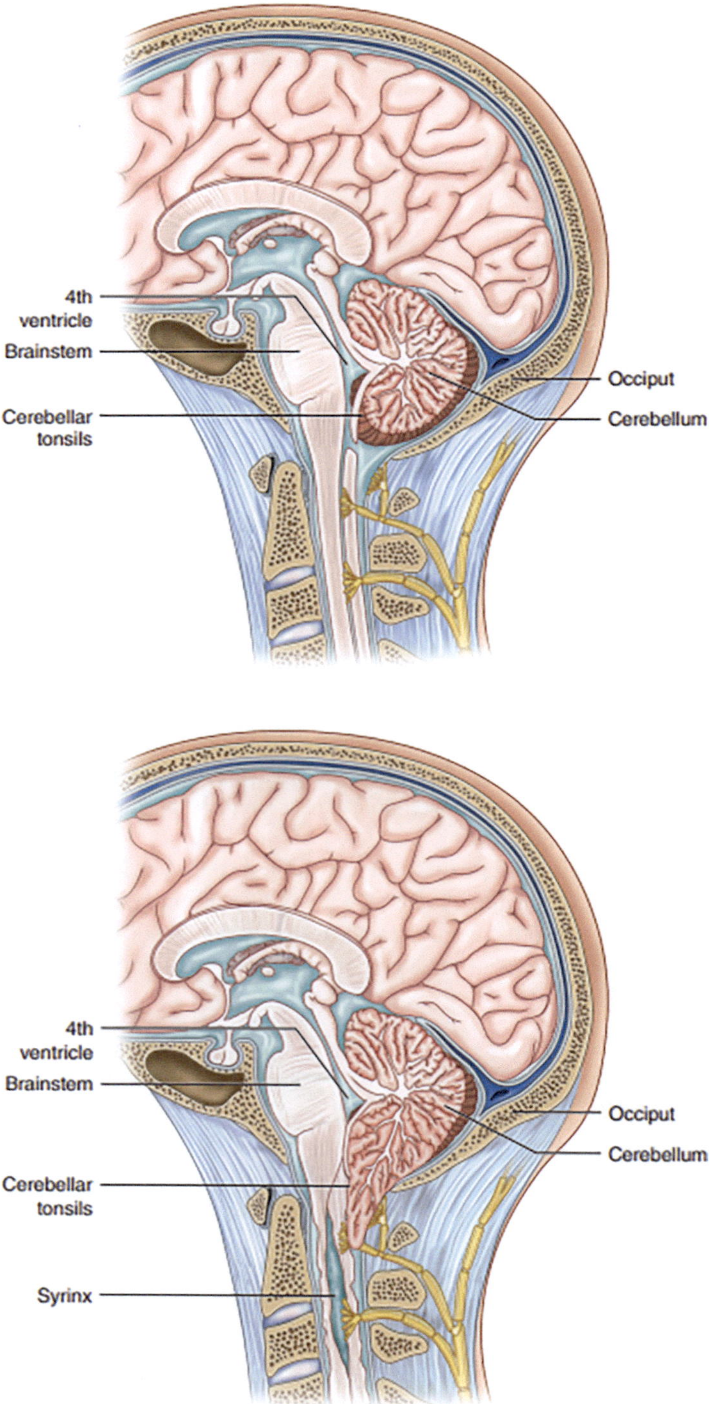

Fig. 1 Illustration of Chiari malformation: Illustration was generated using an artificial intelligence image-generation tool (OpenAI) based on an original prompt created by the author

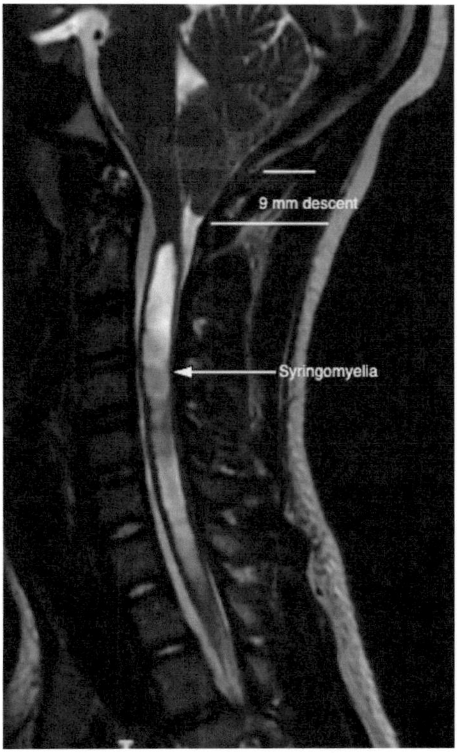

Fig. 2 T2 sagittal MRI and Chiari malformation with the syrinx of the cervical spine. The cerebellar tonsils are 9 mm below the foramen magnum

spinal cord, termed a syrinx or syringomyelia (syrinx = a tube; myelia = spinal cord). Typically, a syrinx is defined as a fluid pocket of 3 mm or more on MRI (Fig. 2).

Roughly, a third of patients with CM1 will have syrinx, and roughly a third of these patients will have associated scoliosis. Treating the Chiari malformation is the best first step at halting or reversing the progression of the syrinx and thus halting or reversing the progression of scoliosis.

Signs and Symptoms

The most common presentation of a CM1 in clinic is an asymptomatic Chiari malformation discovered on imaging obtained for another reason (motor vehicle collision, other trauma, headache workup, etc.). Because of this, it is important to ensure that a patient's symptoms are truly from a Chiari malformation before proceeding with surgery to treat the malformation.

Patient symptoms are not correlated with the severity of the Chiari malformation seen on imaging. Patients with "mild" CM1 on imaging may have debilitating symptoms, while patients with tonsillar descent of several centimeters may be asymptomatic.

Symptoms

For patients with symptoms, symptoms can be categorized into the following groups and are also included in Table 1 along with physical exam findings:

1. Headache
   (a) Headaches can occur in any region of the head
   (b) The classic headache is the back of the head or neck made worse with Valsalva (coughing, sneezing, laughing, having a bowel movement)
   (c) The Valsalva typically will sharply increase the headache, and the intensity of the headache will often reduce significantly after the Valsalva ends
   (d) Typically, headaches are NOT associated with photo- or phonophobia, auras or visual scotomas, or menstrual cycles, as is typical with migraines
2. Cranial nerve symptoms
   (a) Lower cranial nerve dysfunction is more common, likely due to pressure on the lower brainstem from the tonsils
   (b) Difficulty swallowing or choking
   (c) Difficulty breathing, including snoring or sleep apnea
   (d) Hoarse voice
   (e) Facial numbness or weakness
   (f) Vision issues
3. Cerebellar symptoms
   (a) Balance problems/gait ataxia
   (b) Incoordination
   (c) Tremors

Table 1 Summary of symptoms/physical exam findings

Headache	Classic—back of the head or neck, worse with Valsalva maneuvers (coughing, sneezing, bowel movement) Can occur in any region of the head typically NOT associated with photo- or phonophobia, auras or visual scotomas, or menstrual cycles, as is typical with migraines
Cranial nerve (CN) symptoms	Lower CN dysfunction is more common Difficulty swallowing Snoring/sleep apnea Hoarse voice Weak neck rotation Facial numbness or weakness Disconjugate gaze or nystagmus
Cerebellar symptoms	Balance problems/gait ataxia, especially on Rhomberg testing Incoordination Impaired finger–nose–finger or heel–knee–shin Tremors
Spinal cord symptoms	Likely secondary to a syrinx Extremity sensory changes or numbness Extremity weakness Hyperreflexia, Hoffman's sign, Babinski reflex
Scoliosis	Most often secondary to a syrinx

4. Spinal cord symptoms
   (a) Most likely in the presence of a syrinx
   (b) Extremity pain
   (c) Extremity sensory disturbance
   (d) Extremity weakness
   (e) Incontinence—bowel or bladder
   (f) Sexual dysfunction
5. Scoliosis
   (a) Most often secondary to a syrinx

Physical Examination

Most often, patients will have a normal neurological exam. Patients with examination findings can be categorized into the following groups (see Table 1):

1. Cranial nerve signs
   (a) Swallowing issues
   (b) Hoarse voice
   (c) Weak neck rotation
   (d) Face numbness or weakness
   (e) Disconjugate gaze or nystagmus
2. Cerebellar signs
   (a) Ataxia or gait instability
   (b) Impaired finger–nose–finger or heel–knee–shin
   (c) Imbalance on Rhomberg testing
   (d) Nystagmus
3. Spinal cord signs
   (a) Extremity sensory changes or numbness
   (b) Extremity weakness
   (c) Hyperreflexia, Hoffman's sign, Babinski reflex
4. Scoliosis

Labs and Diagnostics

Labs

1. There are no lab studies to confirm or track a CM1

Imaging

1. Patients with an image showing a CM1 should undergo a brain and total spine MRI to evaluate the Chiari malformation, look for other factors that might contribute to a Chiari malformation, and assess for syrinx.

2. X-rays can be considered in patients with scoliosis.
3. A CINE Flow MRI may be considered to look for abnormal CSF flow around the Chiari malformation.

Other studies

1. May consider a sleep study for sleep apnea
2. May consider a swallow study for swallowing issues

Treatment

Medications

1. There are no medications to treat a Chiari malformation.
2. Medications are only beneficial to reduce headaches or pain and usually consist of acetaminophen or ibuprofen for headaches and gabapentin for spinal cord-related pain or sensory issues.

Surgery

Surgery is designed primarily to increase the size of the foramen magnum, thus decreasing the pressure from the cerebellum onto the brainstem and spinal cord (Fig. 3). Additionally, surgery helps improve the flow of CSF. There are several variations on surgery, but the two major groupings are posterior fossa decompression without duraplasty and posterior fossa decompression with duraplasty (see Table 2).

1. Posterior fossa decompression without duraplasty (PFD)
   (a) Some of the bone of the posterior fossa and foramen magnum is removed.
   (b) The back part of the first cervical vertebra is removed (C1 laminectomy).
   (c) Additional levels of laminectomy are performed based on the extent of tonsillar descent.
   (d) The dura is kept intact but may be scored to stretch.
   (e) The bone is left off to prevent bony compression.
2. Posterior fossa decompression with duraplasty (PFDD) (see Video 1)
   (a) a–c above are performed.
   (b) The dura is then opened either in a Y-shape or as a linear opening.
   (c) The outflow of CSF is inspected to make sure there is no scarring or veil of arachnoid blocking fluid flow. These are opened if present.
   (d) A patch is sewn into the dura to increase the space in this area (reduce compression from the dura). This patch may be pericranium from the patient (requires a separate incision but has fewer complications) or a synthetic material [2].
3. Other surgeries
   (a) For complex patients, redo decompressions, fourth ventricular stents, syrinx shunts, ventriculoperitoneal shunts, spinal cord detethering, or spinal fusions may need to be performed.

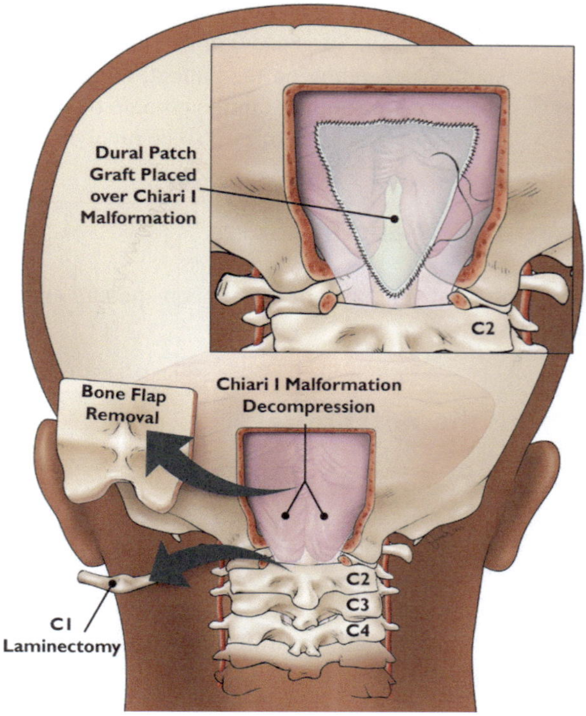

Fig. 3 Reproduced with permission from Springer Nature Publishing: Steps of posterior fossa decompression surgery for CM1. In a PFD, the bone flap and C1 laminectomy portions are removed, and closure is performed. In a PFDD, the dural patch is sewn into the dura after the dura is opened [4]

Table 2 Differences between PFD and PFDD, modified from Akbari et al., 2022 [3]

	PFD	PFDD
Operative time	~2 h	~3 h
Estimated blood loss	Lower	Higher
Approximate length of stay	~2 days	~4 days
Need for revision	Higher	Lower
Syrinx improvement	Lower	Higher
Sign or symptom improvement	Similar	Similar
Complications	Lower	Higher

4. Surgical takeaways
   (a) Both surgeries have similar improvement in signs and symptoms.
   (b) PFD surgeries are shorter and have less blood loss and require shorter hospital stays. While they have a higher revision rate, this may be due to poor patient selection as the subsequent PFDD surgery may have also not generated benefit.
   (c) PFDD is more likely to improve syringes but comes with a significantly higher complication rate including pseudomeningocele, CSF leak, and chemical meningitis. However, PFDD is the only way to visualize the CSF outflow.

(d) The type of surgery performed has been a major debate in neurosurgery with no resolution. Surgeons will be strong advocates of one type of surgery or another depending on the patient, imaging, and the surgeon's own experience. Patients or their families should be made aware of the surgical options and risks so that they may also be involved in decision-making.

Nursing Care and Treatment

Much of what follows will be surgeon-specific and thus may vary on a case-by-case basis.

What Is the Most Critical

1. Level of consciousness
   (a) This is the most important as changes in consciousness indicate the potential for life-threatening complications. Notify a provider immediately.
   (b) Generally, there are no expected deficits from this surgery, though depending on complexity, these may be apparent. Notify a provider immediately if the postoperative neurological exam differs from the preoperative exam in any way.

Immediate Postoperative Care

1. Nausea control
   (a) Nausea and vomiting are expected and normal on postop days (POD) 1–2, especially after PFDD given the presence of the vomiting center of the brain, the area postrema, in the low brainstem.
   (b) Control with anti-emetics.
2. Neck mobility
   (a) Due to the dissection of the neck muscles, muscle tightness, pain, or spasms are common.
   (b) Children will often choose to not move their neck because of pain, but this will increase stiffness and reduce mobility.
      - Encourage mobility; muscle relaxants will help.
   (c) Kids will move to have fun.
      - Adjust the environment to help: Move the bed to side you wish the patient to turn to, this will encourage turning to watch the TV or tablet, grab attention with parents or toys on one side and then the other to stretch the neck; consult physical therapy in severe cases.
3. Pain control
   (a) Schedule acetaminophen and ibuprofen.
      - Some recommend IV Toradol POD 1 for 24 h, unless there is concern for bleeding during the surgery.

(b) Minimize narcotics.
   - Usually not needed for pain control and will often cause constipation, nausea, or emesis.

(c) Schedule diazepam or another muscle relaxer usually needed POD 1–3 and PRN thereafter.

(d) Occasional steroids, especially when a PFDD is performed.

What to Watch for

1. Incision
   (a) Some surgeons will place a dressing, others will not. If one is placed, it will often be removed over the course of 1–3 days.
   (b) Blood: Monitor blood from the incision or on the dressing, notify for constant blood, increase in frequency, change in consistency, or hematoma formation.
   (c) CSF: Monitor and notify for any clear fluid from the wound, as this is likely a CSF leak.
   (d) Purulence: Monitor and notify for any purulent or yellow discharge from the wound, excessive redness, warmth, or pain at the incision that might indicate an infection.
   (e) Openings: Monitor and notify for any openings of the incision.
2. Headaches
   (a) Postoperative and incisional headaches are expected.
   (b) If out of proportion to what is expected, this may indicate the development of intracranial pressure, especially if coupled with nausea, emesis, or a change in the level of consciousness. Notify a provider immediately.
   (c) Positional headaches, especially worse when sitting up or standing, may indicate a low-pressure headache secondary to the expected loss of CSF during the surgery: Notify the provider and likely plan to lay flat with IV fluids.

Wound Care

1. Keep clean and dry—usually ok to start washing the incision by POD 1.
   (a) Do not submerge the incision or have direct pressure from a shower head until a week or two after surgery.
2. Continue to monitor for clear fluid or yellow fluid to indicate either a CSF leak or infection.

Discharge Teaching

Parents should teach back/return demonstrate the following:

1. List reasons to contact Neurosurgery Office.
   (a) Fever.
   (b) Drainage, redness, swelling, warmth, or significant pain from the wound.
   (c) Pain uncontrolled by prescribed medications.
   (d) Changes in neurological examination.
2. Completion of wound care, as described above.
3. Describe any activity restrictions and medication regimen (if any) for home.
   (a) When to take pain medications.
   (b) Steroid wean schedule if applicable.

Suggested Reading

1. Botelho RV, Heringer LC, Botelho PB, Lopes RA, Waisberg J. Posterior fossa dimensions of chiari malformation patients compared with normal subjects: systematic review and meta-analysis. World Neurosurg. 2020;138:521–529.e2. https://doi.org/10.1016/j.wneu.2020.02.182.
2. Yahanda AT, Simon LE, Limbrick DD. Outcomes for various dural graft materials after posterior fossa decompression with duraplasty for Chiari malformation type I: a systematic review and meta-analysis. J Neurosurg. 2021;135(5):1356–69. https://doi.org/10.3171/2020.9.JNS202641.
3. Akbari SHA, Yahanda AT, Ackerman LL, Adeson PD, Ahmed R, Albert GW, Aldana PR, Alden TD, Anderson RCE, Bauer DF, Bethel-Anderson T, Bierbrauer K, Brockmeyer DL, Chern JJ, Couture DE, Daniels DJ, Dlouhy BJ, Durham SR, Ellenbogen RG, Eskandari R, Fuchs HE, Grant GA, Graupman PC, Greene S, Greenfield JP, Gross NL, Guillaume DJ, Hankinson TC, Heuer GG, Iantosca M, Iskandar BJ, Jackson EM, Jallo GI, Johnston JM, Kaufman BA, Keating RF, Khan NR, Krieger MD, Leonard JR, Maher CO, Mangano FT, McComb JG, McEvoy SD, Meehan T, Menezes AH, Muhlbauer MS, O'Neill BR, Olavarria G, Ragheb J, Selden NR, Shah MN, Shannon CN, Shimony JS, Smyth MD, Stone SSD, Strahle JM, Tamber MS, Torner JC, Tuite GF, Tyler-Kabara EC, Wait SD, Wellons JC, Whitehead WE, Park TS, Limbrick DD. Complications and outcomes of posterior fossa decompression with duraplasty versus without duraplasty for pediatric patients with Chiari malformation type I and syringomyelia: a study from the Park-Reeves Syringomyelia Research Consortium. J Neurosurg Pediatr. 2022;30(1):39–51. https://doi.org/10.3171/2022.2.PEDS21446.
4. Butensky S, Rodgers S, Baron S, Schneider S, Mittler M. Comparison of surgical outcomes in patients with Chiari Type I malformation receiving posterior fossa decompression with and without duraplasty. Childs Nerv Syst. 2020;36(7):1399–405. https://doi.org/10.1007/s00381-020-04667-7.

Spinal Dysraphism

Lindsey Tierney and Sara Hartnett-Wright

Description

Spinal dysraphism describes a spectrum of developmental abnormalities in the spinal cord and surrounding meninges, fat, muscle, vertebra (bones), and skin. The normal pattern of development is dependent on the closing of the neural plate into a tube which is subsequently surrounded by bone, muscle, fat, and skin. Spinal dysraphism occurs when there is a disorder in the closure of this tube, resulting in lack of closure or coverage of the neural or spinal elements. Spinal dysraphism is more commonly termed spina bifida and classified into two main types—open (aperta), where the spinal defect is not covered by skin, and closed (occulta), where the defect is covered with a layer of skin. See Fig. 1 for various forms of spinal dysraphism.

Spina Bifida Aperta

The two main spinal anomalies in the category of spina bifida aperta are myelomeningocele and meningocele. Each anomaly describes the anatomic structures which are contained in the defect. Myelomeningocele describes a defect in which the neural structures and meninges protrude through an open defect. Meningocele describes a defect in which only the meninges protrude in a cerebrospinal fluid (CSF) pouch through the skin. Open spina bifida defects are not covered with a layer of skin and

Supplementary Information The online version contains supplementary material available at https://doi.org/10.1007/978-3-032-22664-8_8.

L. Tierney (✉) · S. Hartnett-Wright
Hough Family Institute for Brain Protection Sciences Johns Hopkins All Children's Hospital, Saint Petersburg, FL, USA
e-mail: lcobb5@jhmi.edu

K. Battick et al. (eds.), *Nursing Guide for Pediatric Neuroscience Patients*,
https://doi.org/10.1007/978-3-032-22664-8_8

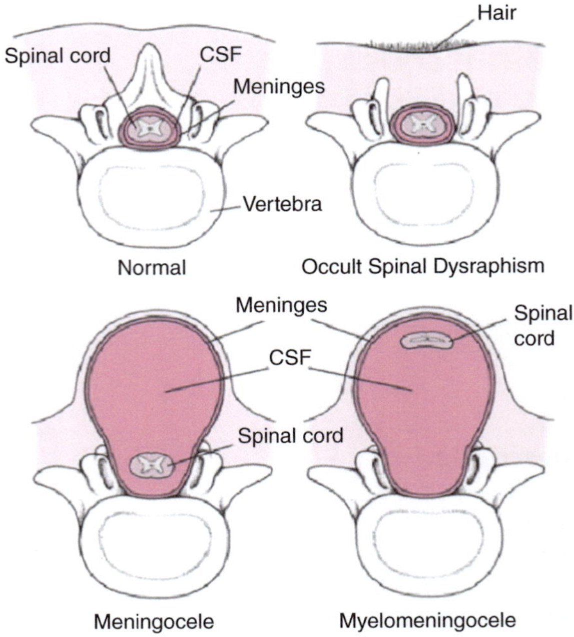

Fig. 1 Representation of the various forms of spinal dysraphism. (From the MSD Manual Professional Version, edited by Sandy Falk. Copyright © 2025 Merck & Co., Inc.)

are therefore at risk for CSF leak, infection, and further neurologic damage due to exposure to the outside environment. Myelomeningocele is associated with Chiari 2 malformation and hydrocephalus which will be discussed in other chapters.

Spina Bifida Occulta

Spina bifida occulta refers to spinal dysraphism in which the defect is covered with a layer of skin. The defects may not be diagnosed at birth. There may be associated skin markings, such as a tuft of hair, or hemangioma, sacral pit or dimple, or fatty mass in the lumbosacral area.

Spinal lipomas are the most common form of occult spinal dysraphism. Spinal lipomas are classified into lipomas of the conus medullaris, spinal lipoma of the filum terminale, and subpial lipomas.

Split cord malformations, or diastematomyelia, are less common and describe a congenital abnormality where there are two spinal cords, either within a single dural sac (Type 2) or in two separate dural sacs, divided by a cartilaginous or bony septum (Type 1).

Sacral dimples may indicate a dermal sinus tract or a connection from the skin to the intraspinal contents via a fibrous tract. The patient is at high risk of meningitis or spinal abscess (see Fig. 2).

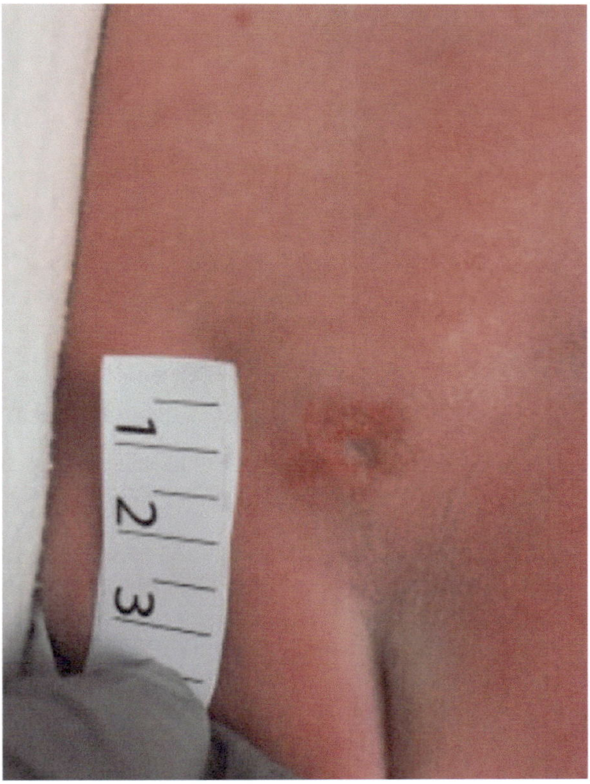

Fig. 2 Image of a sacral dimple with surrounding cutaneous hemangioma, typical stigmata of spina bifida occulta

Tethered Spinal Cord Syndrome

The anatomy of spinal dysraphism will create a tethered cord, where the conus medullaris is lower in position than normal. The pathophysiology of tethered cord syndrome is a stretch-induced injury to the caudal end of the spinal cord. The stretch leads to diminished spinal cord blood flow and altered metabolism. Excessive traction force may result in permanent neuronal damage (see Fig. 3).

Signs and Symptoms

Initial presentation of an open spinal dysraphism will show a sac in the thoracic or lumbar region with a visible neural placode. The infant may have evidence of neurologic dysfunction with club feet or lack of movement in the muscle groups of the lower extremities.

The initial presentation of closed spinal dysraphism may show markings on the skin in the back such as a sacral dimple, tuft of hair in the midline, appendage, fatty mass, or midline hemangioma.

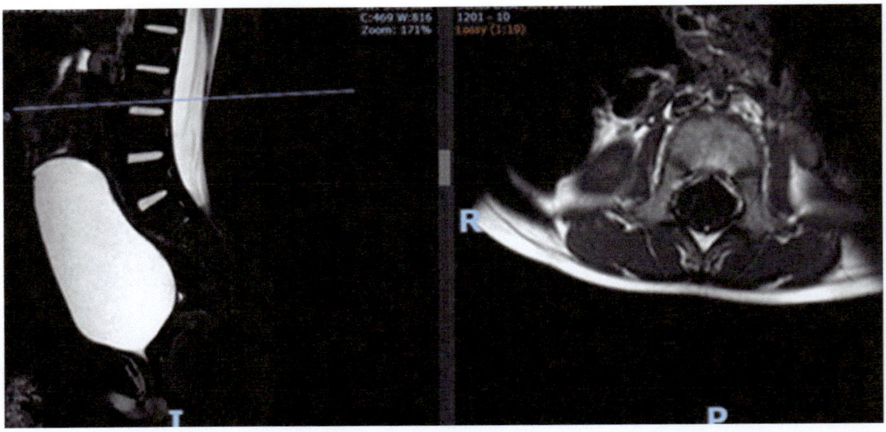

Fig. 3 MRI lumbar spine demonstrating fatty infiltration of the filum terminale and low-lying conus. Note enlarged bladder concerning for urinary retention

In follow-up, patients are monitored for signs and symptoms of tethered cord syndrome. The typical presentation of symptoms of tethered cord syndrome varies with age. Children under 10 years present with gait weakness, urinary incontinence, or re-emergence of nocturnal enuresis after potty training, or club foot deformities (in-turning of feet or curling of toes). Teenage patients may develop scoliosis, back pain, or urinary incontinence. Adult patients are more likely to present with back pain, radicular pain into the legs, or groin pain.

Labs and Diagnostics

Labs

- Labs are not typically needed to diagnose tethered cord syndrome. A urinalysis and urine culture are usually performed prior to surgery or on the day of surgery to treat an occult urinary tract infection.

  Imaging

- MRI lumbar spine or complete spine will be ordered to help confirm the diagnosis and for surgical planning. MRI may show hydromyelia or a syrinx in the cord as an indication of stretch injury.

  Other studies

- If the patient has a shunt, an MRI brain or CT head as well as shunt series X-rays will be performed as a shunt malfunction can also cause similar symptoms.

Treatment

Medications

- Gabapentin may be prescribed preoperatively to assist with pain control before and after surgery. Steroids, such as a Medrol Dosepak or Decadron may also be used before or after surgery to help with inflammation or edema to the spinal cord or nerve roots before and after surgery.

  Surgery

- Open myelomeningocele is repaired at birth within the first 3 days of life to prevent CSF leak and infection.
  - An incision is made above and below the defect in the skin, and the neural placode is separated from the dura and skin, and the layers are then closed.
- Closed spinal dysraphism is typically repaired after 6 months of age or even later, as symptoms of tethered cord syndrome typically do not present until later in life (Video 1).
  - The lumbar spine is localized with intraoperative X-ray, and the incision is planned in the midline at the correct level.
  - Part of the spinous process and the lamina are removed to expose the spinal canal.
  - The dura is opened, and the filum terminale or other tethering points such as lipoma, dermal sinus tract, etc. are exposed and freed from functional nerve roots.
  - The tension on the spinal cord is then released by cutting all points of tethering.
  - Neuromonitoring is used intraoperatively to guide dissection and protect functional nerve roots.
  - The dura is then closed in a watertight fashion.
  - The muscle and skin are closed in multiple layers.
- Re-tethering is common and can occur in up to 70% of myelomeningocele patients and 85% of lipomas. Fatty filum patients are much less likely to re-tether (around 3% of patients). Re-tethering and development of symptoms consistent with tethered cord syndrome may require another surgery to de-tether the spinal cord.
  - The prior skin incision is opened, and dissection is carried down to the spinal canal.
  - The incision may be opened higher up or lower down to assist in the dissection.
  - All points of tethering related to scar tissue are released both extradural and intradural to relieve tension on the spinal cord.
  - The dura is then closed in a watertight fashion, and the muscle and skin are closed in multiple layers.

Nursing Care and Treatment

Much of what follows will be surgeon-specific and thus may vary on a case-by-case basis.

What Is the Most Critical?

1. Motor function, strength, and sensation assessment and ongoing monitoring
   (a) Obtain baseline history from family or patient's chart and monitor for any changes or deviations postoperatively.
   (b) It is sometimes typical for a patient to have a temporary decrease in sensation or motor function postoperatively due to the dissection in surgery. The provider should give a detailed report on any expected temporary deficits.
   (c) Assess for the ability to follow commands, sensation, and motor strength.
2. Level of consciousness
   (a) Mental status change is not typical of cord detetherings; however, if the patient also has hydrocephalus and a shunt, they are at risk of shunt malfunction in the postoperative period.
   (b) Changes in consciousness indicate the potential for life-threatening complications. Notify a provider immediately.
   (c) Generally, there are no expected deficits from this surgery, though depending on complexity, these may be apparent. Notify a provider immediately if the postoperative neurological exam differs from the preoperative exam in any way.

Immediate Postoperative Care

1. Positioning
   (a) Patient may have orders to lay flat for 24 h or longer postoperatively to prevent leakage of spinal fluid from the dural sac. May elevate HOB slightly for meals if permitted.
   (b) May have an indwelling foley catheter while on flat bedrest. Provide daily catheter care with soap and water.
2. Pain control
   (a) Scheduled alternating acetaminophen and ibuprofen.
      - Some recommend IV Toradol POD 1 for 24 h, unless there is concern for bleeding during the surgery.
   (b) Scheduled muscle relaxants (e.g., Valium).
      - Muscles are dissected during the surgery and can cause significant spasms and discomfort.
   (c) Minimize narcotics.
      - Usually not needed for pain control and will often cause constipation, nausea, or emesis.

What to Watch for

1. Incision
   (a) Some surgeons will place a dressing, others will not. If one is placed, it will often be removed over the course of 1–3 days.
   (b) For diapered patients, protect incision and dressing from stool; consider placing a stool/mud flap. This is a plastic dressing with adhesive on one edge and should never touch the incision but only shield it. Covering the incision will allow heat and moisture to be trapped, leading to a wound infection.
      (i) Place the patient on their tummy or side.
      (ii) Trim the plastic to be as wide as the patient's hip and as long as the patient's diaper.
      (iii) Place the plastic face up and the bottom of the sticky part below the incision, close to the butt.
      (iv) Fold the loose portion down over the back of the patient's diaper.
2. Urinary Retention
   (a) Due to the manipulation of spinal cord, patients are at risk for urinary retention.
   (b) After the removal of indwelling foley catheter, monitor for urinary retention by postvoid residual bladder scans. If warranted, patient may need straight intermittent catheterization. Follow hospital protocols for bladder management and retention.
3. Constipation
   (a) Provide daily scheduled stool softeners to prevent constipation. Bearing down can cause harm to the surgical site and/or CSF leak.

Wound Care

1. Keep dressing clean and dry, protecting from stool contamination.
   (a) Remove dressing to inspect incision on POD 2. Cleanse with soap and water, pat dry, and replace dressing. Take a photograph of the incision and place it into the patient's chart for comparison at a postoperative clinic appointment.
2. Monitor for incision and dressing for clear fluid or yellow fluid to indicate either a CSF leak or infection.

Discharge Teaching

Parents should teach back/return demonstrate the following:

1. List reasons to contact Neurosurgery Office.
   (a) Fever.
   (b) Drainage, redness, swelling, warmth, or significant pain from the wound.
   (c) Pain uncontrolled by prescribed medications.

   (d) Changes in neurological examination.
   (e) Inability to void.
2. Demonstrate wound care.
3. Describe the impact of an infection, re-admission, potential for return to the operating room, etc.
4. Describe any activity restrictions and medication regimen (if any) for home.
5. When to take pain medications and differentiating between pain medications versus muscle spasm medication.

References

1. Anderson RCE, et al. In: Jallo GI, Kothbauer KF, Recinos VMR, editors. Handbook of pediatric neurosurgery. 1st ed. New York: Thieme; 2018.
2. Sweet J, Kalhorn CG. Spinal dysraphism: a review of clinical manifestations and surgical treatment options. Semin Spine Surg. 2005;17(1):23–9.
3. Albright L, editor. Principles and practice of pediatric neurosurgery. New York, NY: Thieme Medical Publishers, Inc.; 2015.
4. From the MSD Manual Professional Version, edited by Falk S. Copyright © 2025 Merck & Co., Inc., Rahway and its affiliates. All rights reserved. Available at https://www.msdmanuals.com/professional. Accessed 18 Dec 2025.

Suggested Reading

Mud Flap instructions from Children's of Wisconsin, 2023.

Skeletal Dysplasia

Kira Lurman and Mari L. Groves

These conditions vary in severity, and the neurosurgical needs are a critical area requiring specialized attention. They focus on managing foramen magnum stenosis, cervical spine instability, and spinal stenosis.

Etiology and Pathophysiology

Skeletal dysplasias result from mutations affecting bone and cartilage growth (Table 1). Most are monogenic and inherited in an autosomal dominant, autosomal recessive, or X-linked pattern. The most commonly affected genes include the following:

- *FGFR3* (fibroblast growth factor receptor 3)
- *COL1A1 and COL1A2* (collagen genes)
- *SLC26A2* (sulfate transporter gene)

These mutations interfere with the following:

- *Endochondral ossification* (formation of long bones)
- *Intramembranous ossification* (flat bones like the skull)
- *Bone remodeling and resorption*

K. Lurman (✉)
Johns Hopkins Medicine, Baltimore, MD, USA
e-mail: kmarant1@jhmi.edu

M. L. Groves
Pediatric Neurosurgeon, Johns Hopkins Medicine, Baltimore, MD, USA
e-mail: mgroves2@jhmi.edu

K. Battick et al. (eds.), *Nursing Guide for Pediatric Neuroscience Patients*,
https://doi.org/10.1007/978-3-032-22664-8_9

Table 1 Diagram showing normal versus abnormal endochondral ossification

Mutation type	Bone effect	Clinical outcome
FGFR3 gain-of-function	Inhibited chondrocyte proliferation	Shortened long bones (e.g., achondroplasia)
Collagen mutations	Abnormal collagen formation	Bone fragility (e.g., osteogenesis imperfecta)
Sulfate transporter defects	Disrupted cartilage matrix	Joint deformities, short limbs

Table 2 Common skeletal dysplasias and characteristics

Dysplasia	Inheritance	Features	Gene involved
Achondroplasia	Autosomal dominant	Rhizomelic limb shortening, macrocephaly	FGFR3
Osteogenesis imperfecta	AD/AR	Bone fragility, blue sclera, dentinogenesis imperfecta	COL1A1, COL1A2
Thanatophoric dysplasia	Sporadic	Lethal at birth, narrow thorax	FGFR3
Hypochondroplasia	Autosomal dominant	Milder form of achondroplasia	FGFR3
Diastrophic dysplasia	Autosomal recessive	Cleft palate, hitchhiker thumb	SLC26A2
Campomelic dysplasia	Autosomal dominant	Bowed limbs, ambiguous genitalia	SOX9

Classification of Skeletal Dysplasia

Skeletal dysplasias are classified by clinical, radiologic, and molecular features. The *Nosology and Classification of Genetic Skeletal Disorders (2023 Revision)* lists over 460 entities. Table 2 lists the more common forms and characteristics.

Clinical Presentation

Presentation varies widely by type and severity.

Neonatal Period

- Short limbs
- Macrocephaly
- Thoracic hypoplasia
- Respiratory distress

Infancy to Adolescence

- Delayed motor milestones
- Frequent fractures
- Spinal deformities (e.g., scoliosis, kyphosis)
- Joint pain and stiffness
- Psychosocial impact due to short stature

Assessment and Diagnosis

See Table 3 for key diagnostic tools.

History

- Family history of skeletal dysplasia or consanguinity
- Prenatal history (ultrasound anomalies)
- Developmental milestones

Physical Examination

- Limb proportions (rhizomelic, mesomelic, acromelic shortening)
- Craniofacial features
- Spine curvature
- Joint range of motion

Diagnostic Imaging

- *Skeletal survey*: Full-body X-rays to identify characteristic bone abnormalities
- *CT/MRI*: For complex spinal anomalies or cranial abnormalities

Table 3 Key diagnostic tools for skeletal dysplasia

Tool	Use case	Notes
Skeletal survey	First-line imaging	Consistent with radiologic patterns
Genetic testing	Confirmation, recurrence risk counseling	Requires family sample in some cases
Pulmonary function tests	In thoracic dysplasia	Assess restriction

Genetic Testing

- Targeted mutation analysis
- Gene panels or whole exome sequencing (WES)
- Karyotype if syndromic features are present

Management Strategies

Multidisciplinary Approach

Optimal care involves collaboration among:

- Geneticist
- Orthopedic surgeon
- Pulmonologist
- Physical/occupational therapist
- Nurse care coordinator
- Psychologist

Medical Management

Pharmacologic Therapies

- *Bisphosphonates* (e.g., pamidronate, zoledronic acid)
  - Used primarily in osteogenesis imperfecta (OI)
  - Improve bone mineral density, reduce fracture frequency
  - Administered intravenously, often in a hospital or clinic setting
  - Nursing considerations: Monitor for hypocalcemia, ensure adequate hydration, pain control during infusion
- *Growth Hormone (GH) Therapy*
  - Limited use in skeletal dysplasia; not effective in achondroplasia
  - Some benefit seen in hypochondroplasia and other selected conditions
  - May be used off-label in children with extreme short stature
  - Requires careful monitoring of growth velocity, bone age, and potential side effects
- *Analgesics and Anti-Inflammatory Drugs*
  - Acetaminophen or NSAIDs for chronic joint pain or postoperative discomfort
  - Avoid long-term NSAID use without GI protection
- *Respiratory Support*
  - Noninvasive ventilation (e.g., CPAP or BiPAP) for thoracic insufficiency or sleep apnea
  - Oxygen supplementation in cases with restrictive lung disease

Physical and Occupational Therapy

- Individualized programs to:
  - Enhance gross and fine motor development
  - Maximize independence in activities of daily living (ADLs)
  - Minimize joint contractures and muscle atrophy
- PT/OT are central to improving mobility in children with severe limb deformities or postsurgery

Assistive Devices and Adaptive Equipment

- Wheelchairs, walkers, and crutches tailored to body size and limb proportions
- Modified desks, utensils, and restroom aids
- Custom orthotics for limb support
- Standing frames to assist with bone health and prevent contractures

Surgical Management

Limb Lengthening and Deformity Correction

- *Techniques*: Ilizarov method, PRECICE magnetic intramedullary nails
- Used in achondroplasia, hypochondroplasia, and others to increase height and improve function
- Involves slow distraction osteogenesis (bone cut and gradually lengthened with a fixator)
- Highly specialized procedure with long recovery and high complication risk

Nursing Role

- Pain control and wound care
- Pin site infection monitoring
- Emotional support during extended recovery
- Encourage and monitor participation in PT

Spinal Surgery (Table 4)

- *Indications*: Spinal stenosis, kyphosis, scoliosis
- *Procedures*: Spinal decompression, fusion, growing rods
- In achondroplasia, lumbar stenosis may cause neurogenic claudication

Table 4 Nursing priorities in surgical care

Phase	Key nursing responsibilities
Preoperative	Assess for airway anomalies, educate family, address anxiety
Intraoperative	Assist anesthesia team with positioning; ensure safe transfer
Postoperative	Pain control, wound monitoring, neuro checks, PT coordination
Discharge planning	Equipment setup, home safety, outpatient follow-up scheduling

Postoperative Considerations

- Assess for neurovascular status
- Log-roll technique for turning
- Pain and infection management
- Respiratory care if spinal fusion involves thoracic region

Fracture Fixation and Intramedullary Rodding

- Common in *osteogenesis imperfecta*
- Use of telescoping rods to support long bones and prevent recurrent fractures
- Reduces need for repeated casting and immobilization

Nursing Role

- Postop immobilization care
- Prevention of pressure injuries
- Education for parents on handling and transfers

Cervicomedullary Decompression

- Performed in infants and young children with foramen magnum stenosis (especially in achondroplasia)
- Prevents brainstem compression and sudden death

Critical Nursing Tasks

- Close respiratory and neurologic monitoring, especially in conjunction with administration of narcotics
- Positioning and airway maintenance postoperatively, mindful of pulmonary risk
- Family education regarding symptoms of recurrence (e.g., apnea, weakness)

E. VEPTR (Vertical Expandable Prosthetic Titanium Rib)

- For thoracic insufficiency syndrome
- Expands thoracic cavity to support lung development

Nursing Care (See Table 4 for Priorities)

- Postop pulmonary hygiene (activity, incentive spirometry)
- Pain management
- Activity restriction education
- Infection prevention around hardware

Postoperative Discharge Education (Table 4)

- *The parents should return demonstrate wound care:* Once the bandage is removed, clean the incision daily with water and mild soap. Carefully dry the incision and leave it open to room air. Assess the incision for increased redness, swelling, drainage, or opening of the incision. Avoid swimming or taking baths until the incision is fully healed and free of any scabs
- Review needed follow-up with different specialties
- Reinforce the importance of appropriate activity restrictions if needed, following different surgical procedures
- Request teach back of signs/symptoms, when applicable, for patients at risk for spinal cord compression

Nursing Considerations

Assessment and Monitoring (Table 5)

- Growth charting using dysplasia-specific growth curves
- Respiratory assessments in infants
- Fracture monitoring and mobility checks
- Psychosocial assessments

Table 5 Nursing diagnoses for children with skeletal dysplasia

Nursing diagnosis	Interventions
Impaired physical mobility	Assistive devices, PT coordination
Risk for injury	Safe environment, fall prevention
Ineffective breathing pattern	Respiratory support, positioning
Disturbed body image	Counseling, peer support

Care Planning

- Promote independence with adaptive equipment
- Coordinate physical therapy
- Prevent injury (avoid contact sports)
- Monitor for signs of spinal compression

Family Education and Psychosocial Support

Families require ongoing support and education about:

- Nature and progression of the condition
- Genetic counseling (recurrence risk)
- Adaptive strategies at home and school
- Mental health support for child and parents

Psychosocial Considerations

- Anxiety about social acceptance
- School accommodations (504 plans, IEPs)
- Addressing bullying or social stigma
- Fostering resilience and self-esteem

Prognosis and Long-Term Outlook

The prognosis is highly variable:

- *Achondroplasia*: Near-normal lifespan with supportive care
- *Osteogenesis imperfecta*: May have progressive deformities, but many lead independent lives
- *Lethal dysplasias*: Thanatophoric, campomelic—require palliative care
- *Spinal deformities*: Can impair respiratory and cardiac functions over time
- Provide support during bisphosphonate infusion therapy

Conclusions

Skeletal dysplasias, though rare, present lifelong challenges requiring early identification and comprehensive care. Nurses are essential in managing physical health, advocating for developmental support, and guiding families through complex medical and social landscapes.

References

1. Mortier GR, et al. Nosology and classification of genetic skeletal disorders: 2023 revision. Am J Med Genet A. 2023;191(5):1164–209.
2. Krakow D, Rimoin DL. The skeletal dysplasias. Genet Med. 2010;12(6):327–41.
3. International Skeletal Dysplasia Registry (ISDR), UCLA.
4. Rauch F, Glorieux FH. Osteogenesis imperfecta. Lancet. 2004;363(9418):1377–85.
5. Hoover-Fong J, et al. Achondroplasia: manifestations and management. Curr Opin Pediatr. 2007;19(1):37–43.

Adolescent Idiopathic Scoliosis

Sydney Hyatt and Rajiv R. Iyer

Description

Scoliosis is a spinal condition defined by an abnormal curvature greater than 10° in the coronal plane, typically forming an "S" or "C" shape when viewed from the back. Smaller curve magnitudes may be positional or postural and may simply represent mild spinal asymmetry or spinal alignment effects of a leg length discrepancy. Scoliosis can occur at any age, but it most commonly develops during adolescence, often during the pubertal growth spurt.

Scoliosis is a three-dimensional spinal deformity, typically involving the lateral curvature of the spine from the frontal plane, decreased kyphosis in the sagittal plane, and axial plane rotation, resulting most commonly in a convex rib prominence because of the chest wall interface with the spine.

Because the exact cause of scoliosis is unknown, it is referred to as "idiopathic scoliosis." It is important to note that other types of scoliosis also occur, including congenital scoliosis (caused by disorders of formation/segmentation of the spinal column), syndromic scoliosis (caused by syndromes that have a known association with scoliosis, such as Marfan syndrome), and neuromuscular scoliosis (caused by disorders of the nervous system and muscles). Patients are diagnosed with adolescent idiopathic scoliosis (AIS) between the ages of 10 and 18 years. Scoliosis affecting other age groups may be termed early-onset scoliosis (younger than 10 years old) or adult scoliosis (patients 18 years and older) [1].

S. Hyatt (✉)
Department of Neurosurgery Clinical Neurosciences, Center University of Utah, Salt Lake City, UT, USA
e-mail: sydney.hyatt@hsc.utah.edu

R. R. Iyer
Department of Neurosurgery, University of Utah, Salt Lake City, UT, USA
e-mail: Rajiv.Iyer@hsc.utah.edu

K. Battick et al. (eds.), *Nursing Guide for Pediatric Neuroscience Patients*,
https://doi.org/10.1007/978-3-032-22664-8_10

Incidence

According to Weinstein et al. [2], AIS affects 2% to 3% of the population. Patients are at equal risk of developing AIS regardless of sex, but curve progression (and therefore the need for treatment) is 8–10 times more likely in female patients compared with male patients. Juvenile idiopathic scoliosis is more common in female children, and curves that develop earlier are more likely to require surgical intervention. Factors such as health care access, patient age at the time of presentation, and the genetics of specific patient populations may also affect incidence. AIS has strong genetic and epigenetic components [3].

Signs and Symptoms

Patients with AIS are generally asymptomatic; however, there are signs and symptoms that the practitioner should be familiar with:

- Visible spinal prominences or asymmetries (may not be immediately apparent to the patient, and parents/relatives may not immediately recognize these because many patients have a greater desire for privacy and independence in the adolescent years).
- Asymmetry of shoulders, scapulae, collarbones, hips, or waist.
- Back pain.
- Neurologic symptoms (rare, but warrant advanced imaging such as magnetic resonance imaging (MRI)).
  - Numbness, tingling, weakness in the limbs.
  - Loss of balance or change in coordination.
- In more severe cases, pain or difficulty breathing may result from the compression of lung tissue (otherwise known as thoracic insufficiency syndrome).

Physical Examination

1. Adam's forward bend test
   (a) The Adam's forward bend test is performed by having the patient lean forward at the waist until the spine is horizontal. The patient's feet should be together, with their knees facing forward and not bent; their arms should hang freely. While the patient is in this position, the back is observed for asymmetry, which can be more easily identified when the spine is curved. Asymmetry may be present in the lumbar, thoracolumbar, or thoracic spine. A rib prominence or "rib hump" may be present if the AIS is in the thoracic region (Fig. 1).

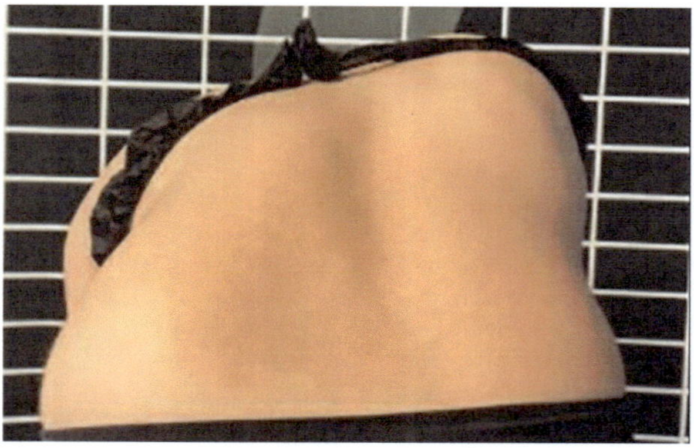

Fig. 1 On Adam's forward bend testing, the patient has a right-sided thoracic rib prominence caused by right thoracic adolescent idiopathic scoliosis convex rotation

   (b) Sensitive evaluations such as this should be completed in the presence of a health care chaperone and/or parent and with the patient's consent to evaluate their spine/body.
2. Scoliometer.
   (a) A scoliometer is a device that can measure axial plane rotational asymmetry. There are smartphone apps that can also be used for a similar purpose.
   (b) The scoliometer is laid perpendicular to the patient's back in a medial–lateral orientation straddling the spinous processes while the patient is in the forward bend position. The ball inside the scoliometer will indicate the angle of trunk rotation [4].

Understanding Skeletal Maturity

Skeletal maturity plays an important role in evaluating AIS because curves tend to progress (increase in magnitude) during the periods of rapid growth. Typically, the pubertal growth spurt in young women occurs during the year before the onset of menses. Understanding where a patient is temporally in their growth is critical in determining how frequently to obtain radiographs to detect potential changes in curve magnitude.

Clinically, the Tanner staging system can be used to objectively evaluate the pubertal stage, and history taking can supplement this [5]. A plain radiograph of the hand can allow for the classification of skeletal maturity with the Sanders Maturity Scale system [6]. Imaging of the hips via spinal radiographs allows for skeletal maturity assessment using the Risser scale score (relative ossification of the iliac crest dorsal apophysis and whether the triradiate cartilage is open or closed) (Fig. 2) [7].

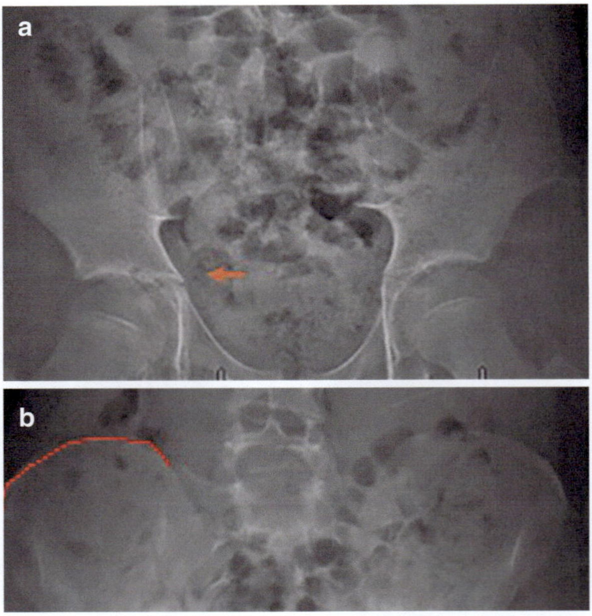

Fig. 2 (**a**) Coronal imaging showing that the triradiate cartilage (orange arrow) is open in this patient, a sign of skeletal immaturity and high growth potential. (**b**) Coronal image showing relative ossification of the iliac crest apophysis (red curved line, unobscured on contralateral ilium) known as the Risser sign. Ossification occurs in a lateral-to-medial direction (Risser stage), which is another marker of relative skeletal maturity

Diagnosis

1. X-ray
   (a) AIS is typically diagnosed with plain radiographs (X-rays) of the spine. These are typically full-length films to evaluate the curvature of the spine in two planes (coronal and sagittal, or posterior–anterior and lateral).
   (b) Ideally, the skull, hips, and knees would be visible to evaluate for limb length discrepancies and compensatory maneuvers that the patient may be using to maintain global balance.
2. Cobb method
   (a) The Cobb method (which uses the Cobb angle) is employed to measure the curve magnitude using the angle between the most tilted vertebra at the rostral and caudal extents of the curve. The curve with the largest magnitude is defined as the major curve, and the remaining curves are defined as minor curves (Fig. 3).
   (b) In addition to the measurement of coronal curvature in patients with AIS, it is important to evaluate the sagittal plane and, indirectly, the axial plane. Thoracic kyphosis can be measured using the angle between the most tilted rostral and caudal vertebral endplates in the sagittal plane. Rotation can be evaluated on frontal views.

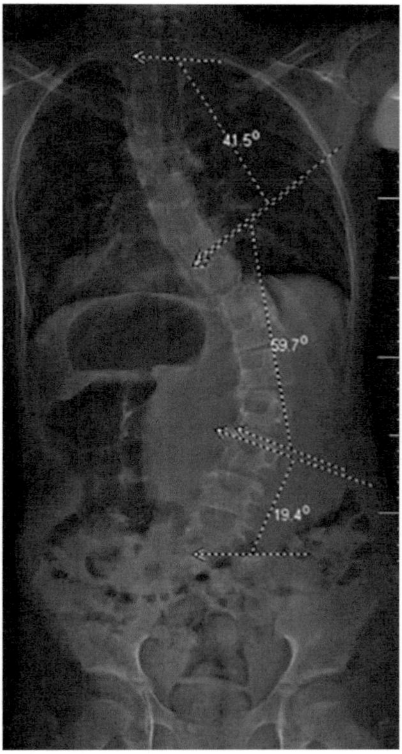

Fig. 3 Curve measurement on a posterior–anterior radiograph. There is a right thoracolumbar major curve with smaller compensatory/minor curves above and below the main curve

3. Advanced imaging
   (a) MRI is sometimes obtained in patients with AIS, but practice patterns vary considerably. Neurological complaints, left thoracic curves, male sex, asymmetric abdominal reflexes, hyperkyphosis, and other atypical curve patterns (broad, sweeping curves) may particularly warrant detailed imaging of the spinal cord with MRI to investigate the presence of any intraspinal anomalies that could contribute to the atypical presentation of scoliosis.
   (b) Computed tomography (CT) is sometimes used to evaluate bony anatomy in detail but can often be avoided preoperatively in AIS.

Prevention

There is no definitive way to prevent AIS; therefore, early detection is key. There is a genetic component to AIS that should be assessed in family history. Earlier diagnosis may allow for closer observation and intervention with bracing or scoliosis-specific exercises, which may obviate the need for surgery. The American Academy of Pediatrics recommends that primary care providers use the Adam's forward bend test to check patients for AIS during annual wellness examinations. This is true for all patients regardless of family history. Pediatricians should start to assess children for AIS at the age of 10 years.

Treatment

Treatment options for AIS range from the observation for mild curves to bracing for moderate cases to surgery for sizeable curvatures. Early detection and management are important in efforts to prevent further curve progression. *Curves of approximately 50° or more are likely to continue to progress despite skeletal maturity (natural history) and are therefore usually treated surgically.* Importantly, the vast minority of AIS cases require surgery. The most common surgical procedure for AIS is posterior spinal instrumentation and fusion (PSIF). In select cases of patients with flexible curves with magnitudes at or near the traditional operative range with continued growth potential, especially in the thoracolumbar/lumbar spine, anterior vertebral body tethering (AVBT) is used.

1. Observation
   (a) When a patient's curvature is less than 20°, no treatment is undertaken outside of regular observation, although scoliosis-specific physical therapy and vitamin D/calcium supplementation may be appropriate.
   (b) Bracing is generally avoided for very mild curves.
2. Scoliosis-specific physical therapy
   (a) Also known as the Schroth method and often used in conjunction with bracing, scoliosis-specific exercises/physical therapy can aid in preventing curve progression.
3. Bracing
   (a) Curves in the 25- to 40-° range in patients with ongoing growth potential may be candidates for bracing. Bracing the spine was shown to effectively decrease the need for surgical intervention in the Bracing in Adolescent Idiopathic Scoliosis trial [8].
   (b) Bracing efficacy is largely dependent on patient compliance. It is recommended that a patient stay in the brace for at least 16–18 h per day for optimal results.
   (c) Bracing is typically discontinued when the patient reaches skeletal maturity.
   (d) Brace types include three-dimensionally corrective braces and standard thoracolumbosacral orthoses.
   (e) If bracing fails and the curve reaches 50°, surgical intervention is considered appropriate.
4. Fusion
   (a) Spinal fusion, or spinal arthrodesis, is the most common surgical intervention for AIS (Fig. 4). Anterior spinal fusion was used historically, but modern techniques most commonly employ the posterior approach today. In rare cases, such as severe curves, anterior fusions or disc releases may still be considered to augment posterior surgery for AIS. Surgery is carried out with intraoperative neuromonitoring to monitor spinal cord and neural element functioning and intraoperative imaging such as fluoroscopy or intraoperative CT.

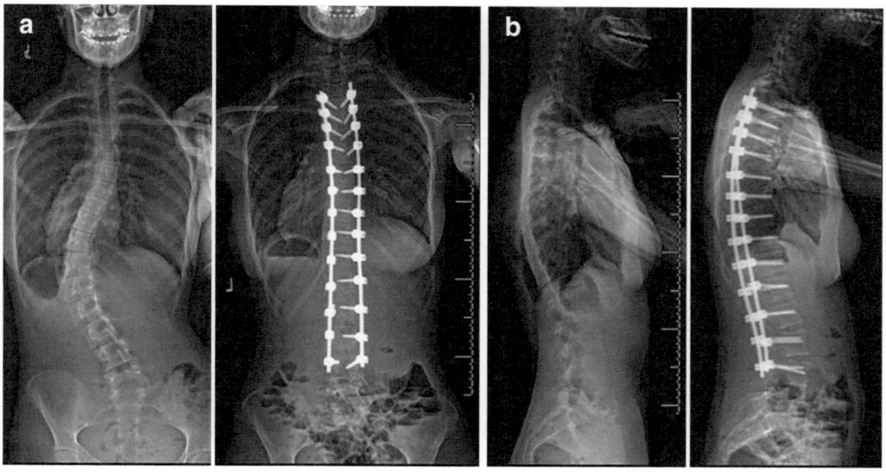

Fig. 4 (**a**) Coronal and (**b**) axial preoperative and postoperative plain radiographs after posterior spinal fusion

   (b) The Lenke classification system classifies operative AIS curves into six subtypes, with modifiers for thoracic kyphosis and distance of the lumbar apex from midline, which helps to guide treatment based on major and minor curves, their relative structurality, and their flexibility [9].
   (c) Instrumentation and fusion of the spine involve placing pedicle screws along the spine in the selected curves (based on the Lenke classification). Osteotomies (bone cuts) are commonly employed to loosen the spine in preparation for correction—usually a facetectomy (removal of the zygapophyseal joints) in the apex of the curvature. Metal rods are then used to translate the spine into a less scoliotic and more kyphotic position (in thoracic curves).
   (d) To achieve fusion, bone graft (obtained locally from the patient (autograft) or cadaveric bone (allograft)) is placed along the spine, typically between the rods but not in the spinal canal, which facilitates fusion.
5. AVBT
   (a) AVBT is a nonfusion option for select patients with curves in the operative range who have failed bracing. Curves must be reasonably flexible and usually cannot be in the severe range. This technique avoids fusion and employs a lateral approach to the spine in either the thoracic region or the thoracolumbar region (an access surgeon is typically used).
   (b) Laterally placed vertebral body screws are implanted and connected by a strong cord, which is then held under tension on the convexity of the curve. Growth modulation occurs in the following months to years, allowing the noninstrumented concavity to continue to lengthen.

(c) This approach has become quite popular given the lack of fusion; however, there is a much higher reoperation rate. There has been a general shift toward the use of AVBT in the thoracolumbar/lumbar region, where more mobility exists in the spine, compared with the more rigid thoracic spine (because of the presence of the rib cage).

Postoperative Nursing Care After Fusion

1. Neurological assessments
   (a) Postoperatively, it is imperative to immediately confirm whether a patient is at their neurological baseline with a wake-up test.
   (b) AIS surgery often entails lengthening the spinal column, which can stretch the spinal cord and cause delayed neurological issues (intraoperative neuromonitoring is used to prevent neurological issues during the procedure). Ongoing assessment of the patient's neurological status is critical.
2. Pain control
   (a) Pain control is one of the most important components of postoperative care. We find that preoperative counseling about expectations can be especially helpful in preparing patients and families for what to expect in the postoperative setting. Spinal fusions can be somewhat painful procedures, and patients often use patient-controlled analgesia (PCA) pumps. Some centers use epidural catheters for instillation of local analgesics.
   (b) Typically, patients will transition off of the PCA or epidural catheter to intravenous and oral medications a day or two postoperatively. Patients will likely need around-the-clock monitoring for adequate pain control. Nonsteroidal anti-inflammatory drugs (NSAIDs) can be very helpful in pain management, but some centers only use NSAIDs in the first 5 days postoperatively or do not use them at all. Use of NSAIDs is controversial after spine surgery because there is a theoretical longer-term risk of bony nonunion or pseudarthrosis.
   (c) Some surgeons opt for a postoperative steroid taper to help control pain. Studies have shown up to 40% lower use of opioids in patients who are on a steroid taper after spinal fusion [10].
   (d) Typical pain regimens are multimodal. Early mobilization protocols may counterintuitively help prevent pain by decreasing muscle stiffness and disuse.
3. Bowel care
   (a) Because anesthesia and analgesics are used for pain control and immobility, the likelihood of a patient developing constipation is high. A strong bowel regimen should be started as soon as the patient tolerates oral medications.
   (b) Consider additional bowel management such as suppositories or enemas when less invasive bowel medications are not successful.
   (c) Early mobilization can help prevent gastrointestinal ileus.

4. Bladder care
    (a) Patients typically have a Foley catheter placed intraoperatively and, depending on the pain management plan, may maintain that Foley catheter until they are able to ambulate safely to the bathroom. When the Foley catheter is discontinued, there is a high chance of urine retention.
5. Incisional care
    (a) Methods of protecting a surgical incision may vary. For some patients, a wound vacutainer or suction drain (Jackson–Pratt drain, Hemovac, etc.) may be used.
    (b) Suction-based drains are used to divert fluid near the surgical site, allowing for optimal wound healing. In other cases, wound closure strips and occlusive gauze dressings (which are typically removed after a few days) are used to cover the incision.
6. Physical therapy/occupational therapy
    (a) Physical therapy and occupational therapy needs are unique to the patient depending on the degree of curvature and comorbidities present.
    (b) It is the goal of these therapies to ensure that the patient can perform their daily activities (including walking, ascending/descending flights of stairs, and body mechanics that protect the surgical incision from mechanical stress) and increase the patient's activity tolerance.
    (c) Practice patterns vary, but at many institutions, patients are encouraged to refrain from bending, lifting, or twisting immediately after postoperative fusion.
    (d) Recommendations for return to sporting activity are highly variable among surgeons, but most patients will be able to return to their sport of choice within months after surgery.
7. Lab work
    (a) After fusion, hematocrit is often tracked to make sure blood loss is not significant enough to require a blood transfusion.
8. Oxygen requirement
    (a) Patients who had thoracic insufficiency preoperatively are likely to see a decrease in oxygen needs once their curve is corrected.
    (b) In the days after surgery, oxygen requirements may increase slightly because of immobility, anesthesia, and analgesia. During this period, it is important to promote frequent usage of incentive spirometers to prevent atelectasis.
9. Immobility
    (a) It is important that patients begin moving as quickly as possible after surgery. When immobility is prolonged, it is vital to initiate a sequential compression device and physical therapy quickly as prophylaxis for deep vein thrombosis.
    (b) When the patient is unable to reposition themselves, they should be repositioned every 2 h to avoid skin breakdown.

10. Fluid
    (a) Blood loss can be substantial after spinal surgery; the body then holds onto fluid as a defense mechanism. It may take a day or two for the patient to undergo diuresis.
    (b) It is important to scan the patient's bladder to assess whether they are experiencing fluid retention or bladder retention.
    (c) Patients should be hydrated according to their intravenous and oral total intake to maximize healing.

Complications

Complications after surgical intervention for AIS may include the following:

1. Infection
2. Bleeding
3. Neurological issues
4. Pain
5. Pseudarthrosis
6. Blood clots
7. Implant-associated complications

Discharge Teaching

Upon discharge, the patient's parent or guardian should be able to:

1. Describe reasons to contact the neurosurgery/orthopedic surgery office
2. Describe activity restrictions
3. Discuss appropriate pain medication scheduling
4. Demonstrate wound care
5. Demonstrate appropriate use of overdose intranasal spray if the patient is being sent home on opioids
6. Explain postoperative steroid taper if pertinent

References

1. Menger RP, Sin AH. Adolescent idiopathic scoliosis. In: StatPearls [Internet]. Treasure Island: StatPearls Publishing; 2025. https://www.ncbi.nlm.nih.gov/books/NBK499908/.
2. Weinstein SL. The natural history of adolescent idiopathic scoliosis. J Pediatr Orthop. 2019;39(6 Suppl 1):S44–6.
3. Aulia TN, Djufri D, Gatam L, Yaman A. Etiopathogenesis of adolescent idiopathic scoliosis (AIS): role of genetic and environmental factors. Narra J. 2023;3(3):e217.
4. Kuznia AL, Hernandez AK, Lee LU. Adolescent idiopathic scoliosis: common questions and answers. Am Fam Physician. 2020;101(1):19–23.

5. Emmanuel M, Bokor B. Tanner stages. In: StatPearls [Internet]. Treasure Island: StatPearls Publishing; 2022. https://www.ncbi.nlm.nih.gov/books/NBK470280/.
6. Tschurl JR, Napiontek W, Żytka Ł, Sławatycka K, Kotwicki T. The Sanders maturity scale for skeletal maturity assessment in idiopathic scoliosis. Chir Narzadow Ruchu Ortop Pol. 2022;87(3):91–8.
7. Troy MJ, Miller PE, Price N, et al. The "Risser+" grade: a new grading system to classify skeletal maturity in idiopathic scoliosis. Eur Spine J. 2019;28(3):559–66.
8. Weinstein SL, Dolan LA, Wright JG, Dobbs MB. Effects of bracing in adolescents with idiopathic scoliosis. New Engl J Med. 2013;369(16):1512–21.
9. Lenke LG, Betz RR, Harms J, et al. Adolescent idiopathic scoliosis: a new classification to determine extent of spinal arthrodesis. J Bone Joint Surg Am. 2001;83(8):1169–81.
10. Fletcher ND, Ruska T, Austin TM, et al. Postoperative dexamethasone following posterior spinal fusion for adolescent idiopathic scoliosis. J Bone Joint Surg Am. 2020;102(20):1807–13.

Traumatic Brain Injury

Theresa Ruddy and Luis F. Rodriguez

Abbreviations

AIS	Abbreviated injury scale
AMS	Altered mental status
AHT	Abusive head trauma
CDC	Center for disease control and prevention
cEEG	Continuous electroencephalogram
CPP	Cerebral perfusion pressure
CSF	Cerebral spinal fluid
CVP	Central venous pressure
DAI	Diffuse axonal injury
ED	Emergency department
EDH	Epidural hematoma
EVD	External ventricular drain
GCS	Glasgow coma scale
HGB	Hemoglobin
HIE	Hypoxic–ischemic encephalopathy
HOB	Head of bed
ICP	Intracranial pressure
LOC	Loss of consciousness
MAP	Mean arterial pressure
Na	Sodium

T. Ruddy (✉)
Pediatric Anesthesiology and Critical Care, Johns Hopkins Hospital, Baltimore, MD, USA
e-mail: truddy1@jhmi.edu

L. F. Rodriguez
Department of Pediatric Neurosurgery, Hough Family Institute for Brain Protection Sciences
Johns Hopkins All Children's Hospital, St Petersburg, FL, USA
e-mail: Luis.Rodriguez@jhmi.edu

K. Battick et al. (eds.), *Nursing Guide for Pediatric Neuroscience Patients*,
https://doi.org/10.1007/978-3-032-22664-8_11

NAT	Non-accidental trauma
PaCO2	Partial pressure of carbon dioxide in arterial blood
PaO2	Partial pressure of oxygen in arterial blood
PbrO2	Brain tissue oxygen
PTA	Post-traumatic amnesia
SAH	Subarchnoid hemorrhage
SDH	Subdural hematoma
TBI	Traumatic brain injury

Incidence and Prevalence

Traumatic brain injury in children remains a critical public health concern globally. Mild traumatic brain injury (mTBI) or concussion in the pediatric population was responsible for two million outpatient visits and three million ED visits between 2005 and 2009 [1]. In 2013, TBI in children aged 0–14 accounted for 640,000 ED visits, 18,000 hospitalizations, and 1,500 deaths [2]. Most TBI is considered mild (70–90% of all ED visits), with 14% of these patients experiencing disability. However, 62% of children who suffer moderate to severe traumatic brain injury experience chronic disability. [2]

Definitions

Traumatic brain injury is divided into *Mild*, *Moderate*, and *Severe,* depending on several factors [3]: (see Table 1)

1. Structural imaging findings
2. Length of loss of consciousness (LOC)
3. Duration of alteration of consciousness or mental state (AMS)
4. Duration of post-traumatic amnesia (PTA)
5. Glasgow Coma Scale (GCS) (best score in 24 h)
6. Abbreviated Injury Scale (AIS)

- *Examples:*
  - *Mild TBI*:

Table 1 Criteria for mild, moderate, and severe TBI

Criteria	Mild	Moderate	Severe
Structural Imaging findings	Normal	Normal or abnormal	Normal or abnormal
Loss of consciousness	< 30 min	30 min to 24 h	>24 h
Alteration of consciousness/mental state	A moment to 24 h	>24 h	>24 h
Post-traumatic amnesia	0-1 day	>1 and < 7 days	>7 days
Best GCS score in 24 h	13–15	9–12	3–8
Abbreviated Injury scale	1–2	3	4–6

    - Child is hit in the head while being tackled; falling in the playground and hitting head; having "bell rung" during sports or play. Imaging shows no abnormalities in the brain, and the patient will have LOC less than 30 min or no LOC at all. Patient has AMS for 24 h or less, and GCS will be 13–15.
  - *Moderate TBI:*
    - Patient in a car accident strikes the dashboard and has LOC of less than 24 h but more than 30 min, may have a structural abnormality on imaging, has AMS of >24 h, and suffers from PTA of 1–7 days. Best GCS within 24 h is 9–12.
  - *Severe TBI*:
    - Patient is struck by a vehicle traveling at a high speed, has a GCS 3–8 (definition of being in a coma), AMS and LOC > 24 h, PTA > 7 days. Most will have structural abnormalities on MRI imaging.

  Key epidemiological insights include the following:

- *Age-related vulnerability*: The highest incidence of TBI is observed in *children under 4 years of age*, followed by *adolescents aged 15–19 years*. These age groups are more susceptible to TBI due to developmental factors, risk-taking behaviors, and dependency on caregivers.
- *Gender disparities*: Boys consistently have a higher incidence of TBI than girls across all age groups, likely due to higher engagement in risk-prone activities.
- *Socioeconomic factors*: Children from low-income or underserved communities are more likely to experience severe TBIs, often due to environmental hazards, lack of access to safety equipment, or delayed medical intervention.
- *Global burden*: In low- and middle-income countries, road traffic injuries, violence, and lack of access to emergency care contribute to disproportionately higher mortality rates from pediatric TBI.

Pathophysiology

- Mechanisms (see Table 2) include penetrating injuries, blast injuries, contact injuries, acceleration–deceleration inertial injuries, or a combination of different mechanisms [4].
- The mechanical impact can cause force dynamics to be transmitted through the dura mater, cerebrospinal fluid, and brain parenchyma. The force can cause

Table 2 Common mechanisms of injury in pediatric TBI

Mechanism of injury	
Age group	Common causes
Infants	Falls, abuse (NAT)
Toddlers	Falls, MVAs
School-age	Sports, bicycle accidents
Adolescents	MVAs, sports, assaults

axons to become dislocated, cell membranes to break down, and fluid shifts resulting in brain tissue swelling [5].

- Neurons transition into impaired metabolism for up to 7–10 days from the initial injury and may alter cerebral blood flow [4].
- During the impaired metabolic state, the brain is vulnerable to repeat injury and impairments in behavior and spatial learning [4].
- Neurons may undergo cytoskeletal damage, altered neurotransmission, and axonal dysfunction [1].
- The primary brain injury occurs at the time of impact. The primary trauma eventually develops into a secondary trauma response [4, 5].
- The secondary brain injury results from a variety of factors such as intracranial hematomas, cerebral ischemia, edema, vasospasm, apoptosis, systemic hypotension, hypoxemia, increased intracranial pressure, and metabolic imbalance [4, 5].
- Secondary brain injury can result in cerebral edema, intracranial hypertension, blood–brain barrier disruption, metabolic dysfunctions, excitotoxicity, oxidative and cellular apoptosis, or necrosis [5].

Glasgow Coma Scale The *Glasgow Coma Scale (GCS)* is an essential tool in assessing the level of consciousness and determining the severity of TBI (see Table 3). In pediatrics, the *modified Pediatric Glasgow Coma Scale (PGCS)* is used to accommodate developmental differences, especially in preverbal children (see Table 4).

Pediatric GCS (PGCS) Modifications

The *PGCS* replaces the verbal component with age-appropriate behavioral responses in preverbal children (see Table 4).

Pediatric TBI is categorized not only by severity but also by the *type of injury* sustained. The type of TBI significantly influences clinical presentation, diagnostic

Table 3 Glasgow coma scale

Eye opening	
Spontaneous	4
To voice	3
To pain	2
None	1
Verbal response	
Oriented	5
Confused, disoriented	4
Inappropriate	3
Incomprehensible	2
None	1
Motor response	
Obeys	6
Localizes	5
Withdraws	4
Flexor posturing	3
Extensor posturing	2
None	1

Table 4 Pediatric Glasgow coma scale

	Infants	Children	Score
Eye opening	Open spontaneously	Open spontaneously	4
	Open to verbal stimuli	Open to verbal stimuli	3
	Open to pain only	Open to pain only	2
	No response	No response	1
Verbal response	Coos and babbles	Oriented and appropriate	5
	Crying, irritable	Confused	4
	Crying to pain	Inappropriate	3
	Moaning to pain	Incomprehensible	2
	No response	No response	1
Motor response	Spontaneous, purposeful movement	Obeys	6
	Withdraws to touch	Localizes	5
	Withdraws to pain	Withdraws	4
	Decorticate or flexor posturing	Decorticate or flexor posturing	3
	Decerebrate or extensor posturing	Decerebrate or extensor posturing	2
	No response	No response	1

Table 5 Summary of pediatric TBI types

TBI type	Pathophysiology	Key features	Imaging	Nursing priorities
Concussion	Functional disruption	Headache, confusion	Normal	Symptom monitoring, rest guidance
Contusion	Cortical bruising	Focal deficits, seizures	CT: hypodensity	Seizure watch, neuro checks
DAI	Axonal shearing	Coma, poor prognosis	MRI (DWI)	Ventilation, poor outcome planning
EDH	Arterial bleed	Lucid interval, fixed pupil	CT: biconvex mass	Rapid OR prep, neuro monitoring
SDH	Venous bleed (NAT common), cortical injury	Bulging fontanel, seizures	CT: crescent shape	NAT reporting, ICP care
SAH	Blood in subarachnoid space	Headache, photophobia	CT or LP	Pain control, vasospasm monitoring
Penetrating injury	Foreign object breach	External trauma, CSF leak	CT, X-ray	DO NOT remove object, antibiotics

strategy, treatment decisions, and prognosis. Below is an expanded classification by *morphological type*, covering both *focal* and *diffuse* injuries (see Table 5).

Concussion (Mild Traumatic Brain Injury)

A *concussion* is a *transient, functional brain injury* caused by biomechanical forces—typically without radiographic abnormalities. It is the most common form of TBI in children and adolescents, especially in sports-related injuries.

Pathophysiology

- No structural damage visible on standard imaging.
- Involves transient neurochemical and metabolic disruption: glutamate release, potassium efflux, and energy crisis.
- Typically resolves within 7–14 days, though prolonged symptoms may occur.

Clinical Features

- Headache, dizziness, nausea.
- Confusion, amnesia (especially retrograde).
- Emotional lability, fatigue, difficulty concentrating.
- *No LOC* required for diagnosis.

Nursing Considerations

- Monitor for postconcussive symptoms.
- Educate family on return-to-learn and return-to-play protocols.
- Refer to pediatric neurology for persistent symptoms (>4 weeks).
- Consider neuropsychological evaluation to identify subtle cognitive deficits.

Cerebral Contusion (Mild-to-Moderate TBI)

A *contusion* is a *bruising of brain tissue*, usually seen at the site of impact (coup) or opposite the impact (contrecoup). Often associated with cortical hemorrhage and edema.

Pathophysiology

- Localized bleeding and inflammation
- Common in frontal and temporal lobes
- May evolve over 24–72 h, increasing ICP

Clinical Features

- Focal neurological deficits (e.g., hemiparesis, speech delay).
- Seizures may occur in 24–48 h post-injury.
- Progressive somnolence or confusion.
- Expanding contusions may lead to elevated ICP requiring surgical intervention.

Imaging

- Serial imaging to evaluate evolution or in the setting of neurological changes or worsening headaches
- CT: Hyperdense regions with associated edema
- MRI: Better for late complications or subtle hemorrhagic changes

Nursing Considerations

- Monitor for seizure activity and rising ICP.
- Frequent neuro assessments.
- Educate family on signs of delayed deterioration.

Diffuse Axonal Injury (DAI) (Mild-to-Moderate-to-Severe TBI)

A *DAI* is caused by *shearing forces* during high-velocity acceleration–deceleration injuries, resulting in widespread axonal disruption.

Pathophysiology

- Involves deep white matter tracts: corpus callosum, brainstem.
- Axonal damage leads to cytoskeletal disruption and apoptosis.
- Often *not visible* on CT; *MRI* (especially DWI) preferred.

Clinical Features

- Immediate loss of consciousness.
- Coma with minimal recovery in severe cases.
- Poor motor and cognitive outcomes in moderate–severe DAI.

Imaging

- CT: Diffuse hyperdense punctate lesions throughout brain seen commonly along the corpus callosum.
- MRI: Much better to delineate the degree of injury. More sensitive for viewing small punctate areas of injury.

Nursing Considerations

- Ventilation support often needed.
- Monitor for autonomic instability.
- Involve palliative care if prognosis is poor.

Epidural Hematoma (EDH)

An *epidural hematoma* is a *collection of blood between the dura mater and skull*, often arterial in origin (e.g., middle meningeal artery).

Pathophysiology

- Usually due to skull fracture in the temporal region.
- Blood collects rapidly, causing brain compression.

Clinical Features

- *"Lucid interval"*: initial unconsciousness → brief recovery → rapid deterioration
- Headaches—continuous or progressively worse in the setting of expanding hematoma.
- Fixed, dilated pupil (ipsilateral) in the setting of large lesion with herniation.
- Vomiting, seizures, Cushing's triad in late stages (hypertension, bradycardia, irregular respirations).
- Brain herniation and death if not treated in a timely fashion.

Imaging

- CT: Biconvex (lens-shaped), hyperdense mass—respects suture lines.
- MRI: Will show the presence of swelling or contusion under the area of injury and possible early findings of brain herniation.

Management

- Neurosurgical emergency: Craniotomy and hematoma evacuation.
- Observation if not growing and not life- or function-threatening.

Nursing Considerations

- Prepare for surgical intervention.
- Headache is a vital sign—masking of headache with narcotics can lead to undetected deterioration and delay in diagnosis.
- Monitor for rapid neurologic decline—baseline neurological exam is important.
- Educate family about the urgent nature and good prognosis with timely treatment.

Subdural Hematoma (SDH)

A *subdural hematoma* is bleeding between the dura and arachnoid layers, typically *venous* in origin. Tearing of veins in convexity denotes more shearing forces applied to brain. Can have cortical injury and worse outcome than epidural hematomas. Prone to clinical and subclinical seizures. Can be caused by rapid deceleration injuries, as well as anticoagulated patients after cardiac procedures. Shunted hydrocephalous patients can develop overdrainage subdurals. Brain tumor patients during and after treatment who develop brain atrophy can also develop them.

Pathophysiology

- Common in infants (especially with abusive head trauma).
  - Shaking of baby leads to tearing of bridging veins from brain surface to dural venous sinuses leading to classic subdural hemorrhages along the falx cerebri (parafalcine subdurals).

  - Degree of injury on imaging does not generally match the story in abusive head trauma (AHT).

- Can be acute (within 72 h), subacute (3–21 days), or chronic (>3 weeks).

Clinical Features

- Altered mental status, vomiting.
- Bulging fontanelle in infants.
- Retinal hemorrhages and rib fractures may suggest Non-Accidental Trauma (NAT).
- Seizures due to the degree of cortical injury and cortical irritation from subdural blood.

Imaging

- CT: Crescent-shaped, crossing suture lines.
- MRI: For chronic SDH or mixed density. Gives info on subdural hemorrhages of different ages and overall degree of brain injury in NAT.

Nursing Considerations

- Report suspected NAT.
- Monitor head circumference in infants.
- ICP monitoring and surgical drainage may be required.
- Frequent neurological exams to detect deterioration/worsening.
- Seizure prophylaxis.

Subarachnoid Hemorrhage (SAH)

Bleeding into the *subarachnoid space* between the arachnoid membrane and the pia mater.

Pathophysiology

- Caused by trauma, AVM rupture, aneurysm, or coagulopathy.
- Irritates meninges, impairs CSF flow.

Clinical Features

- Thunderclap headache, nuchal rigidity, photophobia.
- Possible neurological deficit.
- Seizures or altered level of conciousness.
- Fever due to meningeal irritation.

Imaging

- CT: Most sensitive in the first 24 h.
- LP: If imaging is inconclusive but suspicion is high.
- Vascular study—MRA, CTA: In setting of nontraumatic SAH to rule out vascular etiology.

Nursing Considerations

- Pain management and seizure precautions.
- Monitor for vasospasm and hydrocephalus.

Penetrating Brain Injury

Occurs when an object breaches the skull and dura, damaging brain tissue (e.g., gunshot wound, shrapnel, impaled objects).

Pathophysiology

- Massive localized injury with high risk of infection and hemorrhage.
- May involve multiple lobes or cross hemispheres.
- Low-velocity injuries (impaled objects, dog bites, etc.) have better prognosis and outcomes than high-velocity injuries (gunshot wounds, etc.).
  - Bilateral high-velocity penetrating injuries almost universally fatal.

Clinical Features

- Obvious external wound.
- LOC, seizure, focal deficits.
- CSF leak if dura is breached.

Management

- Emergent neurosurgical consultation.
- Vascular imaging—CTA/MRA.
- Broad-spectrum antibiotics.
- Tetanus prophylaxis.

Nursing Considerations

- Do not remove impaled object.
- Support airway, control bleeding.
- Monitor for meningitis or abscess formation.

Pathophysiological Cascade

Traumatic brain injury initiates a *complex and evolving cascade of molecular, cellular, and physiological events* that contribute to brain damage beyond the initial insult. These changes are categorized into *primary* and *secondary injuries*, and understanding them is essential for effective nursing assessment, monitoring, and early intervention.

Primary Brain Injury

Primary injury refers to the *immediate mechanical damage* that occurs at the moment of trauma and is largely *irreversible*. It includes the following:

- *Skull fractures* (linear, depressed, basilar).
- *Coup–contrecoup injuries*: The brain impacts one side of the skull (coup), rebounds, and hits the opposite side (contrecoup).
- *Tissue disruption*: Lacerations, contusions, and axonal shearing.
- *Vascular injury*: Rupture of arteries or veins, causing hemorrhage (epidural, subdural, subarachnoid).
- *Cerebral edema* begins almost immediately.

Pediatric Implication Due to thinner cranial bones and higher brain water content, infants and toddlers are more vulnerable to skull deformation and diffuse injury even with lower-impact forces.

Secondary Brain Injury

Secondary injury refers to the *subsequent physiological and biochemical processes* that exacerbate brain damage *minutes to days after the primary insult*. These are potentially preventable or modifiable, making them critical targets for clinical and nursing interventions (see Table 6).

Cerebral Edema and Increased ICP

- *Cytotoxic edema*: Cellular swelling from ionic pump failure.
- *Vasogenic edema*: Disruption of the blood–brain barrier (BBB), allowing fluid to leak into interstitial spaces.
- Elevated *intracranial pressure (ICP)* leads to decreased cerebral perfusion pressure (CPP), compromising oxygen delivery.
- Penumbra—area surrounding the area of "primary injury" that can recover.
    - ICP management is directed at preserving the penumbra and avoiding further function- or life-threatening problems.

Table 6 Physiological and biochemical processes specific to pediatric TBI

Pathophysiologic process	Pediatric characteristics	Clinical implication
Skull compliance	More deformable, open sutures in infants	Increased risk of brain distortion, late signs
Water content	Higher brain water fraction	More prone to cerebral edema
Myelination	Incomplete in infants and toddlers	Increased vulnerability to axonal injury
Autoregulation	Immature cerebral autoregulation	Greater risk of ischemia with BP fluctuations
BBB integrity	More permeable in neonates	Higher risk of vasogenic edema, infection

Clinical Correlate A child with rising ICP may exhibit a decreasing GCS, altered pupils, bradycardia, or vomiting. Nursing vigilance in monitoring neuro trends is vital.

Excitotoxicity

- Injury causes *glutamate release*, leading to excessive stimulation of NMDA receptors.
- Results in massive *calcium influx*, mitochondrial dysfunction, and *neuronal apoptosis.*

Immature brains have increased NMDA receptor density, making them especially *vulnerable to excitotoxic damage* even with mild trauma.

Mitochondrial Dysfunction and Energy Crisis

- ATP production declines due to hypoxia and calcium overload.
- Increased *anaerobic metabolism* leads to lactic acidosis.
- Energy failure leads to *cell death cascades.*

Even when CT is normal, brain cells may be undergoing invisible metabolic failure—supporting the use of biomarkers and advanced imaging in clinical trials.

Neuroinflammation

- TBI triggers activation of *microglia* and *astrocytes.*
- Cytokines such as *IL-1β, TNF-α, and IL-6* exacerbate BBB disruption and promote edema.
- Inflammation may persist for *weeks to months*, contributing to chronic neurodegeneration.

Nursing Focus Monitor for secondary fever due to inflammatory cytokines even in the absence of infection. Fever exacerbates brain metabolism.

Seizures and Electrical Instability

- Cellular injury lowers seizure threshold.
- Seizures increase cerebral metabolism, raising ICP and worsening ischemia.

Clinical Practice Initiate seizure prophylaxis in children with moderate or severe TBI. Monitor EEG, especially in comatose patients (risk of subclinical seizures).

Long-Term Implications of the Cascade

- Chronic neuroinflammation may lead to *neurocognitive deficits.*
- Impaired brain development in younger children, especially with injuries under age 2.
- Risk of *post-traumatic epilepsy*, behavioral disorders, and emotional dysregulation.

Key Point In pediatric patients, injury during critical developmental windows can have *lifelong impacts*, making early aggressive management and rehabilitation vital.

Mechanisms of Injury

Accidental Trauma

- Falls (from furniture, stairs).
- Vehicle collisions (improper restraint use).
- Recreational injuries (sports, bicycles, skateboarding).
- Penetrating trauma—low velocity vs high velocity (dog bites, assault, gunshot wounds).

Non-Accidental Trauma (NAT)

- Shaken baby syndrome.
- Blunt force trauma.
- Intentional strikes.

Clinical Presentation (7)

Table 7 Symptoms comparison for mild and moderate/severe TBI

Symptom	Mild TBI	Moderate/severe TBI
LOC	Brief or none	Prolonged
Headache	Common	Severe and persistent
Vomiting	May occur	Frequent, projectile
Seizures	Rare	Common
Pupillary changes	Absent	Present
Irritability	Possible	Marked

Assessment and Diagnosis

Early and accurate assessment of pediatric TBI is critical in preventing secondary brain injury. Nurses play a pivotal role in the identification, monitoring, and escalation of care for neurologically compromised children. Assessment must be rapid, systematic, and developmentally appropriate.

Primary Survey (ABCs + Cervical Spine)

Adopt the *Pediatric Advanced Life Support (PALS)* and *Advanced Trauma Life Support (ATLS)* approaches:

- *Airway*: Ensure patency while maintaining cervical spine immobilization. Signs of obstruction include stridor, drooling, or gurgling sounds.
  - Insert oral/nasal airways if indicated.
  - Jaw thrust maneuver preferred over head tilt.
- *Breathing*: Assess respiratory rate, effort, breath sounds, and oxygen saturation.
  - Hypoxia worsens neurological injury → maintain $SpO_2 > 94\%$.
- *Circulation*: Check heart rate, capillary refill, skin color, and blood pressure.
  - Hypotension doubles mortality in TBI; treat aggressively.
- *Disability*: Rapid neurological screening using *AVPU scale* (Alert, response to Voice, response to Pain, Unresponsive) and *pediatric Glasgow Coma Scale (GCS).*
- *Exposure*: Fully expose child to assess for other injuries; prevent hypothermia.

Neurological Assessment

Pediatric Glasgow Coma Scale (PGCS)

Use the *age-modified GCS* for assessing the level of consciousness, with trends more important than isolated scores. A change in level of consciousness (LOC) is the earliest indicator of a change in neurologic status. A sudden drop in GCS by 2 or more points is an *emergency*.

Pupillary and Cranial Nerve Assessment

- Assess pupil *size, symmetry, and reactivity.*
- Fixed and dilated pupil = possible herniation in the setting of altered or worsening mental status, hypertension, bradycardia.
- Evaluate for cranial nerve palsies (e.g., CN III compression in uncal herniation).

Motor and Reflex Examination

- Look for *asymmetry in movement, decorticate,* or *decerebrate posturing.*

Table 8 Pediatric TBI imaging decision tree (based on PECARN guidelines)

Imaging modality	Case type	Advantages	Limitations
CT scan	Acute injury, bleeding, skull fracture	Fast, widely available	Radiation exposure
MRI	DAI, subacute/chronic injury	High detail, no radiation	Time-consuming, sedation often needed
X-ray	Skull fractures, shunt placement	Quick, inexpensive	Limited soft tissue detail
Ultrasound	Infants with open fontanelles	Noninvasive, bedside use	Operator-dependent

- Check for *abnormal reflexes* in the setting of possible spinal cord injury (Babinksi reflex is normal in infants, not in older patients).

Fontanelle and Head Circumference (Infants)

- *Bulging fontanelle*: raised ICP.
- Serial *head circumference* measurements for infants <1 year.

Diagnostic Imaging (8)

Laboratory and Ancillary Testing

- *Complete blood count*: Anemia, infection.
- *Electrolytes, glucose, osmolality*: Assess for SIADH, DI.
- *Coagulation panel*: Especially important in NAT or bleeding diatheses.
- *Toxicology screen*: If intoxication suspected.
- *Blood gas*: Monitor for hypoxia or metabolic acidosis.

Special Considerations

- *Abusive Head Trauma (AHT)*:
  - Evaluate for *retinal hemorrhages*, *rib fractures*, or *inconsistent history.*
  - Consider *skeletal survey*, *social work consult*, and *reporting to child protection.*
- *Intracranial Pressure (ICP) monitoring*:
  - Indicated for GCS $\leq$ 8 with abnormal imaging or clinical signs of increased ICP.
  - Methods: External ventricular drain *(EVD)*, *intraparenchymal monitor.*

Management of Pediatric TBI

Management is guided by *severity*, *mechanism of injury*, and the presence of *neurological deterioration*. The goal is to *prevent or minimize secondary brain injury* by optimizing oxygenation, perfusion, and intracranial pressure (ICP) (see Table 9).

Table 9 Management of traumatic brain injury and elevated intracranial pressure

Skull "contents"	Causes of increased volume	Treatment strategy	Interventions
Brain	1. Mass lesion 2. Swelling	1. Remove mass lesion 2. Decrease brain swelling 3. "Expand" skull	1. Craniotomy for evacuation of mass lesion, damaged brain 2. Hypertonic saline, head-of-bed 30 degrees, mannitol and hyperventilation for herniation emergencies 3. PRBC'S (osmotic agent like hypertonic saline which improves O2 delivery and avoids hypotension) 4. Decompressive craniectomy
Blood	1. Increased metabolic demand	1. Decrease metabolic demand	1. Sedation 2. Paralytic 3. Temperature control 4. Pentobarbital coma in setting of uncontrolled ICP and maximal medical therapy
CSF	1. Hydrocephalous (obstructive or communicating)	1. Decrease CSF	1. External ventricular drain (temporary) 2. Ventricular shunt (permanent or longer lasting)

- TBI management is based on the principle that the skull is not expandable, and its volume is fixed. The skull "contents" include brain, CSF, and blood.
- Increase in the volume of one of the skull "contents" without decrease in one or both of the other two will lead to *elevation in intracranial pressure (ICP)* and neurological deficit, brain herniation, and possibly death.
- TBI treatment focuses on *treating elevated ICP* by decreasing brain mass or volume, decreasing blood volume (while avoiding hypotension and hypoxia), or decreasing CSF volume.
- ICP monitor helps guide therapy while external ventricular drain can both guide therapy and provide treatment by removing CSF.

Initial Stabilization (0–60 Min)

Follow *ATLS/PALS algorithms* and TBI-specific guidelines:

- *Airway*: Intubate if:
  - GCS ≤ 8.
  - Impending herniation.
  - Poor gag reflex or apnea.
- *Breathing*:
  - Avoid hypoxia and hypercapnia.
  - Target $PaCO_2$ 35–40 mmHg.

- Hyperventilation ($PaCO_2$ 30–35 mmHg) ONLY for signs of herniation (e.g., blown pupil).

- *Circulation*:
  - Treat hypotension based on age-specific SBP thresholds.
  - Use isotonic fluids (normal saline or lactated Ringer's).
  - Avoid overhydration or hypotonic fluids → risk of worsening edema.

Intracranial Pressure (ICP) Management

Normal ICP:
Infants: <5 mmHg.
Children: <10–15 mmHg.
Goal CPP (MAP – ICP): ≥40–50 mmHg in children.

Medical interventions (See Tables 10 and 11)

Table 10 First-tier measures

Measure	Purpose	Nursing actions
Head of bed elevation (30°)	Venous drainage	Maintain neck in neutral position
Sedation and analgesia	Decrease agitation and ICP	Monitor depth, assess pain regularly
Hyperosmolar therapy	Dehydrate brain tissue	Monitor serum sodium and osmolality
Antipyretics	Prevent hyperthermia	Regular temperature monitoring

Table 11 Hyperosmolar Agents and PRBC's

Agent	Dose	Monitoring
Mannitol only used in emergencies to rapidly decrease elevated ICP but not for chronic use	0.5–1 g/kg IV bolus	Serum osmolality (<320), BP, urine output
Hypertonic saline (3%) Hypertonic saline infusion or boluses are first line of treatment PRBC'S—Osmotic agent to decrease swelling while improving oxygen-carrying capacity and avoiding hypotension	3–5 mL/kg bolus or infusion	Serum sodium (target 145–155), CVP "Hemoglobin > 7 (minimum)" [6]

Seizure Prophylaxis and Management

- High-risk patients: GCS ≤ 8, cortical contusions, depressed skull fracture.
- *Phenytoin, fosphenytoin, or levetiracetam* within first 7 days.
- Seizure activity increases ICP and worsens injury.
- Monitor with continuous EEG if altered mental status persists.

Temperature and Glucose Management

- *Fever* increases cerebral metabolism → must be aggressively managed.
- *Glucose extremes* (hypo- or hyperglycemia) are harmful:
  - Maintain glucose: 90–180 mg/dL.
  - Avoid D5 fluids unless hypoglycemia present.

Surgical Interventions (12)

Table 12 Surgical indications for severe pediatric TBI

Indication	Procedure	Notes
Large hematoma (>10 mm)	Craniotomy and evacuation	EDH and SDH
Refractory elevated ICP	Decompressive craniectomy	Controversial but sometimes lifesaving
Hydrocephalus or CSF buildup	External ventricular drain (EVD)	Also for ICP monitoring

ICU Care and Ongoing Monitoring

- Hourly *neuro exams*
- Monitor ICP and CPP
- Ventilator care (PEEP optimization)
- Prevent complications: VAP, SIADH, DVT, stress ulcer

Nursing Insight Anticipate and/or identify changes quickly or before they even happen, important to know the patient's baseline, not just their assessment from the past 12-hour shift. A trending increase in ICP or decreasing GCS should trigger a rapid response and physician notification.

- When ICP monitor or EVD present—sedate +/− paralysis to limit wakeful or agitation periods and decrease metabolic demand.
- MRI imaging is important, but once medically stable for transport, consider a "flat in bed rehearsal" to determine if the patient ICPs can tolerate being flat for MRI, *prior* to transport.
- Systemetic hypotension negatively impacts the outcome in TBI patients [4].
  - Isotonic crystalloids should be used to prevent and correct hypotension [4].
  - Hypotonic fluids should be avoided to prevent volume overload and cerebral edema [5].
  - Large volumes of saline should be avoided to prevent hyperchloremic metabolic acidosis [5].
  - After fluid resuscitation, use inotropes/vasopressors [6].
  - Administer blood transfusion if hemoglobin (hgb) < 7 (minimum). Higher level may be optimal based on advanced monitoring [6].

Severe TBI Insight

- Elevate HOB ≥ 30 degrees. ICP decreases because of the displacement of CSF from the intracranial space and increase of venous outflow [4–6].
- Maintain neck in neutral position and assess cervical collar fit. If the cervical collar is too tight, then it can impede venous outflow [4, 6].
- Administer appropriate analgesics and sedatives to treat pain and agitation [4, 6, 7].
- Maintain adequate oxygenation and PaCO2 35–40 mmHg [4, 6].
- Hyperventilation decreases ICP by lowering PaCO2 leading to vasoconstriction [5]. Routine hyperventilation is not recommended, but in the setting of impending herniation, it is the fastest, short-term method to lower ICP [4].
- Ensure appropriate intravascular volume status [6].
- Maintain hemoglobin >7 (minimum). Higher level may be optimal based on advanced monitoring [6].
- Hyperthermia (> 38 °C) should be avoided [4–6].
- Seizure prophylaxis is recommended for 7 days [6].

- Early (within 72 h from injury) enteral nutrition is suggested to decrease mortality and improve outcomes [6, 7].
- Target normoglycemia/avoid hyperglycemia. Administer insulin if glucose >198 on two consecutive measures [6].
- Treat coagulopathy prior to insertion of ICP or PbrO2 monitors [6].
- Neurosurgery as indicated.
- External ventricular drain (EVD) placement is a standard and common procedure in TBI management [8].
- ICP, CPP, and PbrO2 directed interventions [6].
- CSF drainage through an EVD or lumbar drain may reduce ICP [4, 6, 7].
- Hyperosmolar therapy, such as hypertonic (3% saline) and mannitol, is used to reduce ICP [4, 6, 8, 9]. Recommended initial target Na is between 140 and 150 [6].
- Prophylactic/early moderate hypothermia, corticosteroids, and immune-modulating diet are not recommended [4, 5, 7–9].

Family Engagement and Communication

- Clearly explain procedures, prognosis, and changes in condition.
- Allow parental presence when safe.
- Provide emotional support, involve chaplaincy, or psychology as needed.

Infection Prevention

- Aseptic technique with lines/tubes.
- Monitor for meningitis, pneumonia.

Multidisciplinary Team Approach

- Physical therapy.
- Occupational therapy.
- Speech-language therapy.
- Neuropsychology.

School Reintegration and Support

- IEPs and accommodations.
- Ongoing cognitive assessments.

Prognosis

- Variable outcomes depending on severity.
- Potential for full recovery in mild cases.
- Risk of long-term deficits in severe TBI.

Psychosocial Impact and Family-Centered Care

Family Reactions

- Guilt, grief, fear, confusion.
- Financial and emotional stress.

Role of Nurses

- Advocate for family involvement.
- Coordinate with social work, chaplaincy, psychology.

Family Needs in Pediatric TBI

- Information: diagnosis and prognosis.
- Emotional support: Counseling, support groups.
- Participation: Involvement in care decisions.

Prevention Strategies

- Child safety seats and helmet use.
- Education on fall prevention.
- Public health campaigns against abuse.

Summary and Key Points

- Pediatric TBI is a major cause of morbidity and mortality.
- Presentation varies with age and injury severity.
- Early identification and nursing assessment are crucial.
- Multidisciplinary, family-centered care improves outcomes.
- Prevention strategies and public education are essential.

References

1. Kochanek PM, et al. Guidelines for the management of pediatric severe traumatic brain injury, third edition. Pediatr Crit Care Med. 2019;20(3 Suppl 1):S1–S82.
2. Centers for Disease Control and Prevention (CDC). TBI data and statistics. https://www.cdc.gov/traumaticbraininjury/data/index.html
3. Anderson V, et al. Long-term outcomes from childhood traumatic brain injury. Lancet Neurol. 2009;8(12):1156–66.
4. Haydel MJ, Weisbrod LJ, Saeed W. Pediatric head trauma. In: StatPearls [Internet]. Treasure Island: StatPearls Publishing; 2024.
5. Syzdykbayev M, Kazymov M, Aubakirov M, Kurmangazina A, Kairkhanov E, Kazangapov R, Bryzhakhina Z, Imangazinova S, Sheinin A. A modern approach to the treatment of traumatic brain injury. Medicines (Basel). 2024;11(5):10. https://doi.org/10.3390/medicines11050010. PMID: 38786549; PMCID: PMC11123131
6. Kochanek PM, Tasker RC, Bell MJ, Adelson PD, Carney N, Vavilala MS, Selden NR, Bratton SL, Grant GA, Kissoon N, Reuter-Rice KE, Wainwright MS. Management of pediatric severe traumatic brain injury: 2019 consensus and guidelines-based algorithm for first and

second tier therapies. Pediatr Crit Care Med. 2019;20(3):269–79. https://doi.org/10.1097/PCC.0000000000001737.
7. Kochanek PM, Tasker RC, Carney N, Totten AM, Adelson PD, Selden NR, Davis-O'Reilly C, Hart EL, Bell MJ, Bratton SL, Grant GA, Kissoon N, Reuter-Rice KE, Vavilala MS, Wainwright MS. Guidelines for the management of pediatric severe traumatic brain injury, third edition: update of the brain Trauma foundation guidelines, executive summary. Neurosurgery. 2019;84(6):1169–78. https://doi.org/10.1093/neuros/nyz051.
8. Figaji A. An update on pediatric traumatic brain injury. Childs Nerv Syst. 2023;39(11):3071–81. https://doi.org/10.1007/s00381-023-06173-y. Epub 2023 Oct 6. PMID: 37801113; PMCID: PMC10643295
9. Ben Abdeljelil A, Freire GC, Yanchar N, Turgeon AF, Beno S, Bérubé M, Stang A, Stelfox T, Zemek R, Beaulieu E, Gagnon IJ, Gabbe B, Lauzier F, Labrosse M, Tardif PA, Deshommes T, Gnanvi J, Moore L. Pediatric moderate and severe traumatic brain injury: a systematic review of clinical practice guideline recommendations. J Neurotrauma. 2023;40(21–22):2270–81. https://doi.org/10.1089/neu.2023.0149. Epub 2023 Aug 16

Traumatic Spine Injury

Amanda Johnson and Mari L. Groves

Definition

Pediatric traumatic spine injury is relatively uncommon occurring between 2 and 5% of all traumatic injuries; however, the morbidity and mortality for these types of injuries depending on the location can be very high [1, 2]. Spinal column injuries may result from either nonpenetrating or penetrating injuries and can occur at any level of the spinal column. Nonpenetrating injuries can be caused by falls, diving accidents, motor vehicle crashes, pediatrician accidents, bicycle accidents, and sport-related collisions. Accidents involving acceleration and deceleration or rotational injury can cause ligamentous strain, stretch, or disruption. Fall accidents, diving accidents, or sport collisions can cause an axial loading injury to the bony column. Penetrating injuries are caused by a ballistic injury (unintentional and intentional) or stabbing with a sharp object. Both nonpenetrating and penetrating injuries can be isolated to a bony column injury or be more severe involving the spinal cord.

The anatomy of the pediatric spine throughout growth can predispose children to certain levels of cervical spine injury [3]. Infants have a large head-to-body ratio and have cervical ligamentous laxity that is more likely to apply force and cause injury to the high cervical spine (C1–C3). School-age children are more likely to have upper-to-mid cervical spine injury (C3–C5) as there is the start of ossification of the joints and less ligamentous laxity. Children over 12 years of age have a more skeletally mature spine, with injury to the cervical spine occurring more frequently in the lower cervical spine (C4–C7) as seen in adults. Thoracolumbar injuries can

A. Johnson (✉)
Department of Neurologic Surgery, The University of Chicago Medicine and Biological Sciences, Chicago, IL, USA
e-mail: Amanda.Johnson@bsd.uchicago.edu

M. L. Groves
Johns Hopkins Medicine, St. Baltimore, MD, USA
e-mail: mgroves2@jhmi.edu

K. Battick et al. (eds.), *Nursing Guide for Pediatric Neuroscience Patients*,
https://doi.org/10.1007/978-3-032-22664-8_12

occur in any age group; however, they are more common in school-age children and adolescents due to the patterns of accidents causing injury.

The types of traumatic spine injury can be divided into three categories: ligamentous injuries, bony injuries, and spinal cord injuries (SCI) (Table 1). Ligamentous injuries can occur in either the posterior, anterior, or both. The severity of the ligamentous injury will guide management. Bony injuries can include the whole vertebrae or part and can be isolated to one vertebrae or multiple levels depending on the injury. The type of injury and number of levels involved in the injury will guide management.

Spinal cord injuries can be transient, incomplete, or complete. Transient symptoms are often described with a sport-related injury (i.e., head-to-head contact) causing numbness or weakness in the extremities that often resolves by the time of evaluation in the emergency department. Magnetic resonance imaging (MRI) does not reveal an injury to the spinal cord which is diagnosed as spinal cord injury without radiographic findings (SCIWORA) [4]. Incomplete and complete SCI can be

Table 1 Types of traumatic spine injuries

Ligamentous injuries	Bony injuries	Spinal cord injuries
Anterior ligaments Hyperflexion/extension injury Acceleration–deceleration injury Rotational Stretch Disruption	*Spinous process fracture* Avulsion fracture	*SCIWORA* Sports-related injury Temporary deficits
Posterior ligaments Hyperflexion/extension injury Acceleration–deceleration injury Rotational Stretch Disruption	*Arch fracture* Axial loading, flexion, extension, and rotational injury Jefferson fracture Lateral mass fracture Anterior arch fracture Posterior arch fracture	*Epidural/subdural hemorrhage* Flexion, extension, penetrating injury Compressive Non-compressive Temporary or permanent deficits
Cranio-cervical ligaments Hyperflexion/extension injury Atlanto-occipital dislocation (AOD) Stretch Disruption	*Compression fracture* Axial loading injury Less than 50% of the height loss More than 50% of the height loss	*Contusion* Flexion, extension, penetrating injury Temporary or permanent deficits
	Chance fracture Hyperflexion injury Unstable fracture of the spine	*Infarct/Ischemia* Flexion, extension, penetrating injury Temporary or permanent deficit
	Burst fracture Axial loading, penetrating injury Vertebrae is crushed	*Transection* Penetrating injury Permanent deficit

classified using The American Spinal Injury Association (ASIA) classification scale to help guide management [5, 6]. A patient with a complete SCI will not have any sensation or movement below the level of injury (ASIA A on the classification scale). An incomplete SCI is either the ability to have sensation but no motor below the level of injury (ASIA B) or at least partial motor below the level of injury (ASIA C, sensory incomplete and less than half key muscles still engage or ASIA D, more than half key muscles engage) [5, 6].

Signs and Symptoms

The presentation of a patient with a traumatic spine injury will be dependent on the severity of the accident and the level of the injury. The details of the mechanism of injury are prudent to help guide treatment. The concern for traumatic spine injury is greater for a patient restrained in a high-speed roll-over accident versus a low-speed, no airbag deployment motor vehicle crash. Traumatic spine injury patients might present to the emergency room already intubated and sedated because of various injuries. Documentation of a detailed neurological assessment prior to arrival, at arrival, and ongoing is important to guide management.

Symptoms

For patients who can provide history, symptoms can be divided into these categories:

1. Pain
   (a) Inquire about the onset of pain. Did the pain start immediately or several hours or days after injury?
   (b) Inquire about the location of pain. The location of pain can help guide at what level there might be an injury.
   (c) Does the pain radiate down the extremity? This can help assess dermatomes that can be affected by injury.
   (d) Is the pain limiting activity?
   (e) Medication use for the pain?
2. Weakness
   (a) Do they feel weak in any extremity? Both extremities? Only one side? Only upper extremity? Only lower extremity?
   (b) How long have they been weak?
   (c) Does anything make the weakness better? Worse?
3. Paresthesia/sensation changes
   (a) Different feeling between the extremities?
   (b) Tingling?
   (c) Numbness?
   (d) How long have they been experiencing these sensation changes?
   (e) Anything make it better? Worse?

Physical Examination

The physical examination should include a complete head to toe assessment with a thorough neurological exam. Depending on the acuity of the patient, this exam might be completed in various orders.

1. Constitutional
   (a) Airway
      (i) Any compromise to airway cause for concern with potential cervical injury
   (b) Breathing
      (i) Able to illicit spontaneous breaths prior to sedative or paralytic medications
      (ii) Concern for high SCI if unable to have spontaneous breath
   (c) Circulation
      (i) Heart rate variability particularly bradycardia without other indication concern for high SCI
      (ii) Hypotension/Hypertension without other indication concern for high SCI
   (d) Alertness
      (i) Decreased alertness because of acuity might inhibit neurological exam
2. Neurological
   (a) Cranial nerve exam
      (i) Particular attention to lower cranial nerve exam with concern for high SCI
         1. Cough/gag
         2. Swallow
         3. Shoulder shrug
   (b) Strength exam
      (i) All motor function/strength should be recorded for individual muscle groups of each extremity
   (c) Sensation
      (i) Sensation should be evaluated as light touch and painful touch
      (ii) Dermatome chart should be used as a guide for the level of potential injury
   (d) Reflexes
      (i) Deep tendon reflexes
         1. Knee, ankle, biceps, and triceps can be tested for hypo/hyperreflexia in relation to the level of injury
      (ii) Hoffmann reflex
         1. Middle finger is held while the fingernail is flicked downward
         2. Positive with concern for cervical SCI if thumb or index finger flexes after the flicking of the middle finger

        (iii) Rectal tone
            1. Should be assessed as present or absent
        (iv) Bulbocavernosus reflex
            1. Should only be performed by a care provider who knows how to perform the test
            2. Absence of reflex indicates spinal shock
3. GI/GU
    (a) Distention of abdomen
        (i) Concern for decreased bowel activity with SCI
        (ii) Urinary retention if no foley is in place
    (b) Auscultation
        (i) Assess for bowel sounds which can be decreased or absent with acute SCI
4. Skin
    (a) Assess for abrasions, wounds, or entry and exit points for penetrating trauma
    (b) Document level of external injury if any

Laboratory Values and Diagnostics

Laboratory Values

1. Upon arrival to the emergency department
    (a) Complete blood count (CBC)
    (b) Complete metabolic panel (CMP)
    (c) Coagulation panel
        (i) Might need surgical intervention
    (d) Consider type and screen depending on the acuity of the patient
    (e) Consider arterial blood gas or venous blood gas depending on the acuity of the patient
2. Ongoing laboratory values will be dependent on the acuity of the patient, the level of SCI injury, and type of injury
    (a) Ligamentous injury only
        (i) Consider interval monitoring as needed with other injuries the patient might have sustained
    (b) Bony injury only
        (i) Consider interval monitoring of CBC dependent on possible surgical interventions
    (c) High CSI
        (i) Consider interval of arterial blood gas or venous blood gas to monitor oxygenation and ventilation
        (ii) Consider interval of CMP to monitor electrolyte abnormalities dependent on nutritional status and other injuries
        (iii) Consider interval monitoring of CBC dependent on other injuries the patient might have sustained

(d) Mid and lower CSI
   (i) Consider interval of CMP to monitor electrolyte abnormalities dependent on nutritional status and other injuries
   (ii) Consider interval monitoring of CBC dependent on other injuries the patient might have sustained

Imaging

1. Upon arrival to the emergency department
   (a) Use of a risk stratification score for injury to determine what cervical imaging should be obtained [7, 8].
      (i) NEXUS, PEDSPINE, PECARN
         1. Assess Glasgow Coma Scale (GCS)
         2. Type of injury
         3. Focal neurological deficits
      (ii) Plain radiographic images of cervical spine [7, 8]
         1. Obtained for GCS 9–14
         2. Self-reported neck pain
         3. Head or torso injury
      (iii) Computed topography (CT) scan without contrast [7, 8]
         1. Obtained with GCS 3–8
         2. Abnormal airway, breathing, or circulation
         3. Focal neurological deficits
         4. Mechanism of injury concerning for SCI
   (b) Plain radiographs or CT scan without contrast should be obtained for thoracic and/or lumbar spine based on the mechanism of injury and neurological exam findings
2. After patient is stabilized, additional imaging including vascular imaging and magnetic resonance imaging (MRI) should be considered dependent on injuries sustained
   (a) MRI
      (i) Evaluate ligamentous injury
      (ii) Evaluate cord
   (b) Vascular imaging
      (i) Evaluate for vascular injury
3. Repeat imaging might be needed to re-evaluate healing of injury

Other Studies

1. Consider swallow study for high CSI
2. Consider pressure support trials for patients with high CSI
3. Consider ultrasound to monitor deep vein thrombosis in high CSI

Treatment

Nonoperative

1. Ligamentous injury can occur at any level of the spine. Stretch of the ligaments can cause concern for instability of the spinal column. The amount of ligamentous injury and the age of the patient will determine if the patient can be managed conservatively without operative fusion.
   (a) Bracing for support
      (i) Cervical collar
      (ii) Halo/vest for high ligamentous injuries, i.e., AOD can be used for younger patients
      (iii) Thoracic/lumbar/sacral orthotic (TLSO)
   (b) Medications for pain
      (i) Acetaminophen (10–15 mg/kg/dose) can be used for pain
      (ii) Ibuprofen (10 mg/kg/dose) can be considered if there is no contraindication for use
      (iii) Narcotic might be added for additional short-term pain control
2. Bony injury can occur at any level of the spine. The number of levels affected and the type of bony injury will determine the stability of the spine to be able to be managed conservatively
   (a) Bracing for support and to help decrease pain with mobilization
      (i) Cervical collar
      (ii) Halo/vest for high cervical fractures in younger patients
      (iii) TLSO
   (b) Medications for pain
      (i) Acetaminophen (10–15 mg/kg/dose) can be used for pain
      (ii) Ibuprofen (10 mg/kg/dose) can be considered if there is no contraindication for use
      (iii) Narcotic might be added for additional short-term pain control
3. High CSI injury is considered any injury in the cervical area and/or high thoracic spine. The nonoperative management of high CSI is imperative to help minimize the morbidity and mortality related to these injuries
   (a) Monitor and treat spinal shock
      (i) Maintain mean arterial pressures (MAP) above 80 to perfuse the spinal cord and prevent further ischemia [9].
         1. Consider inotropic support to maintain MAP goal
         2. MAP goal duration will be institution-dependent. Consider 5–7 days
   (b) Ventilatory support
      (i) Assess the ability to initiate breath
      (ii) Pressure support trials
      (iii) Consider consult to otolaryngology for placement of tracheostomy when patient is hemodynamically stable [9]

(c) Monitor for autonomic dysreflexia with the inability to control temperature, blood pressure, and heart rate due to the impairment of the sympathetic pathways [9].
   (i) Treat hyper/hypothermia accordingly
   (ii) Consider TED hose and abdominal binder with position changes to increase vascular resistance
(d) Bracing for support
   (i) Cervical collar might be indicated depending on the injury to support the spinal column and prevent lordosis over time
   (ii) Halo/vest might be indicated depending on the injury
(e) Bowel and bladder management is imperative to help minimize autonomic dysregulation that can be seen with bladder distention and constipation [9]
   (i) At time of initial injury, place foley catheter
      1. Transition to straight catheter regimen every 6 h when able
      2. Avoid over distention and dribbling in between straight catheters
      3. Bladder scan as needed to evaluate bladder fullness
   (ii) Bowel regimen should be initiated by day 3 of hospital stay if able
      1. Daily regimen
      2. As needed regimen
(f) Diet
   (i) Enteral feeds should be initiated within the first 7 days of injury
   (ii) Monitor for abdominal distention with initiation of feeds
(g) Skin
   (i) Monitor for wound breakdown
   (ii) When hemodynamically safe, the patient should be turned every 2 h
   (iii) When hemodynamically safe, out of bed to cardiac chair or equivalent
(h) Medications for pain
   (i) Acetaminophen (10–15 mg/kg/dose) for pain and fever management as needed
   (ii) Gabapentin should be considered for treatment of neuropathic pain
   (iii) Narcotic use as needed for short-term acute pain needs
(i) Consults
   (i) Physical therapy
   (ii) Occupational therapy
   (iii) Social work
   (iv) Rehabilitation.
   (v) Child life.

4. Mid and lower CSI injury include midthoracic and lumbar spine injuries. Cord injuries at these levels will require similar management as high CSI. Autonomic dysreflexia does not occur frequently with these column injury levels but should be monitored.
   (a) Monitor for autonomic dysreflexia with inability to control temperature, blood pressure, and heart rate due to the impairment of the sympathetic pathways [9]

   - (i) Treat hyper/hypothermia accordingly
   - (ii) Consider TED hose and abdominal binder with position changes to increase vascular resistance
- (b) Bracing for support
   - (i) Cervical collar might be indicated depending on the injury to support the spinal column and prevent lordosis over time
   - (ii) Halo/vest might be indicated depending on the injury
- (c) Bowel and bladder management is imperative to help minimize autonomic dysregulation that can be seen with bladder distention and constipation [9]
   - (i) At time of initial injury, place foley catheter
      1. Transition to straight catheter regimen every 6 h when able
      2. Avoid overdistention and dribbling in between straight catheters
      3. Bladder scan as needed to evaluate bladder fullness
   - (ii) Bowel regimen should be initiated by day 3 of hospital stay if able
      1. Daily regimen
      2. As needed regimen
- (d) Diet
   - (i) Enteral feeds should be initiated within the first 7 days of injury
   - (ii) Monitor for abdominal distention with initiation of feeds
- (e) Skin
   - (i) Monitor for wound breakdown
   - (ii) When hemodynamically safe, the patient should be turned every 2 h
   - (iii) When hemodynamically safe, out of bed to cardiac chair or equivalent
- (f) Medications for pain
   - (i) Acetaminophen (10–15 mg/kg/dose) for pain and fever management as needed
   - (ii) Short-term use of NSAID or anti-inflammatories can be helpful and have not been shown to impact long-term bony fusion rates [10]
   - (iii) Gabapentin or other neuroleptic medications should be considered for treatment of neuropathic pain
   - (iv) Narcotic use as needed for short-term acute pain needs
   - (v) Anti-spasm agents such as short-acting benzodiazepines may be helpful for subsequent muscle spasms
- (g) Consults
   - (i) Physical therapy
   - (ii) Occupational therapy
   - (iii) Social work
   - (iv) Rehabilitation
   - (v) Child life

Operative

1. Significant ligamentous injury, i.e., AOD requires stabilization with fusion in older children or children who have failed conservative, nonoperative management. Bony injuries including unstable and burst fractures require stabilization with fusion (Fig. 1).
   (a) Occipital to cervical posterior fusion for AOD
      (a) Incision is made posterior from occiput to cervical level required for stabilization C2 or C3
      (b) Surgical goals include restoration of normal alignment while maintaining good craniocervical alignment (JAW)
      (c) Screw and rod size specific for patient are used to stabilize the spine
      (d) Fluoroscopy or neuronavigation can be used during the surgical procedure to assess hardware placement and alignment
      (e) Incision is closed with preferred surgeons' method
   (b) Posterior fusion typically includes at least one level above and one level below the injury
      (a) Posterior incision is made over the level of injury. Fluoroscopy is used to ensure correct level for incision
      (b) Surgical goals include decompression, restoration of normal cervical alignment, and/or stability

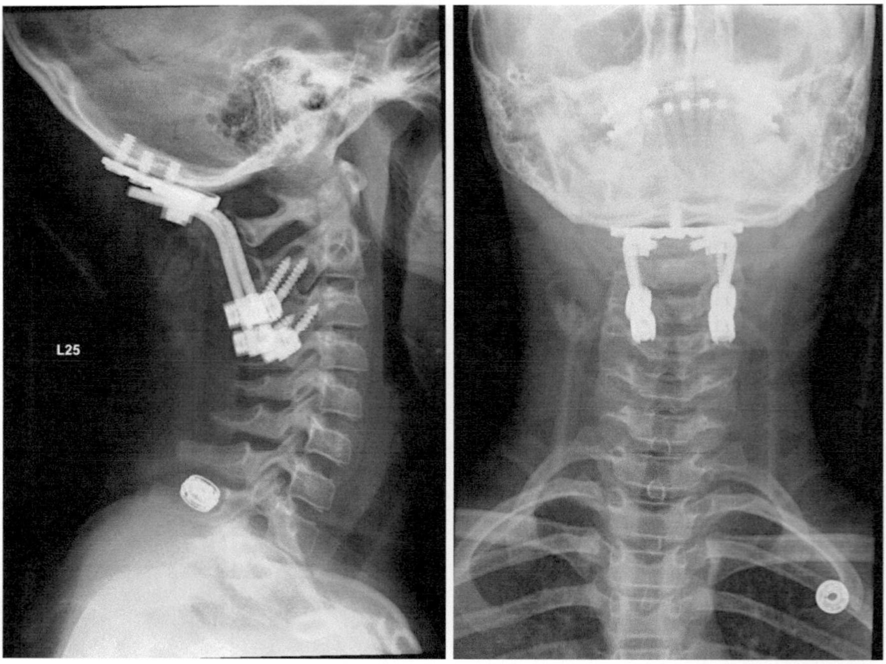

Fig. 1 Plain film radiograph AP/LA of cervical spine revealing occiput to cervical fusion for AOD

   (c) Screws and rods specific for the patient are used to stabilize the spine
   (d) Fluoroscopy is used during the surgical procedure to assess fixation
   (e) Incision is closed with preferred surgeons' method
 (c) Anterior fusion typically includes the level in question
   (a) Incision is fashioned in a small lateral incision over the sternocleidomastoid muscle. Laterality and length of the incision depend on the level of injury
   (b) Decompression may occur with either a discectomy or corpectomy depending on the level of kyphosis, disc involvement, or compression
   (c) Surgical goals include restoration of normal cervical alignment
   (d) Plate and screws are used to hold any graft material in place
   (e) Incision is closed with resorbable sutures
 (d) Anterior/posterior fusion (Fig. 2):
   (a) These may be considered in cases of significant three-column injury that results in gross stabilization or spinal deformity. Principles are similar to those of the isolated procedures listed above.

2. CSI injury might require surgical decompression of either hemorrhage, bone fragments, bullet fragments, or combination.
   (a) Posterior incision is made over the level of injury
   (b) Laminectomy or laminotomy is done to gain access to the spinal cord
   (c) Evacuation of hematoma, bone fragments, and/or bullet fragments from the epidural space or intradural space. Providing hemostasis and secure closure of dura if opened or torn from injury

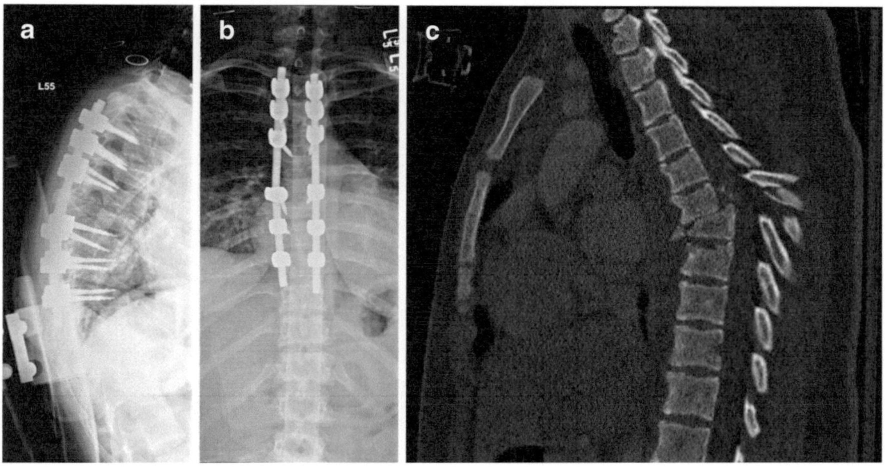

Fig. 2 Plain radiographs of thoracic posterior fusion after anterior subluxation of T6 on T7 and severe compression of T7 vertebral body and bone fragments into the canal. Thoracic CT revealing injury prior to surgery

Nursing Care and Treatment

Diligent nursing care is required for traumatic spine injuries. These patients might present with intact neurological status, however, can decompensate acutely. Care provided will be fluid and be dependent on the type of injury, location of injury, and potential interventions.

What Is Most Critical?

1. Patients arriving following a trauma with concern for traumatic spinal injury should always have their airway, breathing, and circulation initially assessed. For patients admitted from the emergency department or transferred from outside hospitals, there might be further imaging that is needed to assess the full extent of injury
   (a) For high spinal cord injury patients, there is concern for spinal shock, which may manifest with hemodynamic instability
2. Immobilization
   (a) Maintain cervical collar at all times if concern for cervical injury
      (i) Perform collar care based on institutional policy
         1. Assess for skin breakdown
         2. Clean neck with soap and water
         3. Change cervical collar pads and clean as directed by the manufacturer
   (b) Strict spinal precautions are needed until the full extent of injury is assessed
      (i) Log-roll and maintain spinal alignment. Consider 6-person lift for transfer
      (ii) No axial loading until discussed with surgery team

Nonoperative Care

1. Pain control may be required in the acute setting
   (a) Similar pain management
2. Activity:
   (a) Depending on the extent of injury visualized, a collar may be necessary to help protect alignment while ligamentous and bony injuries heal.
   (b) Collar use:
      (i) Should clarify if the collar should be left in place at all times. Special attention should be paid to activities of daily living including bathing and sleeping.
      (ii) Bathing may require a collar that can be dried after or that is relatively waterproof. In some instances, strict spinal precautions to ensure neutral alignment should be implementing with collar changes.
      (iii) Sleeping. In some instances, collar may be able to be removed.

(c) Collar wean:
Once bony and ligamentous healing have occurred the collar may be removed. Depending on the length of collar use, there can be weakening of the paraspinal muscles due to inactivity. As a result, consider collar wean to help patients regain normal activity levels without additional pain. PT may be helpful as well.

Immediate Postoperative Care

3. Pain control
   (a) Scheduled acetaminophen (10–15 mg/kg/dose) every 6 h for the first few days and then consider transitioning as needed.
   (b) Intravenous narcotics can be used as needed 24–48 h after surgery. Once tolerating, oral diet transition to oral narcotic use as needed for another few days.
   (c) Muscle relaxant, i.e., diazepam can be scheduled for the first 24–48 h after surgery and then transition to an as-needed medication. Oral route is preferred to minimize sedating effect.
4. Activity
   (a) Maintain limited elevation of head of bed if the dura was open during surgery for the first 24–48 h.
   (b) Continue bracing with either a cervical collar or TLSO.
   (c) Initiation of physical therapy and occupational therapy should start on postoperative day 1.

What to Watch for?

1. Neurological assessment
   (a) Postsurgical assessments to monitor for any improvements or decline in strength or sensation.
      (i) If laminectomy or laminotomy was performed for hematoma evacuation or bullet/bone fragment removal, it will be important to document any changes in the neurological exam postsurgery.
2. Incision
   (a) Surgical dressing to be maintained per surgeons' preference.
      (i) Most incisions will remain covered for the first 24–72 h.
   (b) Jackson–Pratt (JP drain) to remove excess fluid from near surgical area might be used.
      (i) Monitor JP output every 4 h.
      (ii) Notify surgical service of excessive output.
      (iii) JP drain is removed when drain output is tapering off usually 48–72 h after surgery.

1. Surgical service will remove the drain at the bedside.
2. Exit site for drain may be secured with a stitch and covered with a dressing.
3. Monitor dressing for drainage for the first 24 h after drain is removed.

(c) Assess dressing for drainage (blood or cerebral spinal fluid) at least once a shift.
  (i) Notify surgical service if there is an increase or change in the drainage.

(d) Monitor for infection or wound dehiscence.
  (i) If there is purulent drainage or wound dehiscence from incision, notify surgical service.
  (ii) Place dressing over incision while awaiting surgical service evaluation.

3. Monitor for positional headaches if surgery included laminectomy or laminotomy with a dural opening. Upright positioning can cause headaches if there is a CSF leak through the dural opening.
   (a) If headaches develop with upright positioning, place patient flat.
   (b) Notify surgical service of headache with upright positioning.

Wound Care

1. Keep incision clean and dry.
   (a) Timing of bathing and getting incision wet will be surgeon-dependent.
   (b) No submerging of incision until completely healed. Showering only.
   (c) No swimming in a pool or lake until the incision is completely healed.
2. Bracing with incision.
   (a) Monitor incisions that are under bracing devices closely for breakdown.
   (b) Clean incisions while doing brace care.
   (c) Keep cervical pads on cervical collars dry to help prevent wound breakdown.

Discharge Teaching

Parents should teach back/return demonstrate the following:

1. Demonstrate brace care:
   (a) How to safely remove the front and back of the brace with log rolling
   (b) How to clean skin under the brace with soap and water
   (c) How to clean brace
   (d) How to change pads on the cervical collar
      (i) How to wash cervical pads with soap and water by hand
      (ii) Air dry cervical pads

2. Demonstrate how to put brace on if only wearing while out of bed
   (a) Alignment of front and back of brace
   (b) Secure brace for snug fit
3. Demonstrate wound care
4. Activity limitations
   (a) No lifting
   (b) No gym or recess
   (c) No driving a car while in a cervical collar age dependent
5. Medication use
   (a) Educate on which medications should be used for pain versus muscle spasms
   (b) Dosing of medications and how often to use
6. Contact surgical office
   (a) Concerns for fever
   (b) Concerns for wound dehiscence or wound infection
      (i) Drainage from incision
      (ii) Redness around the incision
      (iii) Incision feels warm to the touch
   (c) Uncontrollable pain even with medication use
   (d) Changes in neurological status

References

1. Floan G, Calvo R, Prieto J, et al. Pediatric penetrating thoracic trauma: examining the impact of trauma center designation and penetrating trauma volume on outcomes. J Peds Surgery. 2020;58:330–6.
2. Gupta S, Hauser B, Zaki M, et al. Morbidity after traumatic spinal injury in pediatric and adolescent sports-related trauma. J Neurosurg Spine. 2020;32:642–38.
3. Herman M, Brown K, Sponseller P, et al. Pediatric cervical spine clearance. J Bone and Joint. 2019;101(e1):1–9.
4. Lemley K, Bauer P. Pediatric spinal cord injury: recognition of injury and initial resuscitation, in hospital management, and coordination of care. J Pediatr Intensive Care. 2015;4(1):27–34.
5. American Spinal Injury Association. International standards for neurological classification of spinal cord injury (SNCSCI). 2019. Retrieved from https://asia-spinalinjury.org/learning/
6. Roberts T, Leonard G, Cepela D. Classifications in brief: American Spinal Injury Association (ASIA) impairment scale. Clin Orthop Relat Res. 2016;475(5):1499–504.
7. Leonard J, Harding M, Cook L, et al. PECARN prediction rule for cervical spine imaging of children presenting to the emergency department with blunt trauma: a multicentre prospective observational trial. Lancet Child Adoldesc Health. 2024;8(7):482–90.
8. Luckhurst C, Wiberg H, Brown R, et al. Pediatric cervical spine injury following blunt trauma in children younger than 3 years the PEDSPINE II study. JAMA Surg. 2023;158(11):1126–32.
9. Sacino A, Rosenblatt K. Critical care management of acute spinal cord injury- part II: intensive care to rehabilitation. Indian Society of Neuroanaesthesiology and Critical Care. 2019;6:222–35.
10. Wheatley BM, Nappo KE, Christensen DL, Holman AM, Brooks DI, Potter BK. Effect of NSAIDs on bone healing rates: a meta-analysis. J Am Acad Orthop Surg. 2019;27(7):e330–6. https://doi.org/10.5435/JAAOS-D-17-00727.

Pediatric Peripheral Nerve and Brachial Plexus Injuries

Jonathan Pindrik, Christy Monson, and Anne Graver

Introduction

Injuries to peripheral nerves and the brachial plexus (BP) carry a wide range of symptom severity, management pathways, and potential long-term sequelae. Pediatric peripheral nerve injuries may result from:

- Direct trauma (blunt, penetrating, or lacerating injury)
- Compression due to external forces
- Iatrogenic injury (during surgery or vascular catheter placement)
- Birthing and delivery (neonatal brachial plexus injury [nBPI])
- Entrapment (compression due to internal, adjacent anatomic structures)
- Stretching during physiologic growth spurts

Epidemiology and Risk Factors

Pediatric peripheral nerve traumatic injuries occur most commonly from penetrating or lacerating injuries, particularly involving the ulnar or median nerve distributions [14]. Upper and lower extremity fractures or subluxations (dislocations) represent another common cause of peripheral nerve injuries in children and adolescents [14]. For instance, supracondylar humerus fractures (above the elbow)

J. Pindrik (✉)
Division of Pediatric Neurosurgery, Nationwide Children's Hospital, Columbus, OH, USA

Department of Neurological Surgery, The Ohio State University College of Medicine, Columbus, OH, USA
e-mail: jonathan.pindrik@nationwidechildrens.org

C. Monson · A. Graver
Division of Pediatric Neurosurgery, Nationwide Children's Hospital, Columbus, OH, USA

K. Battick et al. (eds.), *Nursing Guide for Pediatric Neuroscience Patients*,
https://doi.org/10.1007/978-3-032-22664-8_13

represent a common fracture within the pediatric population, with traumatic neurapraxia (see definition below) as a major sequela (11% of cases) [3]:

- Extension-type fractures mainly involve anterior interosseous nerve (branch of median nerve) injury (34%).
- Flexion-type fractures mainly involve ulnar nerve injury (91%).

Among infants and toddlers, birth-related neonatal brachial plexus injury (nBPI) represents a predominant cause of peripheral nerve-related morbidity. Several studies have reported the incidence and temporal trends of nBPI:

- Overall incidence of birth-related nBPI: 0.4 to 4.6 per 1000 live births [1, 10, 13, 17, 18].
- Temporal trends suggest overall decreasing incidence of nBPI from 1.7 per 1000 live births (1997) to 0.9 per 1000 live births (2012) [2].
- A separate systematic review reported nBPI incidence as low as 0.5 per 1000 live births after year 2000 [7].

Risk factors for birth-related nBPI relate to the mother, fetus, and passage through maternal birth canal. Interestingly, up to 55% of infants impacted by nBPI lack perinatal risk factors [2, 18]. Frequently reported (though debatable) risk factors for nBPI include the following [1, 2, 10, 17, 18]:

- Shoulder dystocia
- Maternal gestational diabetes
- Fetal macrosomia (fetal weight > 4500 gm)
- Complicated delivery requiring vacuum assistance or forceps
- Neonatal hypotonia

Further investigations have questioned the validity of these reported risk factors. For instance, many studies have reported that nearly 1/3 of nBPI cases occur without shoulder dystocia, and majority of nBPI cases occur without complicated delivery [19]. Furthermore, while increasing birth weight has been associated with nBPI, several studies have shown that majority (> 75%) of nBPI cases occur without fetal macrosomia [19]. Intuitively, delivery via a Cesarean section represents a protective factor against birth-related nBPI [2, 7, 19]:

- Incidence of nBPI, birth via vaginal delivery: 1.6 per 1000 live births
- Incidence of nBPI, birth via Cesarean section: 0.3 per 1000 live births
- Delivery via Cesarean section decreases but does not eliminate the risk of nBPI

In contrast to traumatic peripheral nerve injuries, compression and entrapment neuropathies occur rarely in children. Certain themes and patterns characterize the incidence of pediatric traumatic peripheral nerve injuries and compression or entrapment mononeuropathies [8]:

- The most common pediatric upper extremity neuropathy involves the Ulnar nerve, typically due to trauma.
- Neurogenic thoracic outlet syndrome (TOS) (compression of the lower trunk of the brachial plexus) occurs more commonly in adolescents than children (rare).
- Common peroneal nerve compression represents one of the most common pediatric compressive neuropathies.

Risk factors for pediatric compression or entrapment neuropathy include a combination of genetic syndromes, systemic diseases, and conditions related to body habitus [8]:

- Hereditary neuropathy with liability to pressure palsies (HNPP)—genetic condition (autosomal dominant defect on chromosome 17) predisposing patients to multiple, recurrent neuropathies due to minor trauma or compressive forces.
- Low body weight or substantial weight loss, particularly with anorexia.
- Rapid growth (e.g., during puberty), particularly with neurogenic TOS.
- Diabetes mellitus or Vasculitis (due to compromised vascular supply of nerves).
- Childhood obesity may increase risk for meralgia paresthetica.

Peripheral Nerve Anatomy and Neuropathology

Peripheral nerves contain a hierarchical structure which helps characterize and explain the severity of peripheral nerve injuries. Components of peripheral nerves include the following:

- Axons—elongated extensions/processes of neurons transmitting electrochemical signals.
- Myelin—insulating substrate surrounding axons, provided by Schwann cells.
- Endoneurium—supporting connective tissue surrounding nerve fibers within a nerve fascicle.
- Perineurium—supporting connective tissue layer surrounding a nerve fascicle.
- Epineurium—supporting connective tissue layer surrounding a group of nerve fascicles and comprising the circumferential surface of a peripheral nerve.

Peripheral nerve injuries may occur at different levels of this hierarchical structure and involve varying degrees of anticipated recovery (Table 1). Peripheral nerve injuries of moderate severity may lead to formation of a neuroma, an expansile lesion along a nerve consisting of misdirected axons, fibroblasts, and scar tissue (Fig. 1).

Table 1 Neuropathologic description of peripheral nerve injuries [1, 17]

Type of injury	Structures damaged	Description	Expected recovery
Neuropraxia	Myelin	Focal myelin disruption without axonal damage [5] Leads to transient motor or sensory deficits Mildest form of peripheral nerve injury	Full recovery
Axonotmesis	Axons	Preservation of endoneurium and perineurium which fosters peripheral nerve regeneration and spontaneous functional recovery	Full recovery or minor residual functional impairments
Neurotmesis	Axons, endoneurium, perineurium	Compromised ability of regenerating, sprouting axons to re-establish appropriate nerve fascicles to reach end-organ target May lead to neuroma formation	Greater risk of long-term functional impairment May require surgery
Nerve transection or discontinuity	Axons, endoneurium, perineurium, epineurium	Severe nerve injury leading to functional deficit and lack of recovery without peripheral nerve repair	Lack of functional recovery without surgical repair

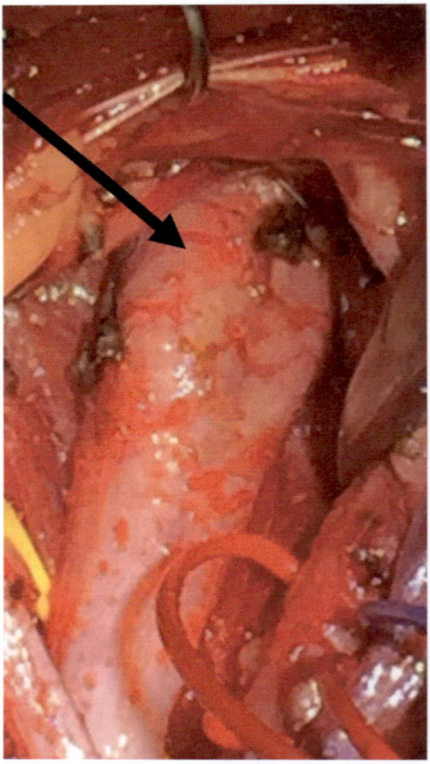

Fig. 1 Intraoperative photograph showing a neuroma along the course of the posterior cord in a patient with traumatic BPI

Brachial Plexus Anatomy

The brachial plexus represents a complex network of peripheral nerve structures organized into nerve roots, trunks, divisions, cords, and branches (Fig. 2). Typically extending from cervical and upper thoracic nerve roots C5-T1, the brachial plexus provides motor and sensory innervation to the ipsilateral upper extremity (Table 2).

Brachial Plexus Injury (BPI)

Brachial plexus injuries (BPIs) deserve special attention among pediatric peripheral nerve injuries. One of the most common types of pediatric peripheral nerve injury, birth-related neonatal brachial plexus injury (nBPI), involves traction to the BP during delivery, often in the setting of shoulder dystocia (trapping of the shoulder under the pelvic brim or pubic symphysis during delivery) [10, 18]. Traumatic BPIs and birth-related nBPIs vary based on the patterns of nerve root or trunk involvement, degree of structural damage, and severity of functional impairment (Table 3). In severe BPI, nerve root avulsion from the spinal cord leads to permanent deficits without surgical repair [17]. Extension of the BPI to nerve roots C4 and C5 may cause phrenic nerve (innervation of diaphragm) injury, leading to respiratory difficulties and asymmetric chest expansion during inhalation [1, 10].

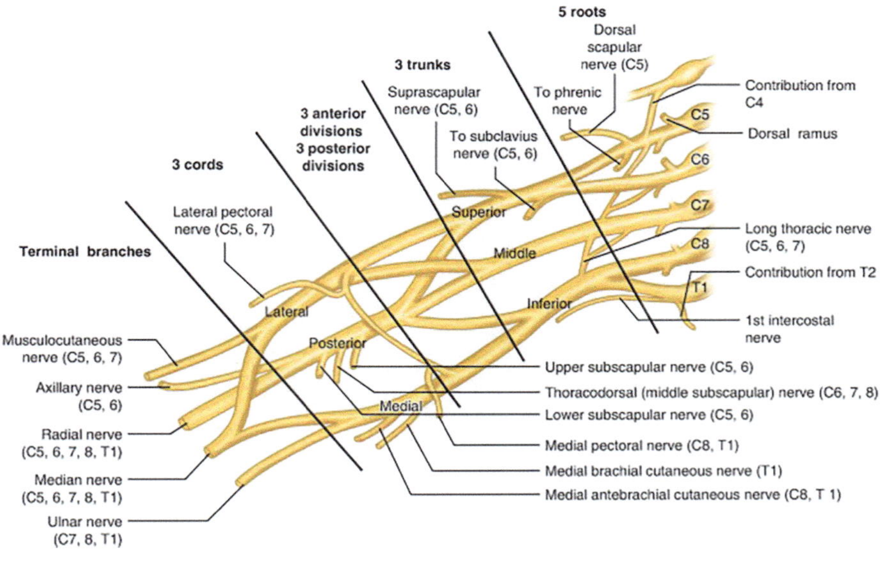

Fig. 2 Diagram of the brachial plexus demonstrating the hierarchical organization into roots (C5–T1), trunks (upper, middle, lower), divisions (anterior, posterior), cords (lateral, medial, posterior), and terminal branches. *Borrowed from*: Borden, S. (2019). Brachial Plexus. In: Abd-Elsayed, A. (eds) Pain. Springer, Cham. https://doi.org/10.1007/978-3-319-99124-5_101

Table 2 Components of the brachial plexus

Organizational level	Components	Location	Important branches
Nerve roots	C5, C6, C7, C8, T1	Extend from spinal cord through neural foramina, between anterior and middle scalene muscles	Dorsal scapular nerve (from C5) Long thoracic nerve (from C5 to C7)
Upper trunk	C5–C6 nerve roots	Above the clavicle, deep to the supraclavicular fat pad	Suprascapular nerve
Middle trunk	C7 nerve root	Above the clavicle, deep to the supraclavicular fat pad Interposed between upper trunk (superiorly) and lower trunk (inferiorly)	
Lower trunk	C8–T1 nerve roots	Above the clavicle, deep to the supraclavicular fat pad Nerve roots C8 and T1 coalesce around T1 rib to form lower trunk	
Anterior divisions	1 anterior division extends from each trunk	Deep to the clavicle	
Posterior divisions	1 posterior division extends from each trunk	Deep to the clavicle	
Lateral cord	Combination of anterior divisions from upper and middle trunks	Deep to clavicle and pectoralis major and minor muscles Named anatomically based on location with respect to axillary artery	Lateral pectoral nerve Musculocutaneous nerve Lateral contribution to median nerve
Medial cord	Extension of anterior division of lower trunk	Deep to clavicle and pectoralis major and minor muscles Named anatomically based on location with respect to axillary artery	Medial pectoral nerve Medial brachial and antebrachial cutaneous nerves Ulnar nerve Medial contribution to median nerve
Posterior cord	Combination of posterior divisions of all three (upper, middle, lower) trunks	Deep to clavicle and pectoralis major and minor muscles Named anatomically based on location with respect to axillary artery	Axillary nerve Radial nerve

Pediatric Compression and Entrapment Neuropathies

Despite their rarity among infants and children, pediatric entrapment neuropathies should be considered in the appropriate context to avoid delayed diagnosis and patient morbidity. Common themes in the etiology and diagnosis of pediatric compression or entrapment neuropathies include the following [8]:

Table 3 Different patterns and types of brachial plexus injury (BPI) [1, 10, 17]

Type of BPI	Nerve components involved	Motor function impairments	Relative frequency
Upper plexus injury (Erb–Duchenne palsy)	C5, C6 nerve roots Upper trunk	Shoulder stability and abduction (supraspinatus, infra-spinatus, deltoid mm) Elbow flexion (biceps brachii, brachialis mm.)	Most common type of birth-related nBPI
Upper and middle plexus injury (extended Erb–Duchenne palsy)	C5, C6, C7 nerve roots Upper and middle trunks	Shoulder stability and abduction (supraspinatus, infraspinatus, deltoid mm.) Elbow flexion (biceps brachii, brachialis mm.) Wrist extension	Results in commonly recognized "waiter's tip" position of upper extremity
Lower plexus injury (Klumpke palsy)	C8, T1 nerve roots	Distal upper extremity deficits including grip and hand intrinsic function	Rare (< 2%) isolated finding in nBPI May result from over-stretching or over-extension at shoulder
Complete or pan plexus injury	C5–T1 nerve roots	Flail upper extremity with proximal and distal impairments May also occur with Horner's syndrome (ptosis, miosis)	Occurs less commonly (approximately 15–20%) among nBPIs

Abbreviations: mm. = muscle

- Pediatric carpal tunnel syndrome (CTS) represents a rare diagnosis in children and may reflect a causative genetic condition or syndrome.
  - Typical age of presentation: 6–8 years.
  - Lysosomal storage diseases (e.g., mucopolysaccharidosis types I, II, III) like Hunter's and Hurler's syndromes account for nearly 1/2 of pediatric CTS cases.
- Ulnar entrapment neuropathy represents an uncommon diagnosis in the pediatric population but most commonly occurs in the cubital tunnel (along the medial aspect of the elbow).
  - Supracondylar fracture of the humerus may lead to delayed ulnar entrapment neuropathy.
  - The proximal edge of the flexor carpi ulnaris represents a potential site of compression.
- Neurogenic TOS (rare in children, more likely but still uncommon during adolescence) may occur due to compression by additional cervical rib (Fig. 3), fibrous band extending from C7 transverse process, T1 rib, hyperostosis or callus formation following clavicular fracture, or adjacent muscular hypertrophy.
- Common peroneal nerve compression typically occurs along the lateral aspect of lower extremity below the knee, along the fibular head.

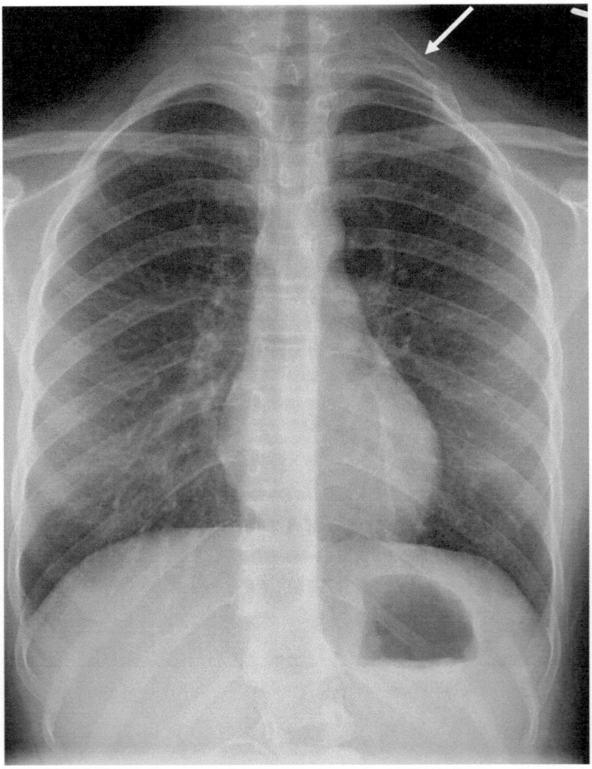

Fig. 3 Anterior–posterior view chest X-ray showing a left-sided (C7) cervical rib causing neurogenic thoracic outlet syndrome (TOS)

- Sciatic neuropathy—one of the more common pediatric neuropathies, typically occurs due to inadequate soft tissue coverage (e.g., gluteal musculature); most common etiologies include trauma or external compression.
- Meralgia paresthetica—rare in pediatric population; arises due to compression of the lateral femoral cutaneous nerve (LFCN) by the inguinal ligament.

Clinical Assessment

General Approach to Pediatric Patients with Peripheral Nerve Injuries

Depending upon the age of presentation, evaluation of pediatric patients with peripheral nerve injuries involves multiple components:

- Comprehensive birth and delivery history (particularly for nBPI).
- Review of past medical history and family history for contributory factors (including history of nBPI in other siblings).

- Detailed evaluation of clinical presentation, including description of traumatic events and timing of symptom onset.
- Characterization of clinical symptoms including pain, motor and/or sensory impairments, severity of deficits, and clinical progression (stagnance, improvement, or worsening of symptoms).
- Observation of global motor deficits or irregularities that may reflect more pervasive underlying central nervous system (CNS) disorder (e.g. cerebral palsy) [10].
- Focused observation of the affected extremity, noting general appearance (e.g., muscular wasting or atrophy), posture or resting position, and spontaneous movements [14].

Physical examination includes inspection of the involved anatomic region, searching for signs of trauma, anatomic deformity or irregularity, muscular wasting or atrophy, and/or abnormal positioning at rest. Neurological evaluation involves full motor and sensory assessment of cranial nerves and upper and lower extremities, with focused examination of motor and sensory functions of the impaired region(s). For older children and adolescents, the Medical Research Council (MRC) scale represents the most commonly used scoring system for motor function [1, 14]:

- MRC 0 = No motor function (no muscle contraction).
- MRC 1 = Minimal muscular contraction with/without subtle movement.
- MRC 2 = Movement in a two-dimensional plane (gravity eliminated).
- MRC 3 = Movement in three-dimensional space (against gravity) with full range of motion.
- MRC 4 = Movement against resistance (with full range of motion) with some weakness.
- MRC 5 = Normal muscular strength against resistance (with full range of motion).

Motor and sensory evaluations determine the location, extent, and severity of injury, while helping to monitor the progress of functional recovery [14].

While less common, pediatric peripheral nerve compression injuries or entrapment neuropathies deserve special attention. Tinel's sign (provoking paresthesias along the distribution of a nerve by digital-tapping a site of nerve compression) represents an important component of the sensory exam [14].

Clinical history and physical examination findings may provide helpful clues to the diagnosis, particularly in pediatric compression and entrapment neuropathy (Table 4).

Table 4 Clinical history and physical examination findings in pediatric compression or entrapment neuropathy [8]

Nerve compression, entrapment, or syndrome	Clinical history findings	Physical examination findings
Pediatric carpal tunnel syndrome (CTS) (median nerve)	Hand clumsiness, decreased manual dexterity Hand pain (less frequently)	Thenar atrophy (lateral aspect of the palmar surface of the hand)
Ulnar nerve	Medial elbow pain Numbness and paresthesias along digits 4–5 (ring and small fingers) Intrinsic hand weakness	Hand motor deficits Positive Tinel's sign along ulnar nerve (percussion of nerve causing sensory symptoms) Ulnar nerve subluxation during elbow flexion
Long thoracic nerve	Compression along the chest wall due to seatbelts, heavy weights (e.g., backpacks), and/or spinal orthotic braces	Scapular winging (elevation of the medial edge of the scapula when pushing against a fixed surface) due to the weakness of the serratus anterior muscle
Neurogenic TOS	Intermittent pain, numbness, and/or paresthesias along the medial (ulnar) aspect of upper extremity extending to digits 4–5 (ring and small fingers) Distal upper extremity weakness (wrist flexion, grip)	Medial (ulnar) wrist flexion weakness Intrinsic hand weakness Sensory impairments along the medial (ulnar) aspect of upper extremity
Common peroneal nerve	Compression due to surgical positioning or splint/brace/cast (iatrogenic) Compression due to prolonged sitting position (knee-crossing) Foot drop	Distal lower extremity weakness involving foot dorsiflexion and eversion
Sciatic neuropathy	Compression due to prolonged sitting position on hard surfaces or heels, or long periods of immobility (supine)	Weakness in distributions of sciatic nerve branches/targets
Meralgia paresthetica	Prolonged prone position (e.g., spine surgery) Dysesthetic (burning) pain and paresthesias along anterolateral thigh	Purely sensory findings (no motor component of LFCN)

Specific Approach to Birth-Related Neonatal Brachial Plexus Injury (nBPI)

Evaluation of infants with nBPI requires patience and close attention given the potential difficulties of engagement or participation and lack of voluntary examination maneuvers. Early evaluation remains critical to identifying the extent of injury, establishing a baseline to monitor recovery, and determining the potential need for peripheral nerve surgery [1, 10]. If possible, examination by a specialty-trained physiotherapist or occupational therapist may augment the evaluation.

Prior to passive manipulation or active movement of the involved extremity, simple observation of resting posture and spontaneous movements may elicit critical details [10]. For instance, recognition of ipsilateral ptosis or miosis (reflecting Horner's syndrome) and flail upper extremity would suggest complete or pan-plexus injury (Table 3). Birth-related nBPI involving the C5–C7 nerve roots (upper and middle trunks) results in a commonly recognized "waiter's tip" position of the affected upper extremity at rest [1, 10, 17] (Fig. 4):

- Shoulder adduction and internal rotation
- Elbow extension
- Forearm pronation
- Wrist flexion
- Finger flexion

Assessment of the involved extremity includes each joint and muscle group, with passive movement (passive range of motion [PROM]) to identify tightness or contractures. Observation of pain during palpation of affected regions—including neck, shoulder, and arm—represents an important component of the exam as well. Infantile expression of pain can be measured objectively with the *FLACC* scale (0—10) [10]:

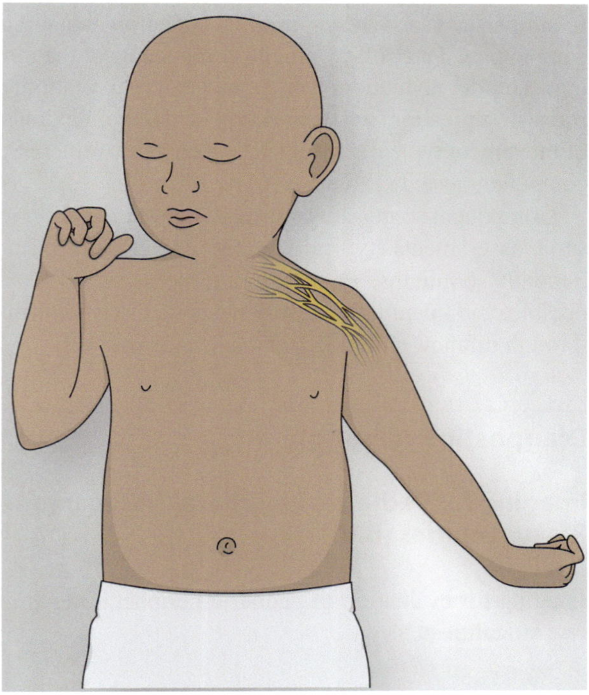

Fig. 4 Artist rendering of left neonatal brachial plexus injury (nBPI) involving the upper and middle trunks. A more realistic depiction may involve a greater degree of left shoulder adduction

Table 5 Active Movement Scale (AMS) for evaluating neonatal brachial plexus injury (nBPI) [9]

Observation/Movement	Gravity contribution	AMS Grade
Absence of muscle tone or contraction	Eliminated (two-dimensional plane)	0
Muscle contraction, no movement	Eliminated (two-dimensional plane)	1
Movement <= 1/2 ROM	Eliminated (two-dimensional plane)	2
Movement >1/2 ROM	Eliminated (two-dimensional plane)	3
Full ROM	Eliminated (two-dimensional plane)	4
Movement <= 1/2 ROM	Against gravity (three-dimensional space)	5
Movement >1/2 ROM	Against gravity (three-dimensional space)	6
Full ROM	Against gravity (three-dimensional space)	7

Abbreviations: ROM = range of motion

- *F*ace—Score 0 (normal), 1 (grimace, frown), or 2 (quivering, jaw clenching).
- *L*egs—Score (normal or relaxed), 1 (restless or tense), or 2 (kicking or hip-flexion).
- *A*ctivity—Score 0 (normal or relaxed), 1 (fidgeting, shifting, or tense), or 2 (rigid or jerking).
- *C*ry—Score 0 (none), 1 (moaning or whimpering), or 2 (frequent or consistent crying).
- *C*onsolability—Score 0 (normal), 1 (intermittently consolable), or 2 (inconsolable).

Evaluation of motor function includes observation of spontaneous movements and provocation of active movements about the shoulder, elbow, wrist, and hand. Exam performance by a specialty-trained physiotherapist may be helpful for these components. Particularly crucial components of the motor exam include the following: shoulder abduction, flexion, and external rotation; elbow flexion and extension; forearm supination; wrist extension; and finger flexion and extension. Quantification of movement typically follows the Active Movement Scale (AMS) for each specific component tested (Table 5).

Component scores are summated, and the total serves as a comparison for future serial assessments (typically at baseline close to birth [2–3 weeks age], then ages 3 months, 6 months, 9 months, 12 months, etc.). The AMS provides reliable, reproducible, and quantitative assessments that may contribute to management planning through infancy, childhood, and adolescence [10]

Diagnostic Evaluations

Imaging for Pediatric Peripheral Nerve Injuries and Brachial Plexus Injuries (BPI)

Imaging for evaluation of pediatric peripheral nerve injuries generally relies upon few modalities:

- Peripheral nerve ultrasound (US)—may demonstrate nerve discontinuity or neuroma formation.
- Magnetic resonance (MR) neurography—may demonstrate neuroma formation, abnormal signal intensity along the course of a peripheral nerve, or muscle signal changes.
- Chest X-ray—may identify cervical rib in the context of neurogenic TOS (Fig. 3).
- Computed tomography (CT)—lower extremity CT may identify osseous tumor or hyperostosis as a cause of common peroneal nerve compression [8].

While US typically requires less time, fewer mandates on patient's lack of motion, and no necessity for sedation or anesthesia in young patients, MR neurography offers greater imaging resolution and detail of nerve and adjacent structures. Muscle signal changes may reflect denervation and/or atrophy, critical for the diagnosis of peripheral nerve injury, decision-making, and timing of repair (if necessary).

Additional imaging studies that may contribute to evaluation of traumatic BPI or nBPI include the following:

- X-ray—determines the presence of clavicular or humeral fracture [1, 10].
- Brachial plexus MR neurography.
- Cervical spine MRI—may demonstrate pseudomeningocele formation (at the lateral aspect of the cervical spinal cord along the vertebral foramen) reflecting nerve root avulsion (Fig. 5).
- Chest X-ray—may demonstrate hemidiaphragm elevation, indicating phrenic nerve involvement.
- Abdominal/Chest US—assess abnormal diaphragm movement and phenic nerve involvement [10, 17].
- Gleno-humeral (shoulder) joint US—may identify joint instability or subluxation.

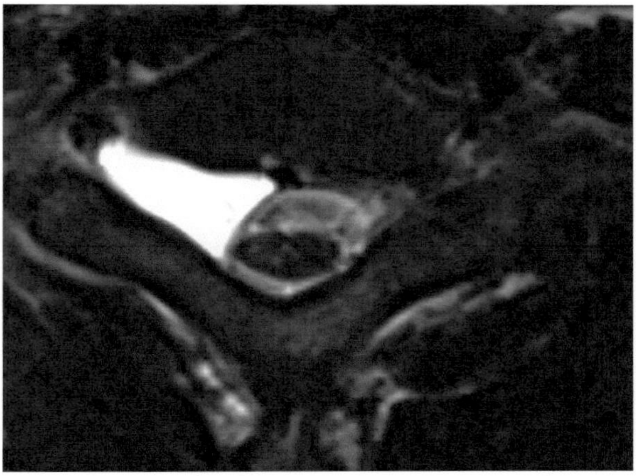

Fig. 5 Cervical spine MRI, with T2 sequence axial image showing right-sided cerebrospinal fluid (CSF) collection extending from dura through the vertebral foramen, consistent with the pseudomeningocele in a patient with traumatic BPI

Other Diagnostic Modalities for Pediatric Peripheral Nerve and Neonatal Brachial Plexus Injuries (nBPI)

Electromyography (EMG) and nerve conduction studies (NCS) serve important roles in the diagnostic evaluation of many pediatric peripheral nerve injuries. As a compliment to peripheral nerve imaging, EMG/NCS offers a thorough assessment of nerve function or electrophysiology. This diagnostic modality offers particular clinical utility in the settings of pediatric entrapment neuropathy and pediatric peripheral nerve trauma [8]. Typically performed as a baseline study approximately 3 weeks after traumatic peripheral nerve injury, EMG/NCS may show [17]:

- Decrease or lack of motor unit potentials (MUPs)
- Denervation changes (fibrillation potentials) in the target muscle
- Stability, worsening, or improvement of findings (particularly regarding MUPs) over serial studies (typically at 3, 6, and 9 months following injury)

Serial studies over time evaluate the progress of peripheral nerve reinnervation and spontaneous functional recovery. Findings on EMG/NCS complement clinical assessments and contribute to surgical decision-making.

In contrast to their important role in pediatric peripheral nerve traumatic injuries and entrapment neuropathies, EMG/NCS have questionable utility in nBPI. For instance, EMG/NCS performed at 3 months of age may not yield reliable or useful data [1, 17]. Additionally, evaluations during neonatal and infant stages may produce false-negative or false-positive results [1, 10]. However, some peripheral nerve surgery groups utilize EMG/NCS at early time points (age 1 month to <3 months) to differentiate between postganglionic nerve rupture and preganglionic nerve root avulsion [16].

Classification of Neonatal Brachial Plexus Injures (nBPI)

Several different grading schemes characterize the severity of nBPI, including the Sunderland and Narakas classification systems. While the Sunderland classification system characterizes injury at the nerve structural level (Table 1), the Narakas grading scale describes injuries at the nerve root and plexus levels [12, 13, 16] (Table 6):

Table 6 Narakas classification system for neonatal brachial plexus injures (nBPI)

Narakas grade	Nerve roots involved	Motor impairments	Proportion of nBPI
I	C5–C6 (upper trunk)	Shoulder stability and abduction (supraspinatus, infraspinatus, deltoid mm.) Elbow flexion (biceps brachii, brachialis mm.)	Narakas groups I and II comprise the majority (approximately 73%) of nBPIs [13]
II	C5–C7 (upper and middle trunks)	Shoulder stability and abduction (supraspinatus, infraspinatus, deltoid mm.) Elbow flexion (biceps brachii, brachialis mm.) Wrist and finger extension	Narakas groups I and II comprise the majority (approximately 73%) of nBPIs [13]
III	C5–T1 (upper, middle, and lower trunks)	Pan plexus injury with flaccid upper extremity	
IV	C5-T1 (upper, middle, and lower trunks, and stellate ganglion)	Pan plexus injury with flaccid upper extremity and Horner's syndrome	

Management of Peripheral Nerve and Neonatal Brachial Plexus Injuries

Conservative Management

Nonsurgical Management of Pediatric Peripheral Nerve Injuries

Conservative management strategies for pediatric entrapment neuropathies (though sometimes unsuccessful) may be applied in the following contexts [8]:

- Ulnar entrapment neuropathy—activity modification, splinting, anti-inflammatory analgesics.
- Long thoracic entrapment neuropathy—activity modifications.
- Radial entrapment neuropathy, in neonates and children.
- Common peroneal nerve compression—typically favorable outcomes (spontaneous recovery) following cessation of predisposing factors (e.g., extrinsic compression).
- Meralgia paresthetica—weight loss, physical therapy, analgesics.

Nonsurgical Management of Neonatal Brachial Plexus Injuries (nBPI)

Within the first few months of birth-related nBPI, management typically involves frequent clinical evaluations, physiotherapy, home stretching exercises, and encouragement of bimanual activities or activities involving usage of the affected upper extremity [10, 17].

- Multidisciplinary BP or peripheral nerve clinic evaluations (if available) with specially trained physiotherapists help optimize and standardize motor function evaluations, assessments of joint mobility or tightness, and family education for home stretching regimens.
- Early mobilization and passive stretching of the affected upper extremity may help foster functional recovery and mitigate risks of joint contracture formation [10, 17].
- Physiotherapy includes active and passive range of motion exercises for the affected extremity.
- Upper extremity changes leading to joint contracture formation may begin within 2–3 weeks of birth, highlighting the need for early intervention [1, 17].
- Additional physiotherapy adjuncts and techniques may include external orthoses, kinesiology taping, electrical stimulation, muscle or sensory re-education, and/or adaptive functional training [20].
- Serial clinic visits (typically within 2 weeks of nBPI and at ages 3 months, 6 months, 9 months, 12 months, etc.) monitor progress and functional recovery, helping with the decision between continued conservative management or operative intervention.
- In addition to serial clinical assessments, other diagnostic modalities (MRI, MR neurography, possible EMG/NCS) at age > = 3 months may help with surgical decision-making.
- Spontaneous functional recovery of elbow flexion (at least anti-gravity, MRC > = 3, AMS > = 5) by age 3 months suggests more favorable prognosis, often precluding the need for surgery [1].

Surgical Management of Pediatric Peripheral Nerve and Neonatal Brachial Plexus Injuries (nBPI)

Indications for Surgery

While neurapraxia and mild peripheral nerve injuries (e.g., axonotmesis) do not require surgical intervention, peripheral nerve injuries of moderate-to-high severity typically require surgical repair to optimize functional recovery. For instance, peripheral nerve discontinuity (e.g., neurotmesis or nerve transection) due to perforating or lacerating injuries requires surgical repair in an early (non-emergent) setting after patient stabilization and management of other acute traumatic injuries. Other indications for considering surgical repair of peripheral nerve injuries and/or birth-related nBPI include the following:

- Imaging or neurophysiologic (e.g., EMG/NCS) evidence of nerve root avulsions. Preganglionic avulsion injuries will not show spontaneous recovery and require surgical repair [1].
- Known or suspected neurotmesis with low likelihood of spontaneous peripheral nerve regeneration.
- Insufficient functional recovery during observation and conservative management.

- Complete (pan-plexus) nBPI, particularly with Horner's syndrome, without functional recovery by 3 months of age [1].
- Birth-related nBPI involving upper ± middle trunks (C5–C6 nerve roots, ± C7 nerve root) without functional recovery of elbow flexion and/or shoulder abduction by age 3 months [1, 17, 18].
  - This warrants consideration of further diagnostic evaluation (MRI or MR neurography, possible EMG/NCS) and possible surgery by age 6 or 9 months, depending on the extent of recovery at serial evaluations.

Importantly, published case reports and series have demonstrated adequate spontaneous functional recovery despite elbow flexion paralysis at age 3 months [17]. Therefore, a conservative but cautious approach with close observation and frequent clinical assessments remains a critical component of nBPI evaluation and management. Equivocal cases (nBPI of moderate severity) with partial spontaneous recovery by 3 months age warrant continued close observation until surgical decision-making around 6–9 months age.

Timing and Techniques of Peripheral Nerve Surgery

The surgical exposures and techniques for repair of traumatic peripheral nerve injuries and birth-related nBPI lie outside the scope of this chapter, but can be found in multiple peripheral nerve surgery texts and published manuscripts. Some critical underlying themes of peripheral nerve surgery timing and techniques include the following:

- Penetrating or lacerating peripheral nerve injuries may be explored early, following stabilization and management of other more serious traumatic injuries. In this context, peripheral nerve repair may be achieved through direct nerve repair, autologous nerve (e.g., sural nerve) grafts, or cadaveric/synthetic nerve grafts (typically up to 30 mm length).
- Optimal timing of surgical repair for traumatic BPI and birth-related nBPI remains controversial.
  - Timing of surgical repair for nBPI typically extends between an age range of 3–6 months (early repair) to 6 months or 9 months (later repair) [6].
  - Timing of surgical repair rarely extends beyond 12 months from injury (except unique circumstances) due to risks for target muscle fibrosis and atrophy.
  - Early repair in nBPI (< 6 months age) may augment functional recovery with hand-to-mouth activities (elbow flexion, forearm supination); however, younger age at repair was not correlated with favorable outcomes in other measures of functional recovery in a large systematic review [21].
  - Most recent studies do not show an impact of earlier age (< 6 months) at surgical repair on outcomes for birth-related nBPI [6].
  - Benefits of mid to later repair include close observation for spontaneous recovery and allowing greater physiologic maturity for anesthetic and surgical safety.

- Blunt or stretch peripheral nerve injuries may result in neuroma formation. Different surgical techniques for managing neuroma-in-continuity include the following:
  - Internal neurolysis (internal dissection around nerve fibers within the neuroma), particularly when intraoperative nerve stimulation suggests conduction across the neuroma.
  - Neuroma resection with nerve grafting across the resulting defect (using autologous nerve grafts or cadaveric/synthetic nerve grafts).
  - Nerve transfer (neurotization) of healthy nerve fascicle(s) from a donor nerve to the recipient (nonfunctional nerve), distal to the neuroma and closer to the target muscle.
- Supraclavicular approaches to the brachial plexus offer adequate exposure for BPIs and repairs involving the roots and trunks (Fig. 6).
- Infraclavicular and medial brachial approaches to the brachial plexus may be required for BPIs and repairs involving the cords and terminal branches.
- Nerve connection or coaptation (during direct nerve repair, grafting, or neurotization) can be performed with small caliber sutures through the epineurium and/or fibrin glue (Fig. 7).
- The surgical management of traumatic BPI or birth-related nBPI involving upper ± middle trunks depends upon the type of nerve injury.
  - Nerve root avulsions typically require nerve root transfers (neurotizations) from functional donor nerves within and outside the brachial plexus.
  - Neuroma-in-continuity may be managed with either neuroma resection and grafting and/or distal nerve transfers (neurotizations).
- Common surgical techniques of nerve transfer (neurotization) in traumatic BPI or birth-related nBPI depend upon the extent and severity of injury and availability of donor nerves (Table 7).

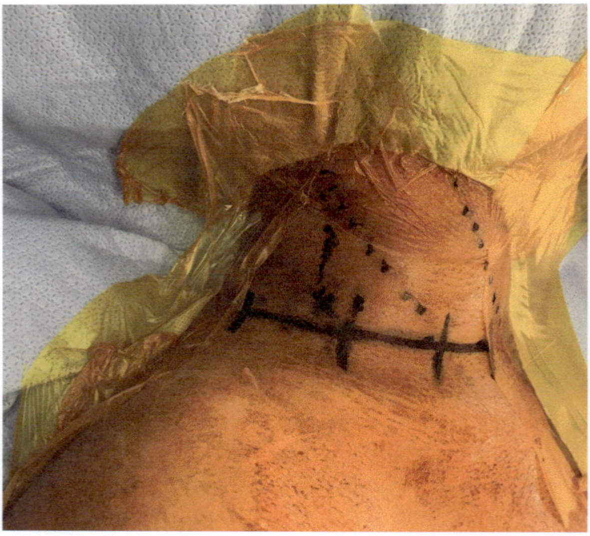

Fig. 6 Intraoperative photograph showing right supraclavicular curvilinear incision used for exposure of the roots and trunks of the brachial plexus. Additional markings include the expected course of the spinal accessory nerve (X) and lateral border of sternocleidomastoid muscle (lateral dotted line)

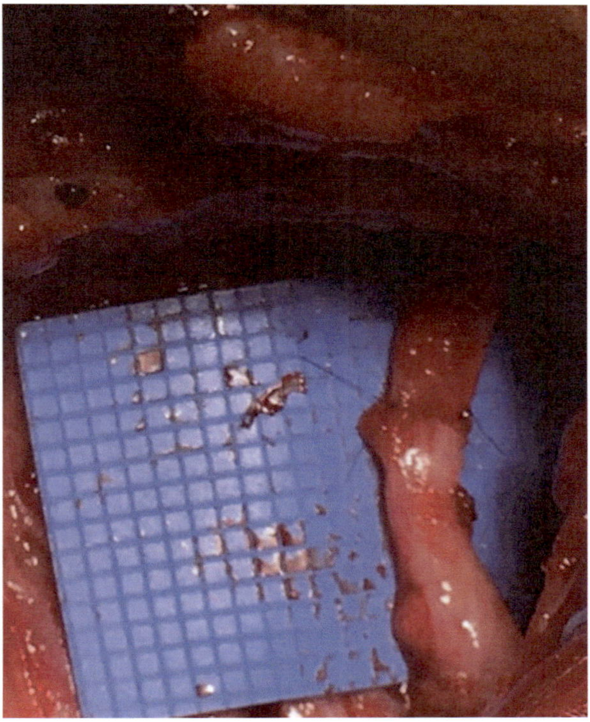

Fig. 7 Intraoperative photography showing end-to-end nerve coaptation in a nerve transfer (neurotization) between the spinal accessory nerve (donor) and suprascapular nerve (recipient) using small caliber sutures against a blue background

Table 7 Common surgical techniques of nerve transfer (neurotization) in traumatic BPI or birth-related nBPI

Extent of injury	Donor nerve	Recipient nerve	Functional goal
Upper ± middle trunks (C5-C6 nerve roots, ± C7 nerve root)	Spinal accessory nerve fascicles(s)	Suprascapular nerve	Shoulder abduction and stability
Upper ± middle trunks (C5–C6 nerve roots, ± C7 nerve root)	Ulnar or median nerve fascicle(s)	Musculocutaneous nerve	Elbow flexion (Oberlin and modified Oberlin techniques)
Upper ± middle trunks (C5–C6 nerve roots, ± C7 nerve root)	Medial pectoral nerve fascicle(s)	Musculocutaneous nerve	Elbow flexion
Upper trunk (C5–C6 nerve roots)	Radial nerve fascicle(s)	Axillary nerve	Shoulder abduction and stability
Complete brachial plexus (C5–T1 nerve roots)	Spinal accessory nerve fascicle(s)	Suprascapular nerve	Shoulder abduction and stability
Complete brachial plexus (C5–T1 nerve roots)	Intercostal nerve fascicles (Fig. 8)	Musculocutaneous nerve	Elbow flexion Effective in 60–70% of cases) [15]
Complete brachial plexus (C5–T1 nerve roots)	Contralateral C7 nerve root [4]	Upper/middle/lower trunks, median nerve, musculocutaneous nerve, radial nerve	Depends on prioritized nerve recipients and target muscle groups

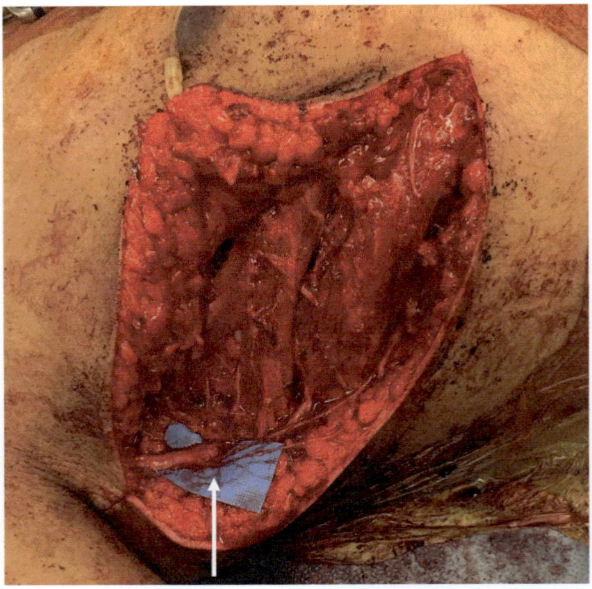

Fig. 8 Intraoperative photograph showing intercostal nerve fascicles to lateral cord nerve transfer (neurotization) in a patient with complete (pan-plexus) traumatic BPI

- Following peripheral nerve surgical repair involving nerve coaptation (e.g., direct nerve repair, nerve grafting, or neurotization), immobilization (typically 3 weeks) at the adjacent joints helps prevent disruption of the repair.
- Awaiting functional recovery following peripheral nerve surgery requires time, patience, and physiotherapy. The accepted rate of peripheral nerve regeneration from the site of injury or repair to the target organ (muscle) approximates 1 mm/day or 1 inch/month.

Following lack of improvement with conservative management, recommendations typically favor operative intervention (peripheral nerve decompression) for less common pediatric entrapment neuropathies [8]:

- Pediatric CTS—carpal tunnel surgical release via transection of the transverse carpal ligament.
- Ulnar entrapment neuropathy—decompression along the cubital tunnel and along the proximal edge of the flexor carpi ulnaris.
- Neurogenic TOS (in the presence of motor impairment or muscular atrophy, or if conservative management fails)—resection of cervical rib or fibrous band, transection of hypertrophied anterior scalene muscle, brachial plexus decompression.
- Common peroneal entrapment neuropathy—decompression at the fibular head, including division of the overlying fascia of the peroneus longus muscle.

Outcomes

Long-Term Outcomes of Birth-Related Neonatal Brachial Plexus Injury (nBPI)

Several studies have assessed outcomes for birth-related nBPI following conservative management. Commonly reported patterns of nonoperative outcomes for birth-related nBPI include the following:

- Low severity nBPIs that involve neurapraxia or axonotmesis typically resolve with full recovery or minor functional impairment, typically within a few weeks (neurapraxia) or 3–4 months (axonotmesis) [17].
- The spontaneous functional recovery rate following birth-related nBPI has been reported as high as 75–95% among several retrospective reviews [1, 13, 18].
- A prospective trial and more recent evidence-based reviews have reported slightly lower rates (65–66%) of complete functional recovery in low severity nBPI (e.g., Narakas groups I and II) by age 6–15 months [10, 13, 18].
- While many instances of birth-related nBPI resolve spontaneously, long-term (> = 12 month) functional impairments occur in up to 10–30% of affected infants [1, 7, 17, 18].
- Among moderate-to-high-severity nBPIs (e.g., Narakas groups III and IV), only 14% of affected infants exhibited complete functional recovery at age 6 months [13].
- Residual long-term functional impairments following nBPI exist within a spectrum from incomplete recovery with minimal deficits to more severe functional limitations [1].

Similarly, multiple studies have investigated outcomes following surgical repair of birth-related nBPI:

- Surgical outcomes for elbow flexion (at least anti-gravity) following nerve transfers remain highly favorable (87–94% success rate) [17].
- Small case series have shown recovery of useful (greater than 50% of range of motion against gravity) shoulder abduction and elbow flexion in 77% and 85% of infants managed operatively for upper nBPI [11, 18].
- Other published studies have reported favorable outcomes for shoulder function in 60–80% of patients with upper nBPI following peripheral nerve surgery [1].
- Infants with complete or pan-plexus nBPI showed less favorable results, with only 20% and 35% achieving useful shoulder abduction and elbow flexion, respectively, following surgical repair [11, 18].

Permanent deficits from birth-related nBPI may cause significant physical, psychological, and psychosocial obstacles for affected children and parents. Long-term sequelae of nBPI may include the following [7, 16]:

- Upper extremity functional limitations and muscle imbalances
  - Incomplete shoulder external rotation, abduction, and/or elevation
  - Incomplete elbow flexion
  - Incomplete forearm supination or rotation
- Joint (e.g., glenohumeral [shoulder]) instability and/or subluxation
- Shoulder deformity
- Joint contractures
  - Shoulder adduction contractures
  - Elbow flexion contractures

These long-term impairments, particularly joint subluxation and/or contractures, may require prolonged physiotherapy, stretching regimens, or secondary surgical correction. With or without peripheral nerve surgical repair, long-term sequelae of nBPI require close attention and care.

Acknowledgments Nationwide Children's Hospital Graphics Support team for production of an illustration.

Disclosures The authors of this textbook chapter have no financial conflicts of interest and no relevant disclosures.

References

1. Abid A. Brachial plexus birth palsy: management during the first year of life. Orthop Traumatol Surg Res. 2016;102:S125–32.
2. Abzug JM, Mehlman CT, Ying J. Assessment of current epidemiology and risk factors surrounding brachial plexus birth palsy. J Hand Surg Am. 2019;44:515.e1–515.e10.
3. Babal JC, Mehlman CT, Klein G. Nerve injuries associated with pediatric supracondylar humeral fractures: a meta-analysis. J Pediatr Orthop. 2010;30:253–63.
4. Bai Y, Han S, Guan JY, Lin J, Zhao MG, Liang GB. Contralateral C7 nerve transfer in the treatment of upper-extremity paralysis: a review of anatomical basis, surgical approaches, and neurobiological mechanisms. Rev Neurosci. 2022;33:491–514.
5. Biso G, Munakomi S. Neuroanatomy, neurapraxia. In: StatPearls. Treasure Island: StatPearls Publishing; 2025.
6. Catena N, Baldrighi C, Jester A, Soldado F, Farr S. Microsurgery in pediatric upper limb reconstructions: an overview. J Child Orthop. 2022;16:241–55.
7. Chauhan SP, Blackwell SB, Ananth CV. Neonatal brachial plexus palsy: incidence, prevalence, and temporal trends. Semin Perinatol. 2014;38:210–8.
8. Costales JR, Socolovsky M, SÁNCHEZ Lázaro JA, Costales DR. Peripheral nerve injuries in the pediatric population: a review of the literature. Part II: entrapment neuropathies. Childs Nerv Syst. 2019;35:37–45.
9. Curtis C, Stephens D, Clarke HM, Andrews D. The active movement scale: an evaluative tool for infants with obstetrical brachial plexus palsy. J Hand Surg Am. 2002;27:470–8.
10. Duff SV, Dematteo C. Clinical assessment of the infant and child following perinatal brachial plexus injury. J Hand Ther. 2015;28:126–33. quiz 134
11. Dumont CE, Forin V, Asfazadourian H, Romana C. Function of the upper limb after surgery for obstetric brachial plexus palsy. J Bone Joint Surg Br. 2001;83:894–900.

12. Eckstein KL, Allgier A, Evanson NK, Paulson A. Brachial plexus birth injuries and the association between pre-procedure and post-procedure pediatric outcomes data collection instrument scores and narakas classification. J Pediatr Rehabil Med. 2020;13:47–55.
13. Foad SL, Mehlman CT, Foad MB, Lippert WC. Prognosis following neonatal brachial plexus palsy: an evidence-based review. J Child Orthop. 2009;3:459–63.
14. Ho ES. Evaluation of pediatric upper extremity peripheral nerve injuries. J Hand Ther. 2015;28:135–42. quiz 143
15. Kline DG. Surgical repair of brachial plexus injury. J Neurosurg. 2004;101:361–3. discussion 363-4
16. Leblebicioğlu G, Pondaag W. Brachial plexus birth injury: advances and controversies. J Hand Surg Eur. 2024;49:747–57.
17. Malessy MJ, Pondaag W. Obstetric brachial plexus injuries. Neurosurg Clin N Am. 2009;20:1–14.
18. Mcneely PD, Drake JM. A systematic review of brachial plexus surgery for birth-related brachial plexus injury. Pediatr Neurosurg. 2003;38:57–62.
19. Ouzounian JG. Risk factors for neonatal brachial plexus palsy. Semin Perinatol. 2014;38:219–21.
20. Skirven TM, Osterman AL, Fedorczyk J, Amadio PC, Felder S, Shin EK. Rehabilitation of the hand and upper extremity. Philadelphia: Elsevier; 2020.
21. Srinivasan N, Mahajan J, Gupta S, Shah YM, Shafei J, Levidy MF, Abdelmalek G, Pant K, Jain K, Zhao C, Chu A, Mcgrath A. Surgical timing in neonatal brachial plexus palsy: a PRISMA-IPD systematic review. Microsurgery. 2022;42:381–90.

Pediatric Brain and Spinal Cord Tumors

Emily Johnson, Paul Klimo, and Nir Shimony

Classification of Pediatric Brain and Spinal Cord Tumors

Pediatric CNS tumors can be classified by their *location*, *histologic type*, and *biological behavior* (benign vs. malignant). Location is often the most clinically relevant factor in initial presentation and treatment planning. While some tumors remain localized, others may spread along the neuroaxis or recur after treatment, necessitating careful monitoring.

By Location

1. *Infratentorial (Posterior Fossa) Tumors*

   Common in younger children and often involve structures such as the cerebellum, brainstem, and fourth ventricle. These tumors may cause hydrocephalus, ataxia, or cranial nerve deficits.

   - *Medulloblastoma*
   - *Ependymoma*

E. Johnson (✉)
Neuroscience Institute, Neurosurgery Department, University of Tennessee Health Science Center, Le Bonheur Children's Hospital, Memphis, TN, USA
e-mail: Emily.Johnson@lebonheur.org

P. Klimo · N. Shimony
Neurosurgery Department, Le Bonheur Children's Hospital, St. Jude Children's Research Hospital, University of Tennessee Health Science Center, Semmes-Murphey Clinic, Memphis, TN, USA
e-mail: pklimo@semmes-murphey.com; nshimony@UTHSC.edu

K. Battick et al. (eds.), *Nursing Guide for Pediatric Neuroscience Patients*,
https://doi.org/10.1007/978-3-032-22664-8_14

- *Pilocytic astrocytoma (cerebellar)*
- *Brainstem gliomas (e.g., DIPG)*

2. *Supratentorial Tumors*

   Occur in the cerebral hemispheres and are more common in older children and adolescents. These may present with seizures, focal weakness, or changes in cognition or behavior.

   - *High-grade gliomas (e.g., glioblastoma)*
   - *Low-grade gliomas*
   - *Craniopharyngioma*
   - *Choroid plexus tumors*
   - *Pineal region tumors*

3. *Spinal Cord Tumors*

   Less common in children but can present with back pain, gait changes, or progressive weakness. These tumors may be intramedullary (within the cord) or extramedullary.
   - *Ependymoma*
   - *Astrocytoma*
   - *Meningioma* (rare in children)

By Biological Behavior

- *Benign Tumors*
  Slow-growing and less likely to invade surrounding tissue. May still cause significant symptoms due to location or compression of vital structures.
  - Pilocytic astrocytoma
  - Craniopharyngioma
  - Meningioma
- *Malignant Tumors*
  More aggressive, often rapidly growing, and may spread through cerebrospinal fluid (CSF) pathways or recur after treatment.
  - Medulloblastoma
  - High-grade glioma
  - Atypical teratoid/rhabdoid tumor (AT/RT)

Molecular Classification and Prognostic Markers

In recent years, molecular and genetic profiling has become an essential part of pediatric CNS tumor diagnosis. These markers help define tumor subtypes more precisely and can influence both prognosis and treatment.

World Health Organization (WHO) classification: Low-grade (I &II) and high-grade (III & IV).

Gliomas/glial cells are cells that support neurons of the brain and spine—astrocytoma, ependymoma, oligodendroglioma, mixed gliomas.

Nonglial cells: Neuronal cells that transmit function of the nervous system—embryonal tumors (medulloblastoma, ATRT), craniopharyngioma, pineal, meningioma, germ cell tumors.

Spinal tumors: Low-grade or high-grade astrocytoma, gangliogliomas, or ependymomas.

Genetic risk factors can include Cowden syndrome, Gorlin syndrome, Li-Fraumeni syndrome, neurofibromatosis type I and II, tuberous sclerosis, Von Hippel-Lindau disease.

Examples

- *Diffuse midline glioma, H3K27-altered*:
  Previously referred to as DIPG, this aggressive tumor is now defined by a mutation in the *H3 K27M histone gene*. Despite its location and sometimes low-grade appearance on imaging, this mutation confers a *poor prognosis*. Standard treatments are often palliative, though clinical trials are ongoing.
- *Low-grade glioma with BRAF mutation*:
  Tumors with *BRAF V600E mutations* may respond to targeted therapies (e.g., BRAF inhibitors). These tumors often behave more favorably than high-grade gliomas and may be managed without radiation or extensive surgery, depending on the location.
- *Medulloblastoma subgroups*:
  Medulloblastomas are now subclassified into molecular groups (e.g., WNT, SHH, Group 3, Group 4), which carry distinct prognostic and therapeutic implications.
  - *WNT subtype*: Excellent prognosis with >90% survival
  - *Group 3 subtype*: Higher risk of metastasis and recurrence
- *Atypical Teratoid/Rhabdoid Tumor (AT/RT)*:
  Defined by *loss of INI1 (SMARCB1)* expression, this is a highly malignant tumor of infancy with a guarded prognosis.

While nurses are not expected to interpret genetic sequencing reports, familiarity with these markers enhances communication with the care team and helps in counseling families about prognosis, anticipated treatments, and clinical trial eligibility.

Signs and Symptoms

The signs and symptoms of pediatric brain and spinal cord tumors vary widely depending on the *tumor's location, size, growth rate*, and *patient's age* (Table 1). Some tumors present acutely with life-threatening signs of elevated intracranial pressure, while others cause subtle, progressive neurologic or behavioral changes.

Table 1 Common presentations of pediatric CNS tumors by location

Tumor location	Examples	Common presenting symptoms
Cerebral hemispheres	Low- and high-grade astrocytomas, oligodendrogliomas	Seizures Hemiparesis or hemisensory loss Visual field deficits Behavioral or cognitive changes
Midline (suprasellar/ pineal/hypothalamic)	Craniopharyngioma, germ cell tumors, optic pathway glioma, hypothalamic tumors	Signs of increased ICP (headache, vomiting) Hydrocephalus Visual field cuts (bitemporal hemianopsia) Endocrinopathies (diabetes insipidus, growth failure, precocious or delayed puberty)
Cerebellum (posterior fossa)	Medulloblastoma, pilocytic astrocytoma	Ataxia and unsteady gait Dysmetria or clumsiness Nystagmus or diplopia Signs of increased ICP
Brainstem	Diffuse midline glioma (e.g., pons), focal brainstem gliomas	Cranial nerve palsies (facial weakness, dysphagia, diplopia) Ataxia Hemiparesis Long tract signs
Spinal cord	Intramedullary ependymoma, astrocytoma	Limb weakness or sensory changes Back or extremity pain (often worse at night) Gait abnormalities Bowel/bladder dysfunction Scoliosis or spinal asymmetry

Nurses are often the first to identify early warning signs and are critical in monitoring for deterioration.

General Symptoms (May Occur with Any CNS Tumor)

- Headache (many times position-dependent; nighttime are red flag)
- Nausea and vomiting (not always associated with eating)
- Lethargy or excessive sleepiness
- Irritability or personality change
- Poor school performance or developmental regression
- Seizures (new-onset or change in pattern)
- Vision changes (blurred vision, double vision, or loss of visual field)
- Failure to thrive or poor weight gain (in hypothalamic or diencephalic tumors)

Infratentorial Tumors (Posterior Fossa)

- Ataxia, unsteady gait, or clumsiness
- Dysmetria (impaired coordination)
- Nystagmus or abnormal eye movements
- Cranial nerve deficits (e.g., facial asymmetry, difficulty swallowing)
- Posterior fossa syndrome (rare, and when it happens, it is usually after medulloblastoma resection)
- Signs of *obstructive hydrocephalus*:
  - Headache
  - Vomiting
  - Papilledema
  - Lethargy or irritability
  - *In infants*: Bulging fontanelle, increased head circumference, sunsetting eyes

Supratentorial Tumors

- Seizures (most common presenting symptom in cortical tumors)
- Hemiparesis or focal weakness
- Sensory deficits or visual field cuts
- Behavioral changes or personality shifts
- Language delays or aphasia
- Endocrinologic symptoms (e.g., precocious puberty, growth failure) in hypothalamic or pituitary region tumors

Spinal Cord Tumors

- Back pain (worse at night or with Valsalva)
- Gait disturbances or foot drop
- Limb weakness or spasticity
- Bowel/bladder incontinence or retention
- Scoliosis or abnormal spinal curvature
- Sensory changes (numbness, tingling)

Red Flags for Nursing Assessment

- Rapid neurologic decline (e.g., sudden confusion, drop in GCS)
- *Increased intracranial pressure* (See Chap. 3, Intracranial Pressure)
  - Headache
  - Vision changes: Abnormal eye movement, reduced vision, double vision
  - Vomiting (particularly upon awakening)
  - Irritability/behavior change

  - Lethargy
  - Bulging fontanelle of infant
  - Increased large head circumference
  - Seizure
- Recurrent unexplained vomiting
- Head tilt or torticollis (especially in infants)
- New seizure activity or changes in seizure frequency/type
- Change in baseline behavior, mood, or alertness
- Change in motor function, especially new asymmetry or coordination issues

Diagnostic Imaging

Imaging plays a critical role in the diagnosis, characterization, and monitoring of pediatric brain and spinal cord tumors. Early and appropriate imaging is often key to timely surgical referral and treatment planning. Nurses support the imaging process by preparing the patient, assisting with sedation planning when needed, and understanding how imaging results inform care.

Magnetic Resonance Imaging (MRI)

Gold standard for evaluating CNS tumors due to its high-resolution soft tissue contrast (Table 2).

- *MRI Brain With and Without Contrast* (Figs. 1 and 2)
  - Identifies tumor size, location, enhancement pattern, and relationship to adjacent structures.
  - Can distinguish between solid, cystic, hemorrhagic, or necrotic tumor components.
  - Gadolinium contrast enhances vascular regions and helps differentiate tumor tissue from edema or inflammation.
  - Advanced sequences (FLAIR, DWI, SWI, spectroscopy) may aid in characterizing tumor type or aggressiveness.

- *MRI Spine* (Fig. 3)
  - Performed when there is concern for spinal cord compression, primary spinal tumor, or *drop metastases* (tumor cells spreading through CSF from brain to spine, especially in medulloblastoma or ependymoma).
  - Complete *craniospinal MRI* is often required in cases of malignant tumors with CSF spread risk.

Table 2 MRI features of common pediatric brain tumors

Tumor type	T1-weighted	T2-weighted/FLAIR	Postcontrast (gadolinium)	DWI/ADC	Notes
Medulloblastoma	Iso- to hypointense	Hyperintense with surrounding edema	*Bright enhancement*, often homogeneous	*Restricted diffusion*(hyperintense DWI, low ADC)	Often midline, posterior fossa; CSF spread common
Pilocytic astrocytoma	Hypo- to isointense	Hyperintense	*Enhancing mural nodule* with large cystic component	No restriction or mild restriction	Common in cerebellum; generally low-grade
Ependymoma	Iso- to hypointense	Heterogeneous; may have cysts or calcifications	Variable enhancement, sometimes *"cap sign"*	May show restricted diffusion	Often near fourth ventricle; may extend through foramina
Craniopharyngioma	Cystic areas may appear hyperintense	Mixed signal with cyst and solid components	Enhancing solid portion; calcifications seen on CT	Typically no restricted diffusion	Suprasellar location; hormonal symptoms common
Diffuse midline glioma (H3K27-altered)	Iso- to hypointense	Hyperintense, often infiltrative	Variable, often *minimal or patchy enhancement*	*Restricted diffusion* common	Located in pons, thalamus, or spinal cord; poor prognosis
AT/RT	Heterogeneous, iso- to hypointense	Heterogeneous, often with necrosis	Strong, irregular enhancement	*Marked restricted diffusion*	Rapid growth; seen in infants and toddlers

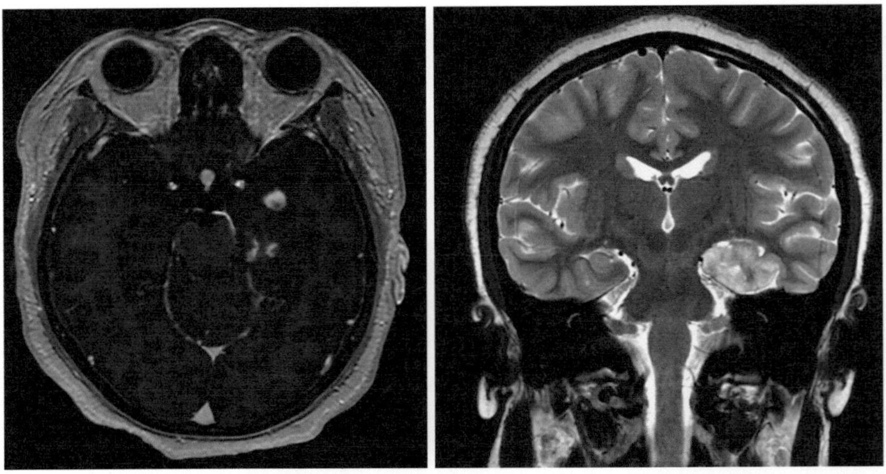

Fig. 1 An 11-year-old female, presented acutely with headaches and seizures. Was found to have left mesiotemporal tumor—angiocentric glioma

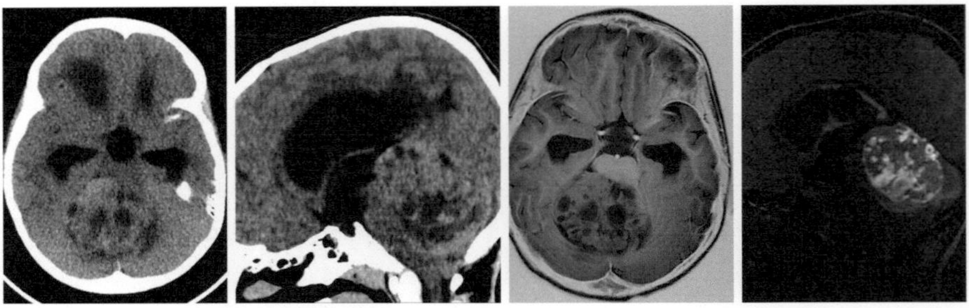

Fig. 2 A 5-year-old male, acutely presented with severe headaches and vomiting. Was found to have large posterior fossa tumor and associated obstructive hydrocephalus (Left to right: axial and sagittal views of head CT showing heterogeneous mass in the posterior fossa with associated obstructive hydrocephalus; MRI of the brain in axial and sagittal views showing the same pictures in a much more detailed way). The patient was operated for complete removal and resolution of the hydrocephalus. Pathology—Medulloblastoma, SHH subtype

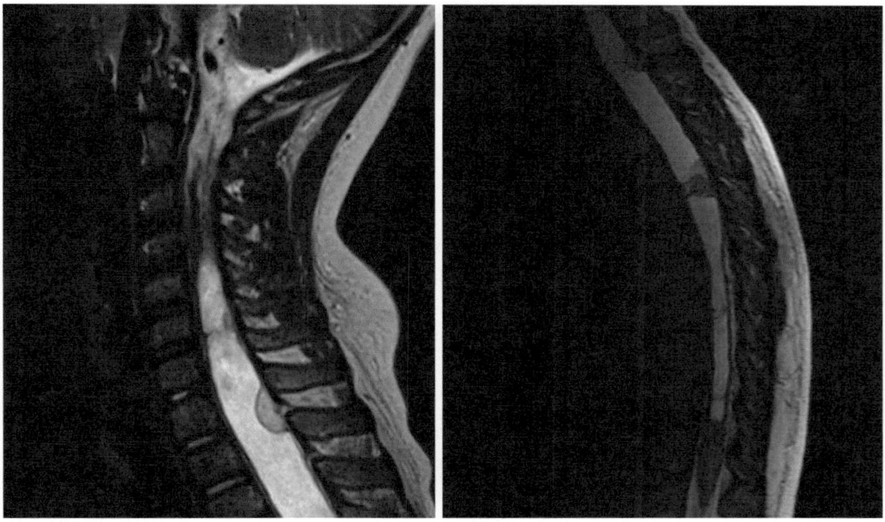

Fig. 3 A 9-year-old male with back pain. Was diagnosed with diffuse spinal cord tumor and associated syringomyelia. Had complete resection with pathology—diffuse leptomeningeal glioneuronal tumor

Computed Tomography (CT Scan) (Fig. 2)

Used primarily in *emergent situations* or when MRI is contraindicated or unavailable.

- *CT Head Without Contrast*
  - Quick, accessible tool to detect acute hemorrhage, hydrocephalus, mass effect, or calcification
  - Common initial imaging in the ER for children presenting with altered mental status or seizures
- *CT With Contrast*
  - Occasionally used to identify enhancing lesions when MRI is delayed
  - Useful for bony abnormalities, calcified tumors, or skull base involvement

Functional and Advanced Imaging

- *MR spectroscopy:* Provides metabolic information about tumor cells; can help distinguish tumor from treatment effects
- *Perfusion MRI or CT:* Evaluates blood flow to the tumor, often used to assess treatment response
- *PET-CT (rarely in pediatrics):* May be used in certain tumor types (e.g., high-grade gliomas, germ cell tumors) or for recurrence detection

Imaging Considerations for Nurses

- *Sedation/Anesthesia:*
  - Many young children will require sedation for MRI due to the length of the study and need to remain completely still.
  - NPO guidelines and anesthesiology coordination are essential.
- *IV Access and Contrast:*
  - Ensure functional IV access before contrast-enhanced studies.
  - Monitor for allergic reaction, although rare with modern agents.
- *Safety Screening:*
  - MRI safety checklist must be completed before the study (screen for implanted devices, braces, prior surgeries).
- *Family Preparation:*
  - Provide age-appropriate explanations of the process.
  - Offer child life support for anxious children or those with sensory sensitivities.

Key

- *T1-weighted:* Good for anatomy; tumors often appear darker.
- *T2-weighted/FLAIR:* Fluid-sensitive; tumors typically appear brighter.
- *Post-contrast:* Shows vascularity; highlights areas of blood–brain barrier disruption.
- *DWI/ADC:* Detects cell density; restricted diffusion suggests high cellularity (often malignant).

Nursing Assessment and Perioperative Role

Pediatric patients with CNS tumors often require complex surgical interventions, prolonged monitoring, and intensive support (Table 3). Nurses play a critical role in the *early assessment*, *preparation for surgery*, and *postoperative care*, including ongoing neurological evaluation, pain management, and coordination of multidisciplinary services.

Preoperative Nursing Assessment and Preparation

- *Baseline Neurologic Assessment:*
  - Document level of consciousness (e.g., using GCS or pediatric coma scales).
  - Evaluate motor strength, symmetry, gait, coordination, and cranial nerve function.
  - Assess for signs of increased intracranial pressure: Headache, vomiting, irritability, papilledema, lethargy.

Table 3 Summary of key points for acute nursing care in pediatric CNS tumor patients

Category	Assessment/intervention	Nursing notes/rationale
Primary assessment	ABCs—Airway, Breathing, Circulation Level of Consciousness	Initial stabilization; frequent neuro checks are essential
Patient history	Gather onset, progression of symptoms, and previous medical history	Establish timeline and potential tumor-related signs
Neurological exam	Age-based assessment (see Chap. 1) Anterior fontanelle in infants Cranial nerve signs Cerebellar signs Spinal cord signs Mobility and voiding status	Helps localize lesion; critical for surgical planning and monitoring postop changes
Management of increased ICP	Support airway Elevate HOB (30°, head midline) Activate critical care team Administer mannitol/hypertonic saline Prepare for EVD	Intervene rapidly to prevent herniation; EVD may be needed to reduce pressure and drain CSF
Psychosocial assessment	Evaluate patient and family anxiety, understanding of diagnosis, coping	Early emotional support reduces distress and improves care engagement
Medications	Corticosteroids (e.g., dexamethasone) GI protection (PPI or H2 blocker) Antiepileptics if seizures Hormone replacement if needed	Manage cerebral edema, prevent GI complications, treat seizures, and support hormonal balance when indicated
Preoperative teaching	Hair shaving and incision expectations NPO instructions Postop location (PICU or PACU)	Reduces fear, sets expectations, and prepares family for postoperative care plan

- *Monitoring for Neurological Changes:*
  - Note any *seizures*, *new or worsening weakness*, or *decline in school performance*.
  - In infants, monitor *head circumference*, *fontanelle status*, and *eye movement* (sunsetting eyes).
- *Hydration and Nutrition:*
  - Maintain hydration, especially if patient has vomiting or decreased intake.
  - Coordinate nutritional support if prolonged fasting or weight loss is a concern.
- *Preoperative Labs and Imaging:*
  - Verify CBC, PT/PTT, type and screen, and imaging completion.
  - Confirm MRI spine if tumor type has risk for CSF dissemination.

- *Family Education and Support:*
  - Explain what to expect before and after surgery using age-appropriate language.
  - Coordinate with child life specialists and social workers.
  - Review informed consent process and surgical goals with caregivers.

Nursing Care for Diagnostic Imaging

(a) Ideal to assess patient prior to imaging to know neurological baseline.
(b) Determine if any metal is implanted or on the body for removal prior to MRI.
(c) Determine if shunt is present, and if so, is there a programmable setting (this must be checked by a provider after MRI because the magnet could change the setting).
(d) Ability to lie still for test and if sedation medication needed.
(e) NPO status.
(f) IV access.

Nursing Care and Seizure Precautions

(a) Patient on centralized monitors
(b) Airway protection (suction and oxygen supplementation)
(c) Rescue medications

Multidisciplinary Approach and Consultations as Indicated

(a) Ophthalmology to look for any visual field deficits, papilledema
(b) Endocrine for hormone function and lab work (serum and urine sodium levels, thyroid studies, ACTH, serum, and CSF tumor markers)
(c) Neuropsychological evaluation for cognitive function and developmental screening
(d) Rehabilitation therapy evaluation (physical, occupational, and speech)

Consulting with child life therapists, social workers, and pastoral care to help the patient and family understand the diagnoses, the physiological component, and coping mechanisms.

Consulting these teams prior to surgery is ideal, so they can also follow-up with the patient and family after surgery to provide comprehensive care.

Surgical Treatment

Surgery is the primary treatment for all newly diagnosed brain tumors. Obtaining pathology with molecular biology will assist in diagnosis. Removal, debulking, or biopsy of the tumor allows for greater efficacy of treatment modalities.

Surgery for placement of external ventricular drain or shunt can provide relief of symptoms of increased intracranial pressure and allow new pathways for CSF circulation.

Surgical approaches and surgical tools, such as intraoperative MRI, are evolving and can be different, with each resection depending on the location and appearance of the tumor.

Complete surgical resection is the goal as survival rates improve for the most aggressive types of tumors. Surgical approaches have become more refined over the years allowing once unresectable tumors to be resected. In patients with suprasellar tumors such as craniopharyngioma, or pontine tumors, surgical efficacy is considered. Resection and quality of life and comorbidities should always be considered with every surgery.

Postoperative Complications and Long-Term Considerations

Vital signs and centralized monitoring (blood pressure management with specific parameters are often provided by the surgeon to prevent postoperative hemorrhage).

Neuro exam and any changes to be reported to the neurosurgery team.

Seizure precautions with oxygen and suction set up at bedside.

Optimize pain control (IV and oral meds with a scheduled and/or prn frequency). Pain after a craniotomy is often felt by the scalp nerves because the brain does not have pain receptors.

Other Med administration: Steroid taper, antibiotic (IV, oral, topical), antiemetic, GI prophylaxis, bowel regimen, antiepileptics.

Strict fluid volume intake and output as indicated.

Advance diet as tolerated with balanced nutrition with protein and fiber.

Wound care: Look at dressing/incision with every assessment, with close attention for CSF leak, bleeding, swelling, or development for pseudomeningocele.

Monitor voiding and bowel movement frequency: Is the patient at risk for development of endocrinopathies such as Diabetes Insipidus (DI), Cerebral Salt Wasting (CSW), or Syndrome of Inappropriate Anti-Diuretic Hormone (SIADH)?

Head of bed elevation and patient positioning as well as activity level.

Rehab therapy (physical, occupational, and speech) for evaluation of neuro impairments: Best to be assessed postop day 1.

(a) Weakness
(b) Dysphagia
(c) Decreased coordination
(d) Ataxia
(e) Visual impairments
(f) Decreased endurance

Neurocognitive effects—the severity depends on the location and size of the tumor.

(a) Visual motor function
(b) Verbal, nonverbal, and visual processing
(c) Executive function: Attention, memory, planning, comprehension, and processing speed

EVD/Shunt (See Chap. 5)

Endocrine deficiency and need for hormone replacement medications, frequent lab work, monitoring strict intake/output.

Posterior fossa syndrome (cerebellar mutism): Collection of symptoms that occur after posterior fossa surgery that can include cerebellar mutism, ataxia, speech and language, swallowing dysfunction, and global intellect decline. These symptoms usually resolve over a few weeks to months. This diagnosis can have variable outcomes of increased risk of neurocognitive impairments of memory, processing speed, and executive function.

Key Points for Postoperative Care

- *Neurologic Monitoring:*
  - Perform frequent neuro checks (e.g., every 1–2 h initially).
  - Monitor level of alertness, speech, motor strength, pupils, and sensory changes.
  - Compare with preop baseline and report any deviations immediately.
- *Monitoring for Complications:*
  - *Increased ICP*: Look for bradycardia, hypertension, altered breathing, decreased responsiveness.
  - *CSF leak*: Watch for clear drainage from incision or nose/ears.
  - *Seizures*: Observe for abnormal movements, eye deviation, or decreased responsiveness.
  - *Hydrocephalus*: Especially after posterior fossa surgery; may require EVD or shunt.
- *Pain Management:*
  - Use age-appropriate scales (FLACC, Wong-Baker, numeric).
  - Provide scheduled and breakthrough analgesia.
  - Avoid excessive sedation to preserve the ability to monitor neurologic status.
- *Positioning and Safety:*
  - Follow neurosurgical orders for head-of-bed elevation (commonly 30°).
  - Maintain spine precautions if spinal surgery was performed.
  - Protect operative site; avoid pressure on craniectomy or spinal wounds.
- *Incision and Wound Care:*
  - Monitor for redness, swelling, drainage, or dehiscence.
  - Keep dressing dry and intact unless otherwise ordered.
  - Note use of staples, sutures, or Dermabond and expected removal timeline.

- *Early Rehabilitation:*
  - Collaborate with PT/OT for early mobilization.
  - Monitor for signs of motor or cognitive regression.

  Evaluate for equipment needs (walker, wheelchair) prior to discharge.

Postoperative Complications and Long-Term Considerations

Children undergoing surgery for brain or spinal cord tumors are at risk for a variety of *neurologic, medical, and functional complications*, both in the immediate post-operative period and throughout long-term recovery. Nurses play a key role in *early detection, intervention*, and in *educating families about what to monitor* as the child transitions from acute care to rehabilitation or outpatient follow-up.

Early Postoperative Complications

1. *Increased Intracranial Pressure (ICP)*
   - May occur due to swelling, blood, or residual tumor obstructing CSF flow.
   - *Signs:* Headache, vomiting, altered consciousness, hypertension + bradycardia (Cushing's triad), pupillary changes, or posturing.
   - *Nursing actions:* Elevate HOB, maintain EVD drainage if present, notify neurosurgery immediately.
2. *Hydrocephalus*
   - Can develop after posterior fossa surgery or if the tumor obstructed CSF pathways.
   - *Signs:* Lethargy, vomiting, irritability, bulging fontanelle, sunsetting eyes.
   - May require *external ventricular drain (EVD)* or *VP shunt* placement.
3. *Seizures*
   - Some tumors or postoperative changes can provoke new-onset seizures.
   - Monitor for abnormal movements, eye deviation, or altered responsiveness.
   - Ensure *seizure precautions* are in place and that rescue medications are available.
4. *CSF Leak*
   - Look for clear drainage from incision, ears, or nose.
   - May require flat bedrest, wound revision, or lumbar drain.
5. *Infection*
   - Risk of meningitis, wound infection, or ventriculitis.
   - Monitor for fever, nuchal rigidity, wound redness, or changes in neurologic status.
6. *Hemorrhage or Hematoma*
   - Rare but serious; presents with rapid neurologic decline or focal deficit.
   - Immediate imaging and surgical intervention may be necessary.

Late or Long-Term Considerations

1. *Endocrine Dysfunction*
    - Tumors near the hypothalamus or pituitary (e.g., craniopharyngioma) may disrupt hormone regulation.
    - Children may require hormone replacement (e.g., cortisol, thyroid, growth hormone).
    - Monitor for *diabetes insipidus*, growth failure, puberty disorders, or fatigue.
2. *Cognitive and Neuropsychological Changes*
    - Attention, memory, and processing speed may be affected by tumor location or treatment (especially radiation).
    - Early neuropsychological evaluation supports school planning and therapy needs.
3. *Motor or Sensory Impairments*
    - Weakness, coordination issues, or spasticity may persist.
    - Long-term *physical and occupational therapy* may be needed.
4. *Behavioral and Emotional Challenges*
    - Anxiety, depression, emotional lability, or PTSD symptoms can emerge.
    - Social work, psychology, and school support services should be involved early.
5. *Hearing Loss*
    - Especially relevant after treatment with platinum-based chemotherapy or posterior fossa radiation.
    - Baseline and follow-up audiology evaluations are important.
6. *Spinal Deformity*
    - Post-laminectomy kyphosis or scoliosis may occur after spinal cord tumor surgery, especially in younger children.
    - Long-term orthopedic monitoring is important.
7. *Tumor Recurrence or Spread*
    - Ongoing surveillance with MRI is required.
    - Nurses should help reinforce the importance of follow-up imaging and clinical appointments.

Neurologic Deficits

New neurologic deficits are a common concern following brain or spinal cord tumor surgery. These deficits may present as changes in *motor strength*, *coordination*, *sensation*, *speech*, *vision*, or *gait*, depending on the tumor's location and the extent of surgical intervention.

Some deficits are *temporary*, resulting from local swelling, surgical retraction, or transient ischemia. Others may be *permanent*, especially if critical brain regions (e.g., motor cortex, brainstem, spinal cord) were involved or damaged by the tumor itself.

- *Location matters*: The specific deficit often corresponds closely to the *anatomical location* of the tumor and surrounding structures:
  - Tumors in the motor cortex or corticospinal tracts may lead to *hemiparesis*.
  - Cerebellar involvement may cause *ataxia* or *dysmetria*.
  - Brainstem lesions may result in *cranial nerve deficits*, *swallowing issues*, or *respiratory instability*.
  - Spinal cord tumors may lead to *limb weakness*, *sensory loss*, or *bowel/bladder dysfunction*.
- *Setting expectations*: It is essential for nurses to work closely with the *neurosurgical team* to understand the expected trajectory of recovery and provide families with accurate, compassionate information.
  - Nurses should clarify whether a deficit is likely *transient or permanent* and help prepare caregivers for both short-term challenges and potential long-term support needs.
- *Early rehabilitation is key*: Prompt initiation of *physical therapy*, *occupational therapy*, and, when appropriate, *speech therapy* can greatly influence functional outcomes.
  - Nursing can advocate for early consults and ensure follow-through with therapy recommendations.
  - Encouraging family involvement in therapy and goal-setting promotes engagement and optimism.
- *Documentation*: Nurses should thoroughly document *baseline function*, *postop changes*, and any *improvements or deterioration* to support care coordination and outcome tracking. Description of baseline in conjunction with postop changes (expected and unexpected) at handoff is critical to determine improvements or deterioration. Performance of a neurologic assessment with the incoming nurse is also very important to infer any changes and confirm current assessment is unchanged since prior assessment. The nurse is key to identifying even slight changes in a patient's neurologic assessment.

Discharge Planning and Family Education

Discharge planning begins early in the hospitalization and should involve collaboration between the *nursing team*, *neurosurgery*, *rehabilitation*, *social work*, and *case management*. Nurses are uniquely positioned to guide families through the transition by reinforcing education, preparing for home care needs, and ensuring follow-up plans are clear. Have care takers teach back and/or return demonstrate instructions as applicable.

When to Call the Neurosurgery Team or Seek Urgent Care

Families should be instructed to contact their neurosurgical provider or return to the hospital immediately for:

- Fever >38.5 °C (101.3 °F)
- Redness, swelling, or drainage from the incision site
- Increasing or severe headache
- Lethargy, confusion, or changes in consciousness
- Vomiting without other cause
- Seizures or abnormal movements
- New or worsening weakness, balance issues, or vision problems
- Clear drainage from the nose, ears, or surgical site (possible CSF leak)

Wound and Incision Care

- Keep incision *clean and dry*; avoid submersion in water (baths, pools) for 3–4 weeks or as directed. Have caretaker return demonstrate wound care (cleaning and drying the wound).
- Follow specific instructions for *staples, sutures, or Dermabond*:
  - Dermabond typically falls off naturally within 1–2 weeks.
  - Non-absorbable sutures/staples are usually removed in the clinic around days 7–10.
- Teach families to observe for:
  - Drainage (especially clear or yellow fluid)
  - Increasing redness or swelling
  - Foul odor or tenderness at the site

Medications

- *Pain Management:*
  - Continue acetaminophen or ibuprofen (if approved).
  - If opioids are prescribed, emphasize secure storage and proper disposal.
- *Seizure Medications:*
  - Review dosing schedule and side effects. Have caretakers teach back.
  - Ensure families know when to call about breakthrough seizures.
- *Steroids, Antibiotics, Hormone Replacement (If Applicable):*
  - Review tapering plans or administration techniques as needed. Have caretakers teach back.

Activity and Recovery

- *Activity Restrictions:*
  - No contact sports or high-impact activities until cleared (usually 4–6 weeks minimum).
  - Gradual return to school; coordinate with neuropsychology or child life for school reintegration plans.

  - Helmet use is required when mobilizing if patient underwent decompressive craniectomy.
- *Supportive Therapies:*
  - Encourage participation in *PT, OT, and/or speech therapy* as recommended.
  - Monitor for fatigue, frustration, or loss of motivation—normalize the recovery process and celebrate small wins.

Follow-Up Appointments

- Families should be given written instructions for:
  - Neurosurgery follow-up (often within 1–2 weeks)
  - MRI or imaging appointments
  - Oncology or neurology consults (if applicable)
  - Endocrinology or audiology (depending on tumor type/location)
  - Rehabilitation follow-up and therapy services

Emotional Support and Resources

- Validate family stress and emotions following diagnosis and surgery.
- Provide information about:
  - Social work and psychology services
  - Local or national brain tumor foundations
  - Support groups for pediatric brain tumor families
- Encourage families to maintain open communication with care teams and advocate for their child's needs.

Chapter Summary

Pediatric brain and spinal cord tumors represent some of the most complex and high-risk conditions managed in pediatric neurosurgery. While the underlying pathology and treatment plans may vary widely, the role of the nurse remains central and consistent: Vigilant monitoring, early recognition of complications, precise communication, and compassionate family-centered care. Nurses are often the first to detect subtle neurologic changes, to support families during emotionally charged conversations, and to reinforce realistic expectations for recovery. A strong understanding of tumor types, imaging patterns, surgical approaches, and postoperative needs equips nurses to advocate effectively and deliver safe, informed care throughout the patient's hospital journey and beyond (Table 4).

Table 4 Quick reference table: nursing priorities in pediatric CNS tumors

Phase of care	Nursing priorities
Initial presentation	Monitor for headache, vomiting, seizures, behavior changes Complete baseline neurologic assessment Support imaging coordination and sedation planning
Preoperative	Review labs and imaging readiness Maintain hydration and seizure precautions Provide emotional support and prepare family
Postoperative	Frequent neuro checks Monitor for increased ICP, CSF leak, seizures, infection Pain management and incision care Initiate rehab services early
Discharge planning	Teach wound care, seizure precautions, and red flags Coordinate follow-up appointments Provide emotional support and connect with resources
Long term	Monitor for recurrence or late effects Encourage ongoing therapy and school reintegration

Suggested Reading

1. Conklin HM, Raches D, Khan RB, Ashford JM, Lin T, Onar-Thomas A, et al. QOL-02. Predicting neurocognitive outcomes among children experiencing varying degrees of postoperative posterior fossa syndrome. Neuro Oncol. 2024;26(Suppl 4):IV171.
2. Ledet D, Battick K, Bess HN, Cartwright C, Pownall A, Scroggins I, Shiers DJ. Care of the pediatric patient with a brain tumor. AANN clinical practice guideline series. J Neurosci Nurs. 2014;46(6):368–9.
3. Pollack IF, Agnihotri S, Broniscer A. Childhood brain tumors: current management, biological insights, and future directions: JNSPG 75th anniversary invited review article. J Neurosurg Pediatr. 2019;23(3):261–73.
4. Shiminski-Maher T. Brain tumors in childhood: implications for nursing practice. J Pediatr Health Care. 1990;4(3):122–30.
5. Weak L, Fecske E, Breedt A, Cartwright C, Crawford D, Forbes A. Reflections on 50 years of pediatric neuroscience nursing. J Neurosci Nurs. 2018;50(5):260–4.
6. Littlejohns L, McNett M, Olson D. AANN core curriculum for neuroscience nursing. 7th ed. American Association of Neuroscience Nurses; 2022.

Pediatric Neurovascular Disease

Blakely Weatherford, Lucas Elijovich, and Nir Shimony

Presenting Symptoms

Pediatric neurovascular disorders can present with a wide range of clinical findings, from subtle behavioral changes to acute, life-threatening neurological emergencies. The nature of the presentation is influenced by the underlying pathology, the location of the lesion, and the presence of associated hemorrhage, ischemia, or mass effect. Prompt recognition of these symptoms is essential to initiate appropriate care.

Clinical Presentations

- *Critically ill presentation*: Some children may present in emergent condition, with an abrupt onset of symptoms such as seizures, decreased level of consciousness, or signs of elevated intracranial pressure (ICP), necessitating immediate stabilization and surgical evaluation.
- *Subtle presentation*: Others may demonstrate more gradual or vague symptoms, including focal neurological deficits (e.g., new limb weakness), progressive

B. Weatherford (✉)
Neuroscience Institute, Neurosurgery Department, Le Bonheur Children's Hospital, University of Tennessee Health Science Center, Memphis, TN, USA
e-mail: Blakely.Weatherford@lebonheur.org

L. Elijovich
Neurosurgery Department, Le Bonheur Children's Hospital, University of Tennessee Health Science Center, Semmes-Murphey Clinic, Memphis, TN, USA
e-mail: lelijovich@semmes-murphey.com

N. Shimony
St. Jude Children's Research Hospital, Le Bonheur Children's Hospital, Semmes-Murphey Clinic, University of Tennessee Health Science Center, Johns Hopkins University School of Medicine, Memphis, TN, USA
e-mail: nshimony@UTHSC.edu

K. Battick et al. (eds.), *Nursing Guide for Pediatric Neuroscience Patients*,
https://doi.org/10.1007/978-3-032-22664-8_15

headaches, lethargy, irritability, or decreased responsiveness. In these cases, clinical suspicion must remain high to avoid delayed diagnosis.

Anatomical Correlation

Symptoms and signs depend heavily on the location of the neurovascular insult:

- A hemorrhagic cavernous malformation in the *internal capsule* may result in contralateral hemiparesis.
- *Brainstem lesions* can affect cranial nerve function, respiratory control, and consciousness.
- Lesions with significant *mass effect* may produce secondary effects such as:
  - *Obstructive hydrocephalus* if cerebrospinal fluid pathways are compressed
  - *Severe elevation in ICP* from hemorrhage, edema, or space-occupying lesions, potentially leading to herniation syndromes or global neurological decline

Each scenario necessitates a tailored diagnostic and management approach, guided by the child's clinical trajectory and imaging findings.

Common Presenting Symptoms

- Sudden, severe headache
- Visual changes (blurred vision, visual field deficits, double-vision)
- Unilateral weakness, numbness, or paralysis
- Facial droop or asymmetry
- Aphasia or slurred speech
- Seizures (focal or generalized)
- Altered mental status (confusion, irritability, lethargy)
- Gait disturbance or ataxia
- Nausea and vomiting (especially with raised ICP)
- Neck stiffness (particularly with subarachnoid hemorrhage)

Additional Signs in Infants and Young Children

- Bulging or full anterior fontanelle
- Persistent vomiting or feeding intolerance
- Hypotonia or decreased spontaneous movement
- Excessive sleepiness or failure to arouse for feeds
- High-pitched or inconsolable crying
- Macrocephaly or rapidly increasing head circumference
- Developmental regression or failure to meet milestones
- Subtle seizure activity (e.g., lip smacking, eye deviation)

Table 1 Age-appropriate neurological findings and red flags

Domain	Infants (<12 months)	Toddlers/young children (1–5 years)	School-age and adolescents
Mental status	Alertness, visual tracking, social smile	Follows simple commands, engages with environment	Oriented (age-appropriate), able to answer questions
Fontanelle	Flat, soft anterior fontanelle	Closed	Closed
Cranial nerves	Symmetrical eye movements, rooting/sucking reflex	Facial symmetry, normal speech articulation	Intact extraocular movements, facial symmetry, gag reflex
Motor function	Symmetric spontaneous movement, normal tone	Walks independently, uses arms/hands symmetrically	Normal strength and tone across all extremities
Posture/tone	Flexed posture, moves all limbs equally	Normal tone, no posturing	No abnormal posturing or tone
Sensory response	Withdraws from touch or painful stimuli	Verbalizes discomfort, localizes pain	Reports sensory changes, localizes stimuli appropriately
Reflexes	Primitive reflexes (e.g., Moro, Babinski present until ~12 mo)	Normal DTRs, Babinski disappears around 12–24 months	Normal DTRs, Babinski absent
Gait/coordination	Not applicable	Walks, may hop, climbs stairs	Tandem gait, heel-to-toe walking, finger-to-nose testing
Red flags	Bulging fontanelle, persistent asymmetry, decreased movement	Unsteady gait, drooling, speech delay, irritability	Focal weakness, cranial nerve deficits, behavior change

Physical Examination

A thorough and systematic neurological examination is critical in the assessment of children with suspected neurovascular disorders. Findings may vary based on the location, extent, and acuity of the lesion. The exam should be adapted to the child's age and developmental stage and repeated frequently in patients at risk for deterioration (Table 1).

General Observations

- Level of alertness
- Interaction with environment
- Responsiveness to voice or touch
- Respiratory effort and pattern (e.g., irregular breathing in brainstem involvement)

Mental Status and Behavior

- Orientation (age-appropriate)
- Mood, behavior, attention span
- Response to caregivers or surroundings
- Irritability or lethargy

Cranial Nerve Examination

- *Pupils*: Size, symmetry, and reactivity to light
- *Eye movement*: Presence of deconjugate gaze, nystagmus, or gaze palsy
- *Facial symmetry*: Observe for droop, flattened nasolabial fold, or asymmetrical smile
- *Visual response*: Tracking, fixation, or blink to threat (age-dependent)
- *Gag reflex and swallowing* (if concern for brainstem lesion)

Motor Examination

- Tone (hypertonia, hypotonia, spasticity)
- Strength (graded movement in all extremities)
- Spontaneous movement vs. weakness or paralysis
- Posturing (decorticate or decerebrate may suggest increased ICP or brain herniation)
- Symmetry of limb use

Sensory Examination

- Light touch, temperature, or pain response (as developmentally appropriate)
- Withdrawal to noxious stimuli in infants
- Parent-reported changes in sensitivity or response

Coordination and Gait

- Ataxia or wide-based gait (in ambulatory children)
- Finger-to-nose or heel-to-shin testing
- Balance with eyes closed (Romberg test, if able)

Reflexes

- Deep tendon reflexes: Hypo- or hyperreflexia
- Babinski reflex (extensor response may be abnormal after infancy)

Signs of Elevated Intracranial Pressure

- Bradycardia, hypertension, irregular respirations (Cushing's triad)
- Papilledema (if funduscopic exam is possible)
- Full or bulging fontanelle in infants
- Vomiting without nausea
- Decline in Glasgow Coma Scale (GCS) or other validated coma scores

Diagnostic Imaging

Neuroimaging is essential in the evaluation of pediatric neurovascular disease, guiding diagnosis, monitoring, and surgical planning. The selection of modality depends on acuity, clinical suspicion, patient stability, and the level of anatomical detail required. Nurses play a vital role in preparing patients, supporting sedation or anesthesia, and recognizing post-imaging complications.

Non-contrast Computed Tomography (CT Head)

- *Purpose*: Initial study for children presenting with acute neurologic deterioration, suspected hemorrhage, hydrocephalus, or trauma.
- *Advantages*: Fast, widely available, highly sensitive for detecting acute blood.
- *Limitations*: Lower sensitivity for small vascular malformations or early ischemia; radiation exposure is a concern in pediatric patients.

Findings by Pathology

- *AVMs*: May appear as hyperdense serpentine structures, sometimes with calcification. Hemorrhage into the surrounding brain tissue is often the first visible sign.
- *Cavernous malformations*: Often missed unless calcified or if there is recent bleeding. Acute hemorrhage appears hyperdense.
- *Hydrocephalus*: Dilated ventricles; possible transependymal CSF flow (periventricular lucency).
- *Subarachnoid hemorrhage*: Blood layering in sulci, cisterns, or ventricles.

Magnetic Resonance Imaging (MRI Brain with and Without Gadolinium)

- *Purpose*: Gold standard for characterizing vascular malformations, detecting hemorrhage (acute and chronic), ischemia, and parenchymal changes
- *Key Sequences:*
  - *T1-weighted*: Useful for anatomy and subacute hemorrhage
  - *T2-weighted*: Detects edema and chronic changes
  - *FLAIR*: Enhances visualization of edema and subarachnoid blood
  - *DWI/ADC*: Critical for early ischemia detection
  - *Gradient Echo (GRE) or Susceptibility-Weighted Imaging (SWI)*: Highly sensitive for blood products (especially microhemorrhages)
  - *Post-contrast (T1 + gadolinium)*: Enhances vascular lesions and helps differentiate tumor vs vascular pathology

Findings by Pathology

- *AVMs* (Fig. 1):
  - Flow voids (signal absence) on T2 due to rapid blood flow
  - Enlarged feeding arteries and draining veins
  - Surrounding gliosis or hemosiderin from prior hemorrhage
  - Enhances strongly with gadolinium
- *Cavernous malformations* (Fig. 2):
  - "Popcorn" or "berry-like" appearance with mixed signal intensity from blood at various stages
  - Hemosiderin rim (dark on T2 or SWI) from prior bleeding
  - No significant enhancement or large feeding vessels (low-flow lesion)

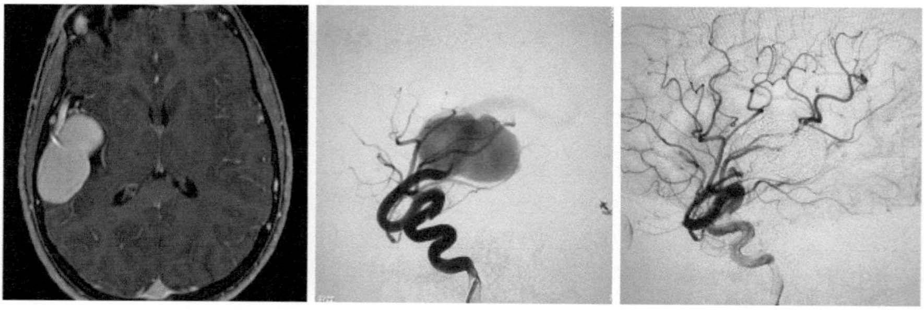

Fig. 1 A 14-year-old male presented acutely with headaches. Has a family history of HHT, was diagnosed with right pial AVM that was being supplied by the inferior division of M2. Diagnostic studies angiogram for diagnosis and treatment using coils and glue (left—MRI T1 with contrast; middle—diagnostic angiography; right—post coiling with no residual filling of the AVM)

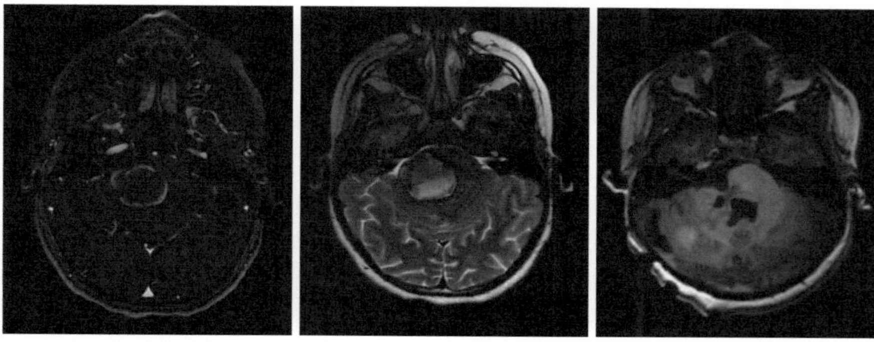

Fig. 2 A 10-year-old female presented acutely with severe consciousness deterioration and cranial nerves deficits. MRI showed suspected pontine cavernous malformation. She had a successful surgery for complete removal of the cavernoma

- *Moyamoya disease:*
  - Areas of ischemia or infarct
  - Prominent basal collaterals ("ivy sign" on FLAIR)
  - Vessel narrowing best appreciated on MRA

Magnetic Resonance Angiography (MRA) and Computed Tomography Angiography (CTA)

- *Purpose*: Noninvasive techniques used to evaluate vessel anatomy, patency, and detect stenosis, aneurysms, or AVMs
- *MRA:*
  - Often performed with MRI
  - Preferred for patients needing repeat imaging (no radiation)
  - Limited resolution for small distal vessels
- *CTA:*
  - Faster, higher resolution for vessel visualization
  - More sensitive than MRA for detecting aneurysms and calcified lesions
  - Requires iodinated contrast—monitor for allergy or renal function in high-risk patients

Cerebral Angiography (Digital Subtraction Angiography, DSA)

- *Purpose*: Gold standard for diagnosing vascular malformations, evaluating flow dynamics, and guiding endovascular therapy
- *Indications:*
  - Characterizing AVMs or fistulas
  - Pre-operative planning
  - Evaluating aneurysm morphology
  - Post-treatment follow-up (e.g., embolization, radiosurgery)

Procedure Overview

- Performed in a specialized neurointerventional suite.
- Requires general anesthesia or deep sedation in pediatric patients.
- A catheter is introduced through the *femoral artery* (commonly), advanced under fluoroscopy into the cerebral circulation.
- Contrast is injected into the internal carotid, external carotid, and vertebral arteries to visualize intracranial and extracranial vasculature.
- Imaging is timed to arterial, capillary, and venous phases.

Nursing Considerations

- *Pre-procedure:*
  - NPO status per sedation protocol.
  - Ensure IV access and baseline labs (especially coagulation profile).
  - Consent signed and questions addressed with family.
- *Intra-procedure:*
  - Monitor sedation and vitals.
  - Support positioning and comfort.
- *Post-procedure:*
  - Bedrest with affected leg straight (usually 4–6 h).
  - Monitor vascular access site for bleeding, hematoma, or swelling.
  - Neurovascular checks of distal pulses and limb color/temp.
  - Monitor for allergic reaction to contrast (rash, respiratory changes).
  - Assess for headache, nausea, or new neurologic deficits.

Findings by Pathology

- *AVMs* (Fig. 1):
  - Tangle of abnormal vessels with early draining veins
  - Clearly visualized arterial feeders and venous outflow
  - Used to guide embolization planning (e.g., staged treatment)
- *Cavernous malformations* (Fig. 2):
  - Often *angiographically occult* (not visible), especially if small and low flow
- *Aneurysms:*
  - Identified by saccular outpouching of vessel wall
  - Shape, neck, and location guide decisions for coiling vs clippi

Imaging Preparation: Nursing Considerations

Nurses play an essential role in preparing pediatric patients and families for diagnostic imaging. Proper preparation minimizes delays, improves image quality, and enhances patient safety—especially in cases involving contrast administration or invasive procedures.

General Preparation for All Imaging Modalities

- *Explain the procedure:*
  Use developmentally appropriate language. Younger children may benefit from visual aids or support from child life specialists.
- *Emotional support:*
  Imaging environments can be intimidating. Offer reassurance to both patient and caregivers. Include familiar comfort items (e.g., blanket, stuffed animal) when possible.
- *Immobilization support:*
  Children who cannot remain still may require physical support or swaddling for brief imaging studies (CT). Inform the team if immobilization aids will be needed.
- *Assess for medical devices or implants:*
  Confirm the presence of any implanted medical devices (e.g., VP shunts, programmable valves, pacemakers) before MRI. Notify radiology to assess MRI safety and compatibility.

IV Contrast Studies (CT or MRI with Contrast, CTA, MRA)

- *IV access:*
  Confirm patent IV access in advance. A 22-gauge or larger peripheral IV is typically preferred. For contrast studies, ensure IV site is secure and has been recently flushed.
- *Screen for allergies and renal risk:*
  - Assess for *iodine or contrast allergies* for CT/CTA.
  - For patients with underlying renal disease, recent *creatinine or GFR* may be required (particularly before iodinated contrast).
- *Hydration:*
  Encourage oral fluids (if not NPO) pre- and post-contrast to support renal clearance of contrast agents.

MRI-Specific Considerations

- *MRI safety checklist:*
  Complete and review institutional safety screening for metal exposure, implants, surgical history, or prior foreign body injuries (e.g., metal in the eye).
- *Remove external devices or metallic items:*
  Ensure all jewelry, hearing aids, hairpins, and removable orthodontics are removed prior to entering the MRI suite.
- *Coordinate with radiology:*
  Verify ordered sequences and need for contrast. Communicate known clinical concerns (e.g., "rule out AVM," "known CCM with new symptoms"), so appropriate protocols are used.

Cerebral Angiography-Specific Preparation

- *NPO status:*
  Ensure patient is NPO per protocol (typically 6 h for solids, 2 h for clear liquids).
- *Pre-procedural labs:*
  Verify that coagulation profile (PT, PTT, INR) and CBC are available and within safe ranges. Platelet count should be sufficient for vascular access.
- *Baseline assessments:*
  Document neuro exam, vital signs, and distal pulses before transport. Establish a comparison point for post-procedure monitoring.
- *Pre-procedure checklist:*
  Confirm signed consent, appropriate sedation orders, IV access, allergies, and emergency contacts.

Laboratory Studies

Laboratory evaluation complements imaging and clinical assessment in pediatric neurovascular disorders. Labs are often needed urgently in the acute setting or preoperatively and may help identify underlying etiologies, guide surgical planning, or assess risk for complications such as bleeding or infection.

Routine Laboratory Studies

- *Complete Blood Count (CBC):*
  - Evaluates hemoglobin/hematocrit levels, especially important in hemorrhagic presentations.
  - Assesses white blood cell count in cases of suspected infection or inflammation.
  - Platelet count helps assess bleeding risk before surgical or interventional procedures.

- *Basic or Comprehensive Metabolic Panel (BMP/CMP):*
  - Monitors electrolytes, renal function, and glucose levels—all critical in acutely ill children.
  - Important before administration of IV contrast (renal function).
  - Liver function tests (if CMP) may be relevant for patients with metabolic or genetic syndromes (e.g., HHT).
- *Coagulation studies:*
  - *Prothrombin Time (PT), Partial Thromboplastin Time (PTT), and International Normalized Ratio (INR):*
    - Required before surgical interventions or cerebral angiography.
    - Prolonged values may suggest underlying coagulopathy or require correction prior to invasive procedures.
- *Type and screen/crossmatch:*
  - Prepares for potential transfusion in cases of hemorrhage or expected intraoperative blood loss.
  - Crossmatch is often ordered to hold units for high-risk procedures (e.g., AVM resection).

Additional or Condition-Specific Tests

- *Erythrocyte Sedimentation Rate (ESR)/C-Reactive Protein (CRP):*
  - May be elevated in vasculitic or inflammatory causes of stroke (e.g., autoimmune arteritis)
  - Helps in evaluating Moyamoya or other secondary vasculopathies
- *Procalcitonin (PCT):*
  - May assist in distinguishing infectious from non-infectious causes of systemic symptoms when infection is on the differential
- *D-dimer:*
  - Occasionally used in the evaluation of venous sinus thrombosis or hypercoagulable states, though not specific in children
- *Platelet function testing:*
  - Provides information on the *functional capacity of platelets*, especially in patients with normal platelet count but suspected bleeding tendency
  - May be used preoperatively for patients with a history of easy bruising, abnormal bleeding, or antiplatelet medication exposure (e.g., aspirin, NSAIDs)
  - May involve PFA-100 testing or platelet aggregation studies
- *Genetic or specialty testing:*
  - May be indicated in cases of suspected syndromic associations:
    - *ENG/ACVRL1 mutations* in suspected Hereditary Hemorrhagic Telangiectasia (HHT)
    - *RNF213 mutation* in familial Moyamoya disease
    - Coagulation panel in children with stroke or thrombotic event

Nursing Considerations

- Ensure timely drawing and labeling of stat labs for emergent cases (e.g., stroke alert).
- Monitor venipuncture sites, especially in coagulopathic or anticoagulated patients.
- Clarify any anticoagulation history (e.g., low-molecular-weight heparin in sickle cell patients) before invasive procedures.
- Prepare families for the potential need for additional blood draws for transfusion crossmatch, platelet function studies, or specialty genetic panels.

Surgical Intervention

Surgical management of pediatric neurovascular disorders is often required for hemorrhage control, lesion resection, decompression, or revascularization. The timing and type of intervention depend on the lesion's nature, location, hemorrhagic status, hydrocephalus, and the child's clinical condition. Coordination between neurosurgery, neurocritical care, and nursing is essential for perioperative success.

Hematoma Evacuation and Decompression

- *Indication*: Life-threatening intracranial hemorrhage (intraparenchymal, subdural, or epidural) with mass effect, midline shift, herniation syndrome, or rapid neurological decline
- *Procedure:*
  - *Craniotomy* or *burr hole evacuation*, with or without placement of an external drain.
  - In *rare but critical cases* with severe cerebral swelling or refractory intracranial hypertension, a *decompressive hemicraniectomy* may be performed. This involves removing a large bone flap to allow for brain expansion and reduce life-threatening pressure.
- *Goal*: Relieve mass effect, remove clot burden, restore cerebral perfusion, and prevent secondary brain injury

Cerebrospinal Fluid (CSF) Diversion for Acute Hydrocephalus

- *Indication*: Obstructive hydrocephalus due to intraventricular hemorrhage, mass effect, or compression of CSF pathways (e.g., aqueduct, foramen of Monro)
- *Initial Intervention*: Placement of an *external ventricular drain (EVD)* to relieve intracranial pressure and monitor CSF output
  - EVDs provide *temporary CSF diversion* and allow for ICP monitoring in the acute phase.

  - Drain height and output are adjusted based on ICP targets and clinical status.
- *Long-Term Management*: If hydrocephalus persists, a *permanent CSF diversion procedure* such as a *ventriculoperitoneal (VP) shunt* may be required.
  - Some patients may be candidates for *endoscopic third ventriculostomy (ETV)* depending on etiology and anatomy.
- *Nursing Considerations:*
  - Maintain strict sterile technique when handling the EVD.
  - Monitor and document output volume and quality regularly.
  - Monitor for signs of infection, catheter obstruction, or worsening hydrocephalus.

Vascular Lesion Resection

Vascular malformations such as arteriovenous malformations (AVMs) and cavernous malformations may require surgical removal, particularly when symptomatic, hemorrhagic, or associated with neurological deficits. The decision to proceed with resection is based on lesion size, location, hemorrhagic risk, and patient stability.

- *Arteriovenous Malformations (AVMs):*
  - Surgical resection is the definitive treatment for accessible lesions with prior hemorrhage, progressive symptoms, or high rupture risk.
  - The goal is complete removal of the *nidus* (tangle of vessels) and associated feeders and drainers to eliminate future bleeding risk.
- *Cavernous Malformations:*
  - Often surgically removed if located in non-eloquent brain and associated with seizure, hemorrhage, or focal deficit.
  - Unlike AVMs, cavernomas are low-flow and typically do not require preoperative embolization.

Angiographic Embolization

- *Definition*: Endovascular technique in which embolic agents are delivered via catheter directly into the feeding arteries of a vascular lesion to reduce blood flow
- *Roles in AVM Management:*
  - *Preoperative embolization*: Often performed 24–72 h prior to surgery to:
    - Reduce intraoperative blood loss
    - Decrease nidus flow and complexity
    - Facilitate safer surgical dissection
  - *Definitive therapy (stand-alone):*
    - In select cases, especially small AVMs or single-feeder lesions, embolization alone may achieve complete obliteration.
    - Success depends on lesion angioarchitecture and accessibility.

- *Postsurgical embolization:*
  - Rarely, residual AVM components may be identified after surgery and treated endovascularly.
- *Agents used:*
  - Liquid embolics (e.g., n-butyl cyanoacrylate, Onyx)
  - Coils or particles in certain vascular patterns
- *Nursing considerations:*
  - Monitor for post-procedural neurologic changes.
  - Observe vascular access site for bleeding, hematoma, or limb ischemia.
  - Assess for signs of embolic complications (e.g., stroke, headache, seizure).
  - Maintain flat bedrest post-procedure (typically 4–6 h).

Expanded Surgical Management of Moyamoya Disease

Moyamoya disease is a progressive cerebrovascular disorder characterized by stenosis or occlusion of the intracranial internal carotid arteries and their proximal branches, resulting in the development of fragile collateral vessels. Without intervention, these collaterals are prone to thrombosis, hemorrhage, and ischemia. Surgical revascularization is the mainstay of treatment and aims to augment cerebral blood flow and reduce stroke risk.

Surgical Techniques

1. *Indirect revascularization (e.g., Pial Synangiosis):*
   - Most commonly used in children.
   - Involves placing a donor extracranial artery (typically the superficial temporal artery) directly onto the surface of the brain.
   - Over time, new collateral vessels form between the donor artery and cortical vessels.
   - Advantage: Technically simpler; avoids deep brain dissection.
   - Disadvantage: Delayed onset of flow improvement (weeks to months).
2. *Direct revascularization (e.g., STA-MCA bypass):*
   - Involves direct anastomosis between a scalp artery and a cortical branch of the middle cerebral artery
   - Less common in young children due to small vessel size
   - Provides immediate blood flow augmentation
3. *Combined procedures:*
   - Incorporate both direct and indirect techniques for both short- and long-term benefit.

Nursing Considerations in Moyamoya Patients

Patients with Moyamoya disease are uniquely vulnerable to perioperative ischemic and hemorrhagic events due to impaired cerebral autoregulation. Strict perioperative protocols must be followed to prevent stroke.

- *Hydration and volume management:*
  - Maintain *euvolemia* or slight hypervolemia to support cerebral perfusion.
  - Avoid dehydration at all times, including during pre-op fasting or GI illness.
  - Continue *IV fluids preoperatively* and postoperatively until full oral intake is restored.
- *Blood pressure control:*
  - Avoid hypotension and hypertension, both of which can precipitate ischemia or hemorrhage.
  - Continuous BP monitoring is required in the perioperative period.
  - Notify the neurosurgical team of deviations from target BP ranges.
- *Pain control:*
  - Adequate pain management is essential; pain-induced sympathetic stimulation can elevate BP and increase metabolic demand.
  - Use scheduled analgesics when appropriate; avoid undertreatment.
- *Fever and hypermetabolism:*
  - Fever increases cerebral metabolic demand and may exacerbate ischemia.
  - Treat fevers promptly and monitor for infection.
- *Early mobilization:*
  - Mobilize cautiously; ensure volume and pressure stability before activity.
  - Monitor for signs of transient ischemic attack (TIA) with exertion: Limb weakness, dysarthria, facial droop.

Radiosurgery (e.g., Gamma Knife) (Table 2)

- *Indications*: Small, deep, or surgically inaccessible AVMs or cavernomas.
- *Goal*: Deliver focused radiation to obliterate the lesion gradually.
- *Timeline*: Obliteration occurs over 1–3 years.
- *Risks*: Radiation necrosis, delayed hemorrhage, incomplete resolution.

Table 2 Comparison of open resection versus radiosurgery

Feature	Radiosurgery	Surgical resection
Procedure type	Noninvasive, outpatient	Invasive, requires craniotomy
Time to effect	Delayed (months to years)	Immediate resolution of lesion and symptoms
Best for	Small, deep, or eloquent-location lesions	Accessible, symptomatic, or ruptured lesions
Risks	Radiation effects, incomplete obliteration	Bleeding, infection, neurological deficits
Recovery	Minimal downtime	Hospital stay and rehabilitation as needed

Endovascular Surgery

Endovascular techniques are increasingly used in the management of pediatric neurovascular disorders. These minimally invasive procedures involve navigating microcatheters through the vascular system to target lesions within the brain or spinal cord. They may serve as a primary treatment, an adjunct to surgery, or an emergency intervention.

Indications

- Arteriovenous malformations (AVMs)
- Intracranial aneurysms
- Vein of Galen malformations
- Dural arteriovenous fistulas
- Tumor embolization (pre-resection)
- Acute hemorrhage or vascular injury control

Common Endovascular Treatments (Table 3)

- *Embolization of AVMs or fistulas:*
  - Reduces or eliminates blood flow through the lesion
  - Can be staged over multiple sessions for complex AVMs
  - May serve as definitive therapy or preoperative adjunct
- *Aneurysm coiling:*
  - Involves placement of soft platinum coils within an aneurysm sac to induce thrombosis and prevent rupture or re-bleeding
  - Used primarily for saccular aneurysms, especially those not accessible via open surgery
- *Stent placement:*
  - Metal mesh tubes are placed to reinforce weakened vessel walls or maintain vessel patency.
  - Often used in conjunction with coiling for wide-necked aneurysms.
- *Use of embolic agents:*
  - *Liquid embolics* (e.g., Onyx, n-butyl cyanoacrylate): Delivered through microcatheters into high-flow lesions like AVMs.
  - *Particles or coils* may also be used depending on anatomy.

Table 3 Summary of endovascular procedures in pediatric neurovascular disorders

Procedure	Indications	Mechanism	Role	Considerations
AVM embolization	AVMs, AV fistulas	Injection of embolic agents into feeding arteries to reduce flow	Pre-operative adjunct or stand-alone treatment	May require staged treatment; risk of bleeding or ischemia
Aneurysm coiling	Saccular aneurysms (ruptured or high-risk unruptured)	Platinum coils inserted into aneurysm sac to induce thrombosis	Prevents rupture or rebleeding	Often used with stents in wide-neck aneurysms; may require follow-up angiography
Stent placement	Wide-neck aneurysms, vessel narrowing	Metal mesh tube deployed to scaffold vessel walls or support coiling	Structural reinforcement	Antiplatelet therapy may be required; rarely used in young children
Tumor embolization	Highly vascular tumors pre-resection	Reduces blood flow to tumor to minimize surgical bleeding	Preoperative hemostasis	Timing critical—usually within 24–72 h before surgery
Venous malformation embolization	Vein of Galen malformation, dural AV fistula	Closure of abnormal connections or flow shunting with coils or glue	Definitive or staged treatment	Requires specialized pediatric neurointerventional team

Procedure Overview

- Performed under general anesthesia in pediatric patients.
- Femoral artery is most commonly used for catheter access.
- Real-time fluoroscopy and contrast injection guide catheter positioning.
- Catheters are navigated into cerebral arteries or veins to deliver treatment precisely.

Nursing Considerations: Pre- and Post-procedure

- *Pre-procedure:*
  - Ensure NPO status and IV access.
  - Confirm signed consent and relevant labs (CBC, PT/PTT, creatinine if contrast is used).
  - Baseline neurologic exam and distal pulses.
- *Intraprocedure support:*
  - Monitor for anesthesia or sedation-related changes.
  - Assist with positioning and patient stability.

- *Post-procedure:*
  - *Neuro checks*: Monitor closely for changes in level of consciousness, new focal deficits, or seizures.
  - *Access site care*: Maintain flat bedrest (typically 4–6 h). Monitor puncture site for bleeding, hematoma, or limb perfusion changes.
  - *Vital signs and I/O*: Monitor for signs of contrast reaction, embolic complications, or reperfusion symptoms.
  - Educate caregivers on signs of delayed complications, including stroke-like symptoms or recurrence of symptoms.

Nursing Care and Management

Pediatric neurovascular patients require vigilant, comprehensive nursing care across all phases of treatments. Nurses are essential to early recognition of neurologic decline, coordination of multidisciplinary care, family education, and emotional support.

Preoperative Nursing Care

- *Baseline neurological assessment:*
  - Perform and document a full neurologic exam, including level of consciousness, cranial nerve function, motor strength, sensation, and gait (as age-appropriate).
  - Note any pre-existing deficits to guide postoperative comparison.
- *Preprocedural preparation:*
  - *Skin prep*: Chlorohexidine bath or wipes per institutional protocol (if not contraindicated).
  - *IV access*: Secure at least one large bore IV for fluids, medications, and contrast if imaging is needed.
  - *Hydration*: For Moyamoya patients or those at risk of stroke, maintain euvolemia with IV fluids to avoid hypotension and minimize cerebral ischemia.
  - *Labs and imaging*: Ensure all preoperative labs (CBC, PT/INR, type and screen, etc.) and imaging are completed and available for review.
- *Family and emotional support:*
  - Involve child life specialists to reduce anxiety and improve cooperation.
  - Facilitate family discussions with the surgical and anesthesia teams.
  - Address spiritual or cultural needs (involve chaplaincy or interpreters if applicable).

Postoperative Nursing Care

- *Neurologic monitoring:*
  - Conduct frequent neuro checks per protocol or neurosurgical orders (e.g., every 1–2 h).
  - Compare with preoperative baseline to identify new deficits or deterioration.
  - Monitor for:
    - Changes in the level of consciousness
    - Cranial nerve changes (e.g., pupil reactivity, facial asymmetry)
    - New or worsening motor/sensory deficits
    - Seizures or posturing
    - Signs of raised ICP (headache, vomiting, bradycardia, hypertension, decreased responsiveness)
- *Pain management:*
  - Use age-appropriate pain scales (FLACC, Wong–Baker, numerical).
  - Administer medications as ordered:
  - *IV acetaminophen* routinely for the first 24 h.
  - *Opioids* for moderate to severe pain.
  - *NSAIDs* are used cautiously based on surgeon preference and the patient's bleeding risk.
    - Some advocate avoiding NSAIDs in the immediate postoperative period due to concerns about platelet inhibition and increased risk of postoperative hemorrhage, particularly after intracranial surgery.
- *Nausea and vomiting:*
  - Treat prophylactically or as needed with:
    - *Ondansetron* (Zofran)—safe across most age groups
    - *Promethazine* for older children (>2 years) when indicated
- *Hydration and fluids:*
  - Continue IV fluids until patient tolerates oral intake.
  - Pay special attention to Moyamoya patients: avoid hypovolemia or hypotension.
- *Wound care:*
  - Dressing type and removal instructions vary:
    - Some surgeons apply occlusive dressings (removed after 5–7 days).
    - *Dermabond* may be used and typically flakes off naturally in 1–2 weeks.
  - Monitor incision for:
    - *Erythema*
    - *Drainage or bleeding*
    - *Edema or fluctuance*
- *Mobilization and rehabilitation:*
  - Early physical and occupational therapy involvement (usually postop day 1).
  - Begin with passive range of motion, progressing to ambulation as tolerated.
  - Evaluate for durable medical equipment (walker, wheelchair) if needed for discharge.

Special Considerations

- *Patients with External Ventricular Drains (EVDs):*
  - Maintain head-of-bed at ordered height (typically 30°).
  - Ensure the EVD system is level with the external auditory meatus.
  - Monitor for:
    - Obstruction or kinking of tubing
    - Infection (fever, redness at site, cloudy CSF)
    - Over-drainage (headache, collapsed ventricles)
  - Document CSF output and appearance hourly.
- *Decompressive hemicraniectomy patients:*
  - Protect surgical site—no pressure on the craniectomy side.
  - Helmet use as ordered once mobilizing.
  - Watch for paradoxical herniation if patient becomes hypotensive.
- *Moyamoya patients:*
  - Strict BP monitoring to avoid hypotension or hypertension.
  - Maintain hydration and avoid rapid fluid shifts.
  - Monitor closely for signs of stroke or transient ischemic attack postoperatively.

Discharge Teaching

Discharge planning begins early in the postoperative course and involves collaboration among nursing, neurosurgery, rehabilitation, and social work. Family education is essential to ensure safe recovery at home, minimize complications, and prepare for follow-up care. Caretakers should teach back and/or return demonstrate applicable elements of discharge teaching.

When to Contact Neurosurgery or Seek Immediate Medical Attention

Caregivers should be instructed to call the neurosurgical team or seek emergency care for any of the following:

- Fever >38.5 °C (101.3 °F)
- Redness, swelling, or drainage from the incision site
- Worsening or uncontrolled pain
- Persistent vomiting or signs of dehydration
- Lethargy, new confusion, or difficulty waking
- New or worsening weakness, numbness, or visual changes
- Seizures or abnormal movements
- Bulging at the incision site or head (for patients with craniectomy or shunt)

Wound Care Instructions

- *Dressings:*
  - If a dressing was placed, follow surgeon instructions for removal (typically after 5–7 days).
  - Keep dry and intact until removal unless otherwise instructed. Have caretaker Return demonstrate cleaning of wound
- *Dermabond or skin adhesive:*
  - Will peel off naturally in 1–2 weeks.
  - Do not scrub or pick at the surgical site.
- *Bathing:*
  - Avoid submerging the incision in water (bathtub, pool, hot tub) for **3–4** *weeks*.
  - Gentle shampooing may be allowed once cleared by the provider.
- *Sutures or staples:*
  - Most sutures are dissolvable.
  - If nondissolvable, return to clinic for removal per instructions (typically days 7–10).

Medication Instructions

- *Pain medications:*
  - Continue scheduled or as-needed acetaminophen.
  - Use prescribed opioids sparingly for breakthrough pain.
  - Discuss safe storage and disposal of opioids with caregivers.
- *Antiemetics (if prescribed):*
  - Ondansetron or promethazine can be given for persistent nausea or vomiting.
- *Anticonvulsants:*
  - If the child was discharged on seizure medications, ensure dosing and follow-up with neurology are understood.
- *Other medications:*
  - Review all prescribed medications, dosing schedules, and possible side effects. Have caretaker teach back this information.

Activity and Restrictions

- Avoid high-impact activity, contact sports, or playground use until cleared by neurosurgery (typically 4–6 weeks).
- Gradual return to school or daycare may be recommended based on energy level and neurocognitive recovery.
- Protect head if craniectomy was performed (helmet required when out of bed or mobilizing).

Follow-Up Planning

- Provide specific date, time, and location for:
  - Neurosurgery follow-up (typically within 1–2 weeks)
  - Imaging (if post-op scans are needed)
  - Physical, occupational, and speech therapy evaluations (if applicable)
  - Neurology or genetics, if involved in ongoing care
- Encourage caregivers to bring a written list of questions to follow-up visits.

Chapter Summary

Pediatric neurovascular disorders present with a diverse range of clinical challenges, from silent malformations discovered incidentally to life-threatening hemorrhages requiring urgent intervention. Accurate diagnosis, timely surgical or endovascular management, and meticulous perioperative care are essential to optimize outcomes. Nurses play an irreplaceable role across the care continuum—performing frequent neuro checks, recognizing early signs of deterioration, managing postoperative pain and hydration, and providing family-centered education and support. With attention to neuroanatomy, surgical technique, and patient-specific needs (as in Moyamoya disease), pediatric neurosurgical nurses serve as critical advocates and protectors of neurologic function and recovery.

Suggested Reading

1. Wilseck ZM, Lin LY, Chaudhary N, Rivas-Rodriguez F. Newer updates in pediatric vascular diseases. Semin Roentgenol. 2022;57(1):46–56. https://doi.org/10.1053/j.ro.2022.09.002.
2. Sinha R, Ramji S. Neurovascular disorders in children: an updated practical guide. Transl Pediatr. 2020;9(6):867–78. https://doi.org/10.21037/tp-20-205.
3. Al-Dasuqi K, Orbach DB, Rispoli J. Introduction: neurovascular disease across the pediatric age spectrum. Neuroimaging Clin N Am. 2024;34(4):481–90. https://doi.org/10.1016/j.nic.2024.08.024.
4. Scott RM, Smith ER. Moyamoya disease and moyamoya syndrome. N Engl J Med. 2009;360(12):1226–37. https://doi.org/10.1056/NEJMra0804622.
5. Fullerton HJ, et al. Pediatric arterial ischemic stroke: acute management, risk factors, and prevention. Lancet Neurol. 2022;21(4):302–12. https://doi.org/10.1016/S1474-4422(22)00030-0.
6. Albright AL, Pollack IF, Adelson PD. Principles and practice of pediatric neurosurgery. Thieme Medical Publishers; 1999.
7. Littlejohns L, McNett M, Olson D. AANN core curriculum for neuroscience nursing. 7th ed. American Association of Neuroscience Nurses; 2022.

Seizures and Epilepsy

Amy L. Sullivan and Angel W. Hernandez

Description

- Seizure: A sudden, temporary disruption in the brain's electrical activity that can cause changes in behavior, movement, sensation, or consciousness. Seizures occur when a group of brain cells (neurons) fire abnormally, sending out excessive electrical impulses. This can lead to a variety of symptoms, including the following:
  - Muscle contractions or spasms
  - Loss of consciousness
  - Confusion or altered awareness
  - Changes in sensation, such as tingling, numbness, or hallucinations
  - Emotional disturbances
- Seizures can be caused by a wide range of factors, including epilepsy, brain injury, stroke, brain tumors, and certain medications. They can also be triggered by stress, lack of sleep, or flashing lights.
- Seizure types include the following (See Figs. 1, 2, and 3):
  - Focal
  - Generalized
  - Unknown

A. L. Sullivan (✉)
Hough Family Institute for Brain Protection Sciences, Johns Hopkins All Children's Hospital, Saint Petersburg, FL, USA
e-mail: asulli16@jhmi.edu

A. W. Hernandez
Johns Hopkins University, Hough Family Institute for Brain Protection Sciences, Johns Hopkins All Children's Hospital, Saint Petersburg, FL, USA
e-mail: aherna82@jhmi.edu

K. Battick et al. (eds.), *Nursing Guide for Pediatric Neuroscience Patients*,
https://doi.org/10.1007/978-3-032-22664-8_16

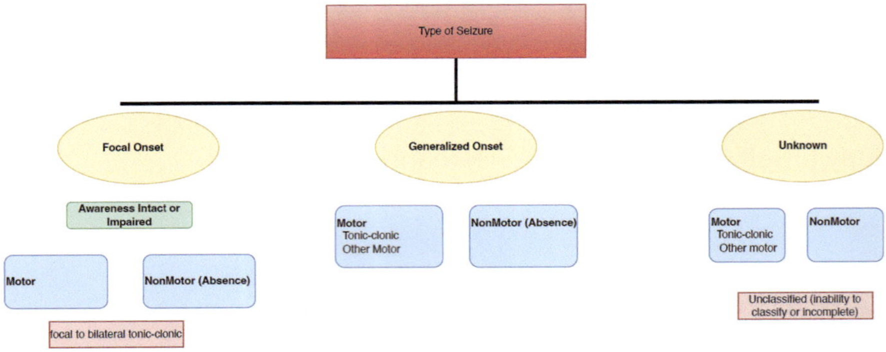

Fig. 1 Adapted from International League Against Epilepsy (ILAE)Operational 2017 Classification of basic seizure types

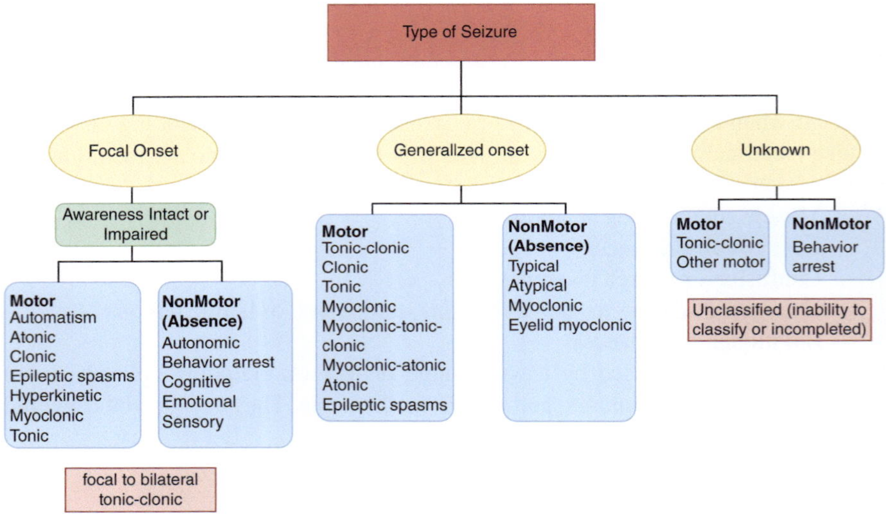

Fig. 2 Adapted from International League Against Epilepsy (ILAE)Operational 2025 Classification of seizure types with expanded information

- Epilepsy
  - Definition: Epilepsy is a disease of the brain defined by any of the following conditions—at least two unprovoked (or reflex) seizures occurring >24 h apart, one unprovoked (or reflex) seizure and a probability of further seizures similar to the general recurrence risk (at least 60%) after two unprovoked seizures, occurring over the next 10 years or diagnosis of an epilepsy syndrome.
  - Epilepsy is considered to be resolved for individuals who had an age-dependent epilepsy syndrome but are now past the applicable age or those who have remained seizure-free for the last 10 years, with no seizure medicines for the last 5 years.
- Epilepsy syndromes (see Fig. 3)
  - Definition: An epilepsy syndrome as a cluster of features that incorporates seizure type, EEG, and imaging features that tend to occur together, often with age-dependent features such as age at onset and remission (where applicable), seizure triggers, diurnal variation, sometimes prognosis, and distinctive comorbidities such as intellectual and psychiatric dysfunction.
  - Common epilepsy syndromes (see Fig. 3):
    - Infantile Epileptic Spasm Syndrome (IESS):
      - (West Syndrome) triad of epileptic spasms, hypsarrhythmia on EEG, and developmental plateauing or regression
      - Age of onset: 4–6 months
      - Clinical: Cluster of flexor, extensor, and mixed spasms
      - EEG: Hypsarrhythmia
      - Etiology:

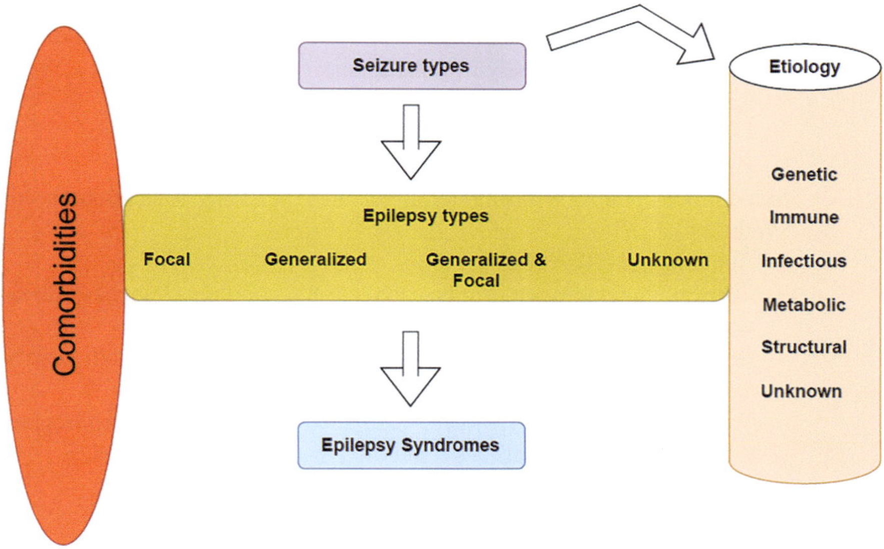

Fig. 3 Adapted from International League Against Epilepsy (ILAE) classification of epilepsies

    - Structural brain abnormalities, both developmental and acquired (e.g., tuberous sclerosis Aicardi syndrome, or hypoxic–ischemic encephalopathy)
    - Chromosomal disorders, e.g., Down syndrome or Miller–Dieker syndrome
    - Gene abnormalities, e.g., ARX, CDKL5, SPTAN1, STXBP1, TSC1, TSC2
    - Metabolic etiologies
  - Treatment: ACTH (high dose: 150 U/m^2), prednisone (high dose 4–8 mg/kg), vigabatrin (tuberous sclerosis complex)
- Severe myoclonic epilepsy of infancy (Dravet syndrome):
  - Age of onset: First year of life.
  - Clinical: Recurrent and prolonged febrile seizures, evolve into myoclonic, atypical absence, and focal clonic seizures.
  - Etiology: SCN1A in 90%.
  - Treatment: Refractory to medications (drugs of choice: valproic acid, clobazam, stiripentol, fenfluramine); other medications: felbamate, topiramate, levetiracetam, ketogenic diet, VNS. Disease-modifying treatments: ETX101, a potential one-time, disease-modifying gene regulation therapy. STK-001, Zorevunersen (STK-001) is intrathecal injection, not a one-time therapy; will likely need to be administered every several months. Antisense oligonucleotide or ASO. CRISPR. Contraindicated: Carbamazepine, oxcarbazepine, phenytoin, lamotrigine.
- Self-Limited Epilepsy with Centro-temporal Spikes (SeLECTS) (benign rolandic epilepsy of childhood):
  - Age range: 3–15 years.
  - Clinical: Focal motor seizures with or without secondary generalization. Seen in sleep, rarely in wakefulness.
  - EEG: Centro-temporal spike waves.
  - Treatment: Drug of choice: Carbamazepine and oxcarbazepine.
  - Prognosis: >90% of patients remit 10–15 years of age.
- Self-limited epilepsy with autonomic seizures (SeLEAS) (Panayiotopoulos syndrome):
  - Age range: 3–10 years.
  - Clinical: Panayiotopoulos type early-onset autonomic changes (nausea/vomiting/mydriasis), eye deviation, and ictal vomiting.
  - EEG: Unilateral or bilateral occipital spike wave. Some with centro-temporal spike waves.
  - Treatment: Drug of choice: carbamazepine and oxcarbazepine. Prognosis: >90% of patients remit after 2–4 years of diagnosis.
- Childhood absence epilepsy:
  - Age range: 3–11 years.
  - Clinical: Staring spells may or not be associated with automatisms (eye blinking, chewing, head jerks).

- Diagnosis: Hyperventilation at bedside.
- EEG: Generalized 3 Hz spike waves.
- Other: 36% exhibit attention deficits despite otherwise intact neurocognitive functioning.
- Treatment: Drug of choice: Ethosuximide; Others: Valproic acid and lamotrigine.

- Epilepsy with myoclonic–atonic seizures (Doose syndrome):
  - Age range: 6 months–8 years.
  - Boys > girls.
  - Clinical: Sometimes begins with febrile seizures. Seizures: myoclonic, atonic, atypical absence, rarely tonic, GTC.
  - EEG: Generalized spike waves.
  - Treatment: Valproic acid, rufinamide, lamotrigine, topiramate, felbamate, clobazam, levetiracetam, high-dose steroids, ketogenic diet, VNS.
- Lennox-Gastaut syndrome:
  - Age range: 18 months and 8 years of age (peak 3–5 years)
  - Around 10–30% of cases of Lennox-Gastaut syndrome evolve from a prior epilepsy syndrome, e.g., infantile epileptic spasms syndrome or early-infantile developmental and epileptic encephalopathy
  - Clinical: Intellectual disability, multiple seizure types (atonic, myoclonic, tonic*, GTC, atypical absence, partial)
  - Treatment: Drugs of choice: Valproic acid, rufinamide, lamotrigine, topiramate, felbamate, clobazam. Others: Levetiracetam. Alternatives: Ketogenic diet, VNS, corpus callosotomy
- Juvenile myoclonic epilepsy:
  - Age range: 10–17 years
  - Clinical: Myoclonic seizures (am), absence seizures, and GTC
  - EEG: Generalized spike/polyspike wave, activated with photic and hyperventilation
  - Treatment: Drugs of choice: lamotrigine, levetiracetam, brivaracetam, topiramate, valproic acid; Others: benzodiazepines, felbamate, zonisamide; alternatives: VNS, MAD
- Juvenile absence epilepsy:
  - Age of onset: 9–13 years
  - Clinical: Seizure description: Absence and GTC (20% present in absence status epilepticus). EEG: generalized 3–5 Hz spike waves
  - Treatment: Valproic acid, lamotrigine, ethosuximide (usually in combination)

- Drug-resistant epilepsy: May be defined as failure of adequate trials of two tolerated and appropriately chosen and used AED schedules (whether as monotherapies or in combination) to achieve sustained seizure freedom.
  - Labs and diagnostics (standard of care):

  - Labs: Genetic and metabolic testing should be considered depending on presentation.
  - Imaging:
    - Magnetic Resonance Imaging (MRI): High-resolution 3 T MRIs are ideal. It is considered standard: Best 1 mm cuts throughout the brain for subtle cortical dysplasias.
    - Functional Magnetic Resonance Imaging (fMRI): Functional MRI is typically performed in patients to map areas of eloquent cortex like language, motor, sensory, vision, and auditory cortices.
    - Positron Emission Tomography (PET): 18F-fluorodeoxyglucose (18F-FDG-PET), help identify the epileptogenic zone (the area of the brain causing seizures) by measuring regional cerebral glucose uptake, a marker of neuronal activity.
    - Single-Photon Emission Computer Tomography (SPECT): Help pinpoint the seizure onset zone by visualizing blood flow changes during seizures and compare between seizures, aiding in surgical planning.
      - Ictal: During seizure
      - Inter-ictal: Between seizures
  - Video EEG
    - Standard: Class I evidence
    - Standard: Evaluation of patients being considered for epilepsy surgery
    - Helps: Exclude non-epileptic events; electroclinical/semiology correlation
  - MEG:
    - MEG is a noninvasive test. MEG measures magnetic fields naturally generated by brain cells. Magnetic fields are analyzed to localize the activity within the brain and are superimposed on an MRI. Superconducting Quantum Interference Device (SQUID) magnetometer; cryogenic refrigeration (helium)
- Other studies:
  - Neuropsychological evaluation

Treatment

- Anti-seizure medications:
  - Valproic acid/Divalproex (Depakene/Depakote®): Used to treat generalized epilepsies. Common side effects: Weight gain, hair loss, increase appetite. Others: Thrombocytopenia, leukopenia. Consider weaning 2–3 weeks prior to surgery due to increased bleeding time. Requires blood monitoring.
  - Lamotrigine: Used to treat generalized and focal epilepsies. Start slow due to increased risk of rash or Stevens-Johnson syndrome.
  - Oxcarbazepine: Used to treat focal epilepsies. Start slow, with weekly titration for better tolerability. Others: Rash, headache.

  - Carbamazepine: Used to treat focal epilepsies. Start slow, with weekly titration for better tolerability. Others: Rash, headache. Narrow therapeutic window, requires blood monitoring.
  - Lacosamide: Used to treat focal epilepsies primarily but also generalized epilepsies. Start slow, with weekly titration for better tolerability. Others: Rash, nausea, vomiting.
  - Levetiracetam: Used to treat focal epilepsies and generalized epilepsies. Start slow, with weekly titration for better tolerability. Others: Behavioral side effects (aggression). Sometimes Vitamin B6 started at the same time.
  - Ethosuximide: Used to treat absence seizures. Common side effects: Nausea, vomiting, abdominal pain. Others (rare): Thrombocytopenia, leukopenia. Requires blood monitoring.
- Acute/rescue medications:
  - Intranasal: Diazepam (Valtoco®); Midazolam (Versed®) (Nayzilam®)
  - IV: Lorazepam, Diazepam, Midazolam
  - Oral: Clonazepam ODT
- Diet therapy: See below
- Epilepsy surgery:
  - Phase 1 and 2 monitoring:
    - Phase 1 monitoring: Initial (noninvasive) evaluation of a patient to determine epilepsy surgery candidacy. It requires capturing of seizures on video EEG and additional tests to support hypotheses like: MRI, PET, SPECT, MEG, neuropsychology.
    - Phase 2 monitoring: Also known as invasive evaluation. It involves placing electrodes directly on or into the brain to record seizure activity and pinpoint the seizure focus, often using techniques like stereoelectroencephalography (SEEG) or subdural/depth EEG. Phase 2 evaluation is crucial for precisely identifying the area of the brain where seizures originate, which is essential for planning safe and effective surgery. It helps map critical brain functions (like language, motor, or vision) to ensure that the surgical removal of the seizure focus does not cause significant functional deficits.
  - Resective/disconnection surgery:
    - Temporal lobectomy: It is a surgical procedure that involves removing a portion of the temporal lobe, typically anterior and sometimes mesial temporal structures. This procedure is primarily performed to treat drug-resistant temporal lobe epilepsy.
    - Extra-temporal resection or extratemporal cortical resection: It is a surgical procedure to remove brain tissue that contains a seizure focus but is located outside the temporal lobe, such as in the frontal, parietal, or occipital lobes.
    - Hemispherotomy: It is a surgical procedure where one-half (hemisphere) of the brain is either removed or disconnected from the rest of the brain. Hemispherotomy is typically performed to treat severe, intractable epilepsy that originates in one hemisphere of the brain. Typically performed

in patients with: Hemimegalencephaly, Sturge–Weber syndrome, Rasmussen's encephalitis, stroke.

- Palliative surgery:
  - Corpus callosotomy: It is a surgical procedure that involves severing the corpus callosum, a thick band of nerve fibers that connects the two hemispheres of the brain. This procedure is primarily performed to treat atonic, tonic, and sometimes generalized tonic–clonic epilepsy.
  - Other resection to reduce seizure frequency: Aims to reduce seizure frequency and severity, rather than cure the condition.
- Neuromodulation:
  - Vagus Nerve Stimulator (VNS): It is an open-loop system, meaning it does not receive feedback from the brain; therefore, it is intermittently stimulating depending on parameters programmed. It is a surgical procedure that involves implanting electrodes on the vagus nerve to deliver electrical stimulation. This therapy can be used to treat refractory epilepsy.
  - Responsive Neuro Stimulator (RNS): It is a closed-loop system, meaning that it continuously monitors brain activity and delivers stimulation only when needed. It is primarily used to treat: Drug-resistant focal epilepsy (seizures that originate in a specific area of the brain) that is not controlled with medication.
  - Deep Brain Stimulator (DBS): It is an open-loop system, meaning it does not receive feedback from the brain; therefore, it is intermittently stimulating depending on the parameters programmed. It is a surgical procedure that involves implanting electrodes in specific areas of the brain to deliver electrical stimulation. This therapy can be used to treat refractory epilepsy.

Nursing Care and Treatment

- *What is Most Critical:*
  - Patient safety:
    - Seizures can occur at any time and are often unpredictable.
    - Falls can occur during or after seizure activity and result in serious injuries.
      - Fall risk identification
      - Socks with grips
      - Assist patient out of bed and during ambulation
      - Use of gait/safety belts
      - Raised, padded siderails
      - Clean, uncluttered room
      - Hourly rounds
      - Supervision by parent/guardian
    - Emergency equipment available and ready to use

    - Suction-cannister, connection tubing, and suction catheter or oral suction tip
    - Source of oxygen
    - Manual ventilation bag
    - Appropriately sized mask or nasal cannula
- *Care of the patient in the Epilepsy Monitoring Unit (EMU)*
  - Acute seizure management
    - Seizure first aid
      - ABCs of seizure first aid
        - Position the patient in the lateral decubitus position to ensure a patent airway and prevent aspiration.
        - Provide suctioning as needed to remove excess oral secretions or gastric contents if vomiting occurs.
        - Assess respiratory status and provide support as needed.
          - If breathing is impaired, intubation may be required to protect the airway and allow for mechanical ventilation.
        - Administer oxygen to maintain oxygen saturation and initiate continuous pulse oximetry to monitor the patient.
        - Establish IV access.
        - Administer anticonvulsant medication as ordered.
        - Protect patient from injury.
          - Ensure siderails are up.
        - Stay with the patient and call for help if needed.
    - Seizure assessment
      - Turn the lights on.
      - Remove covers to visualize patient.
      - Ensure camera is focused on patient.
      - Push event button to mark the record.
      - Note the time the seizure started.
      - Describe aloud what you see.
      - Perform ictal testing.
        - Aura: "What are you feeling?"
        - Level of consciousness: "Tell me your name. Where are you? What day is it?"
        - Motor assessment: "Lift up your arms"
          - Assess extremities for tone and sensation.
        - Verbal memory testing: "Remember these code words: purple cow"
        - Object recognition: "What is this?"
      - Post-ictal testing
        - Seizure recall: "Do you remember what happened? What did you feel?"
        - Level of consciousness
        - Motor assessment

    - Verbal memory testing: "Do you remember the code words I gave you?"
    - Object recognition
  - How to remember all the elements while your patient is seizing?
    - Dr. Neel Parikh at Johns Hopkins All Children's Hospital created an acronym: PUSH—NURSE
      - *PUSH:*
        - *P*: Push event button
        - *U*: Uncover patient
        - *S*: Side/Suction/Speak
          - Turn patient on their side.
          - Suction PRN.
          - Speak out loud what the patient is doing.
        - *H*: Have oxygen mask/rescue med ready.
      - *NURSE:*
        - *N*: Name
          - Ask the patient their name (checking responsiveness, speech, and orientation).
        - *U*: Raise Arms UP
          - Motor testing, assess symmetry, drift, following commands
        - *R*: Remember
          - Memory testing
          - State a code word (purple cow, pink pineapple, red dog)
        - *S*: Say it back
          - Testing recall
          - Show a toy/object and ask "what is this"
        - *E*: Examine
          - Examine tone and sensation, all four extremities for numbness, tingling, pain
- Physician notification:
  - Prolonged seizures that do not respond to anticonvulsant medications or per orders
  - Any injuries incurred during seizure

- *Testing during EMU stay:*
  (i) Brain MRI: Used to identify lesions (i.e., tumors, dysplasias, or gliosis) or structural abnormalities (i.e., brain malformations) that could be the source for abnormal excitability. MRI can help pinpoint the location in the brain where seizures are originating from.
  (ii) Functional MRI: Used to map eloquent cortex like language, motor, sensory, vision, and auditory cortices.
  (iii) PET (Positron Emission Tomography) scan: Used to measure brain metabolism by detecting the distribution of radioactive tracers injected into the blood stream. Areas of the brain that generate seizures may have altered metabolism. PET scans can help identify these abnormal areas and localize where seizures originate from.

1. Patients should follow a low-carbohydrate, high-protein diet the day prior to their PET scan. On the day of the PET scan, patients should have water only and no IV dextrose for 6 h prior to the injection of the radioactive tracer.

(iv) SPECT (Single Photon Emission Computed Tomography) scan: A nuclear medicine test used to assess brain function and cerebral blood flow and can help identify the specific area in the brain that seizures originate from. During and after seizures, the brain's blood flow changes in response to abnormal electrical activity. SPECT scans can help identify these changes and localize where the seizure originates.

1. Ictal SPECT: Performed during seizure activity to detect blood flow changes during a seizure.
   (a) This test is completed during the EMU stay. Anti-seizure medications may need to be weaned in order to illicit a seizure.
   (b) The goal is to inject the radioactive tracer within 30 s of the seizure onset in order to demonstrate the area of the brain involved in the onset of the seizure.
2. Interictal SPECT: Performed in-between seizures (at least 24 h after a seizure has occurred) to assess brain activity when the patient is not having a seizure.
   (a) This test is typically completed outpatient, separate from the EMU admission.
3. Ictal and interictal SPECT are subtracted to localize the seizure focus.

(v) MEG: In some instances, MEG may be performed inpatient while the patient has been weaned off medication or medication doses have been lowered to increase the yield of finding epileptiform abnormalities and in some cases record a seizure.

(vi) Neuropsychological testing: In some instances, neuropsychological testing may be performed while the patient is in the EMU.

- *Patients on dietary therapy:*
  - Classic Ketogenic Diet (CKD): High-fat, adequate-protein, low-carbohydrate diet
    - Initiated in the hospital under the care of a dietician.
    - CKD is the most restrictive in terms of calories and carbohydrates.
    - Typical ratios: 3:1 and 4:1
      - 3 or 4 g of fat for every 1 g of protein and carbohydrate
      - 80–90% of calories from fat, 6–8% from protein, and 2–4% from carbohydrates
    - Food is weighed on a gram scale
    - Fluids are not restricted
    - Urine ketones and blood glucose will typically be monitored twice daily and as needed for symptomatic management

- Modified Atkins Diet (MAD):
  - Typically started outpatient with the assistance of a dietician.
  - Carbohydrates are limited to 10–15 g per day for children and 15–20 g per day for adolescents.
  - Food portions are typically estimated.
  - MAD focuses on limiting carbohydrates and encouraging fats.
- Low glycemic index diet:
  - Carbohydrates are limited to 40–60 g per day.
  - Food choices must be <50 on the glycemic index.
- Nursing considerations for patients on diet therapy:
  - Monitor for side effects of diet (i.e., constipation, diarrhea, nausea, vomiting, reflux, hypoglycemia).
  - Monitor for signs of electrolyte imbalances and dehydration.
  - Monitor for intolerance of ketosis (i.e., vomiting, severe lethargy, Kussmaul's respiration).
  - Patients that need to be NPO will require frequent blood glucose checks.
  - Patients on diet therapy, specifically CKD, should not take any liquid, chewable, or dissolvable medications as they may contain carbohydrates, unless approved by an epileptologist.
  - Patients should not receive dextrose in IV fluids.
  - All IV medications should be screened by pharmacy to ensure they do not contain carbohydrates or dextrose that exceeds the patient's keto diet recipe.

– *Intracranial monitoring (patients with intracranial electrodes in Phase 2 of epilepsy surgery evaluation):*
  - Invasive monitoring is performed using intracranial electrodes such as subdural grid or strip electrodes or depth electrodes. This allows EEG recording directly from the surface of the brain or from deeper cortical structures.
    - Patient assessment:
      - Monitor neurological status.
      - Assess and manage postoperative pain.
        - Administer analgesics as ordered.
      - Observe and document seizure activity:
        - Follow ABCs of seizure first aid.
        - Perform seizure assessment.
        - Administer rescue medication as ordered.
      - Monitor for complications:
        - Infection
        - Bleeding
        - Dislodged, broken or kinked electrode
      - Monitor head dressing/head wrap:
        - Bleeding
        - Leaking
        - Dislodgement of dressing and/or electrodes

- Cortical stimulation and mapping: A type of electrocorticography that involves an invasive procedure with the goal to localize the function of specific brain regions through direct electrical stimulation of the cerebral cortex. Cortical stimulation is used during Phase 2 for functional mapping, to define the epileptogenic zone, and/or to induce a typical seizure. Cortical stimulation and mapping typically happen at bedside but may also be done in the operating room.
  - Communication with the epileptologist is vital (e.g., goals for stimulation and mapping, rescue medication parameters, and patient safety concerns).
  - Ensure emergency equipment is available and ready for immediate use.
  - Ensure IV access is established and maintained.
  - Rescue medicine should be readily available for use.
  - Provide education regarding procedure for patient and family.
  - In the event of a seizure, follow the ABCs of seizure first aid, perform seizure assessment, administer rescue medicine as directed/ordered by physician, and document seizure activity and any interventions performed.

- *Patients with implanted neuromodulation devices:*
  - Vagus Nerve Stimulation (VNS):
    - Patients are provided a magnet that can be swiped over the device to manually activate the VNS during a seizure to stop the seizure or lessen the severity and duration of a seizure. During an EMU stay, parameters for using the magnet should be discussed with the epileptologist.
  - Responsive Neurostimulation (RNS):
    - Patients are provided a magnet that can be held over the RNS to activate the device during a seizure. This provides an additional stimulation to stop the seizure or lessen the severity and duration of a seizure. During an EMU stay, parameters for using the magnet should be discussed with the epileptologist.
    - Follow-up care is essential for the patient with an implanted RNS device. Routine visits are required for device maintenance, setting adjustments, and overall epilepsy management and care.
  - Deep Brain Stimulation (DBS):
    - The DBS device is programmed by a doctor or nurse using a computer and a wand, and it delivers stimulation continuously or on a pre-set schedule.
    - Unlike VNS and RNS, DBS is not typically triggered by a magnet, though some newer devices may incorporate this feature.
    - Follow-up care is essential for the patient with an implanted DBS device. Routine visits are required for device maintenance, setting adjustments, and overall epilepsy management and care.

- MRI for the patient with an implanted neuromodulation device:
  - Verify device brand and model.
  - Communicate with radiology regarding device location, brand, and model: Some devices are not MRI-safe, and others may require specific MRI protocols.
  - Most neuromodulation devices need to be turned off prior to MRI and then turned back on and reprogrammed once MRI is complete.
- *Neurological emergencies:*
  - Status epilepticus: Seizures lasting longer than 5 min or recurrent seizure activity without the return to baseline
    - Follow ABCs of seizure first aid.
    - Initiate rapid response team or code blue if warranted.
    - Obtain IV access, blood glucose, cardiac monitoring.
    - Administer rescue medications as ordered.
    - Follow facility-specific status epilepticus pathway.
  - Trauma: Any injury as a result from seizure activity (i.e., head injury, facial fractures, aspiration, choking, and drowning)

Discharge Teaching

Parents should teach back/return demonstrate the following:

- Teach back medication education and return demonstration of medication administration:
  - Administer maintenance ASDs as ordered with respect for timing to maintain therapeutic blood level.
  - Do not stop ASDs without communication and instruction from provider.
  - Medication side effects and signs of toxicity.
  - When/how to give rescue medication.
- List common seizure triggers:
  - Missed medication doses
  - Sleep deprivation
  - Anxiety and stress
  - Fever and illness
- Describe safety precautions:
  - Water safety:
    - An adult should be watching at all times when a child is swimming.
    - Adults should be trained in CPR and appropriate actions to take if a child has a seizure in the water.
    - Showers and baths should be closely monitored.
  - Recreational activities:
    - Helmets should be worn appropriately (biking, skating, skateboarding, etc.).

- Review seizure action plan:
  - A seizure action plan is a document to utilize for when a seizure happens, at home, with caretakers, at school, etc. It includes information on seizure types, triggers, medications, and who to contact. A seizure action plan provides clear instructions on how to respond to a seizure, reducing harm, and providing consistency and facilitates communication to all involved. The plan should be reviewed and updated at least once a year.
  - Seizure first aid:
    - Stay with the child until they are awake and alert after the seizure.
      - Stay calm.
      - Time the seizure.
      - Check for medical ID bracelet/necklace.
    - Keep your child safe.
      - Guide them or move them away from harm.
    - Turn the child onto their side if they are not awake and aware.
      - Keep airway clear.
      - Loosen tight clothes around neck.
      - Put something small and soft under their head.
    - Give rescue medicine as directed.
      - Swipe magnet for VNS (if applicable).
    - Call 911 for the following reasons:
      - Seizure that lasts longer than 5 min.
      - Child does not return to their usual state.
      - Child is injured or sick.
      - Repeated seizures.
      - First time seizure.
      - Difficulty breathing.
      - Seizure that occurs in water.
    - Do NOT restrain.
    - Do NOT put any objects in the mouth.
- List reasons to contact provider:
  - Increase in seizure frequency or intensity.
  - Change in seizure type or pattern.
  - Child does not return to usual behavior.
  - Medication side effects.
- Discuss follow-up care:
  - Importance of scheduling and attending regular follow-up appointments for ongoing seizure and epilepsy management
  - How to contact provider for questions and/or concerns
  - How to cancel or reschedule appointments

Suggested Reading

1. Hickey JV. The clinical practice of neurological and neurosurgical nursing. 7th ed. Wolters Kluwer/Lippincott Williams & Wilkins; 2014.
2. Olson D, McNett M, Littlejohns LR, editors. AANN core curriculum for neuroscience nursing. 7th ed. American Association of Neuroscience Nurses; 2022.
3. Fisher RS, Acevedo C, Arzimanoglou A, Bogacz A, Cross JH, Elger CE, Engel J Jr, Forsgren L, French JA, Glynn M, Hesdorffer DC, Lee BI, Mathern GW, Moshé SL, Perucca E, Scheffer IE, Tomson T, Watanabe M, Wiebe S. ILAE official report: a practical clinical definition of epilepsy. Epilepsia. 2014;55(4):475–82. https://doi.org/10.1111/epi.12550.
4. Fisher RS, Cross JH, French JA, Higurashi N, Hirsch E, Jansen FE, Lagae L, Moshé SL, Peltola J, Roulet Perez E, Scheffer IE, Zuberi SM. Operational classification of seizure types by the international league against epilepsy: position paper of the ILAE Commission for Classification and Terminology. Epilepsia. 2017;58(4):522–30. https://doi.org/10.1111/epi.13670. https://epilepsydiagnosis.org/.
5. Zuberi SM, Wirrell E, Yozawitz E, Wilmshurst JM, Specchio N, Riney K, Pressler R, Auvin S, Samia P, Hirsch E, Galicchio S, Triki C, Snead OC, Wiebe S, Cross JH, Tinuper P, Scheffer IE, Perucca E, Moshé SL, Nabbout R. ILAE classification and definition of epilepsy syndromes with onset in neonates and infants: position statement by the ILAE task force on nosology and definitions. Epilepsia. 2022;63(6):1349–97. https://doi.org/10.1111/epi.17239.
6. Specchio N, Wirrell EC, Scheffer IE, Nabbout R, Riney K, Samia P, Guerreiro M, Gwer S, Zuberi SM, Wilmshurst JM, Yozawitz E, Pressler R, Hirsch E, Wiebe S, Cross HJ, Perucca E, Moshé SL, Tinuper P, Auvin S. International league against epilepsy classification and definition of epilepsy syndromes with onset in childhood: position paper by the ILAE task force on nosology and definitions. Epilepsia. 2022;63(6):1398–442. https://doi.org/10.1111/epi.17241.
7. Riney K, Bogacz A, Somerville E, Hirsch E, Nabbout R, Scheffer IE, Zuberi SM, Alsaadi T, Jain S, French J, Specchio N, Trinka E, Wiebe S, Auvin S, Cabral-Lim L, Naidoo A, Perucca E, Moshé SL, Wirrell EC, Tinuper P. International league against epilepsy classification and definition of epilepsy syndromes with onset at a variable age: position statement by the ILAE task force on nosology and definitions. Epilepsia. 2022;63(6):1443–74. https://doi.org/10.1111/epi.17240.
8. Hirsch E, French J, Scheffer IE, Bogacz A, Alsaadi T, Sperling MR, Abdulla F, Zuberi SM, Trinka E, Specchio N, Somerville E, Samia P, Riney K, Nabbout R, Jain S, Wilmshurst JM, Auvin S, Wiebe S, Perucca E, Moshé SL, Tinuper P, Wirrell EC. ILAE definition of the idiopathic generalized epilepsy syndromes: position statement by the ILAE task force on nosology and definitions. Epilepsia. 2022;63(6):1475–99. https://doi.org/10.1111/epi.17236.
9. Joshi CN, Karakas C, Eschbach K, Samanta D, Auguste K, Desai V, Singh R, McGoldrick P, Wolf S, Abel TJ, Novotny E, Oluigbo C, Reddy SB, Alexander A, Price A, Reeders P, Mcnamara N, Romanowski EF, Mutchnick I, Ostendorf AP, Shaikhouni A, Knox A, Aungaroon G, Olaya J, Muh CR. Pediatric neuromodulation for drug-resistant epilepsy: survey of current practices, techniques, and outcomes across US epilepsy centers. Epilepsia Open. 2024;9(2):785–92. https://doi.org/10.1002/epi4.12902.
10. Cross JH, Reilly C, Gutierrez Delicado E, Smith ML, Malmgren K. Epilepsy surgery for children and adolescents: evidence-based but underused. Lancet Child Adolesc Health. 2022;6(7):484–94. https://doi.org/10.1016/S2352-4642(22)00098-0.

Spasticity

Katherine Rogers, Jac-lyn Mela, and James Chinarian

What Is Spasticity?

- Increased muscle tone (hypertonia) and tightness due to prolonged or excessive muscle contraction.
- "Velocity-dependent resistance of a muscle to stretch."
- The degree can vary from mild muscle stiffness to more severe uncontrollable spasms and muscle contracture.
- Includes both positive (clonus, hypertonia, hyperreflexia and spasms) and negative (muscle fatigue and weakness, incoordination, impaired mobility and motor control) signs/symptoms.
- A symptom of damage to brain or spinal cord.
- Associated with
  - Cerebral palsy (CP)
  - Traumatic brain injury (TBI)
  - Spinal cord injury (SCI)
  - Brain injury (stroke, birth trauma, asphyxia, non-accidental trauma)

Supplementary Information The online version contains supplementary material available at https://doi.org/10.1007/978-3-032-22664-8_17.

K. Rogers (✉) · J.-l. Mela · J. Chinarian
Pediatric Rehabilitative Medicine, Hough Family Institute for Brain Protection Sciences, Johns Hopkins All Children's Hospital, Saint Petersburg, FL, USA
e-mail: kroger31@jhmi.edu; jmela1@jhmi.edu; jchinar1@jhmi.edu

K. Battick et al. (eds.), *Nursing Guide for Pediatric Neuroscience Patients*,
https://doi.org/10.1007/978-3-032-22664-8_17

Table 1 Modified Ashworth Scale used to measure spasticity

0	No increase in tone
1	Slight increase in tone, catch/release at the end of ROM
1+	Slight increase in tone, catch/release through the rest of ROM (1/2 ROM)
2	More marked increase in tone through ROM; the affected part moves easily
3	Considerable increase in tone; passive movement becomes difficult
4	Affected part in rigid flexion and extension

How Is It Diagnosed?

- Spasticity is diagnosed based on a clinical exam. When hypertonia is present, it can be caused by spasticity, dystonia, rigidity, or a combination.
- The degree of spasticity is based on Modified Ashworth Scale (MAS) (Table 1).

Modified Ashworth Scale

Treatment (Table 2)

- Not all spasticity needs treatment.
  - For patients with chronic spasticity, some spasticity may be beneficial to the patient to aid in movement.
  - Severe spasticity, which impairs function and hinders hygiene and/or care, causes limb and spine deformities, pressure injuries, or severe pain requiring treatment.
  - *Conservative treatment:*
    - Stretching, range-of-motion exercises, positioning, therapy (first-line treatment)
    - Splinting to prevent contractures or maintain the range of motion
      - AFOs (ankle foot orthoses)
      - SMOs (supramalleolar orthoses)
      - prAFOs (pressure-relieving AFOs)
      - WHO (wrist hand orthosis)
      - Elbow or knee immobilizers
  - *Medication management:*
    - Baclofen (oral)
      - Side effects: Lowers seizure threshold, drowsiness, constipation
      - Caution: Taper off, do not stop abruptly
      - Withdrawal symptoms: Seizures, hallucinations, rebound spasticity
    - Tizanidine (oral)
      - Side effects: Drowsiness, dizziness, constipation
      - Caution: Requires liver enzyme levels every 6 months to monitor for hepatotoxicity

Table 2 Spasticity treatment review

Treatment type	Description	Nursing considerations	Discharge teaching
Nonsurgical conservative:	Stretching, range of motion exercises, positioning, therapy (first-line treatment) Splinting to prevent contractures or maintain range of motion with AFOs (ankle foot orthoses)	Inspect devices when on patients for signs of pressure injury, as the child grows, they will need to be resized for new devices	Parent to provide teach back to ensure understanding the need to inspect devices for pressure/appropriate sizing to prevent injury
Nonsurgical/ medications	Baclofen (oral/enteral)	Give with food or milk if nausea occurs Do not stop abruptly, must taper off Withdrawal symptoms: Seizures, hallucinations, rebound spasticity If patient is NPO, discuss plan with provider to allow administration or provide an IV equivalent to prevent withdrawal symptoms	Parent to provide teach back to ensure understanding of: Reason for medication Side effects/ withdrawal symptoms Any necessary precautions to take
	Tizanidine (oral/enteral)	Side effects: Drowsiness, dizziness, constipation Requires liver enzyme levels every 6 months to monitor for hepatotoxicity	
	Gabapentin (oral/enteral)	Side effects: Brain fog, drowsiness Do not rapidly titrate due to risk of drowsiness; recommendation is for Qday→ BID→ TID	
	Dantrolene	Side effects: Fatigue, dizziness, diarrhea, GI upset, flushing, shortness of breath, trouble swallowing Can cause muscle weakness of the diaphragm and accessory respiratory muscles Requires liver enzyme levels every 6 months to monitor for hepatotoxicity	
	Benzodiazepines (oral/enteral) Diazepam, clonazepam, lorazepam	Side effects: Drowsiness, fatigue, impaired cognition Taper off, do not stop abruptly, Class 4 schedule medication can cause dependence or respiratory depression	
	Neurotoxin injections Botulinum toxins: Botox, Dysport, Xeomin	Used in conjunction with oral medications or alone Dosing based on weight Used for severe focal limb spasticity, not general spasticity Temporary, can be repeated every 12 weeks as needed Not an acute treatment, therefore, usually performed outpatient Commonly used in conjunction with serial casting for ankle spasticity	
	Nerve block (phenol or alcohol injection)	Used in conjunction with oral medications, botulinum toxin, or alone Targets motor nerves Used with electrical stimulation guidance	

(continued)

Table 2 (continued)

Treatment type	Description	Nursing considerations	Discharge teaching
Surgical intervention: Baclofen pump	Surgically implanted device with medication reservoir, implanted into the abdomen that delivers medication Programmable—Continuous dose with the ability to add custom boluses or variable rate Candidacy typically determined by intrathecal baclofen trial (test dose) Requires surgical replacement at the end of battery life (~7 years) Contraindications: Insufficient body mass or space Spinal anomalies preventing catheter placement Poor follow-up—requires regular refills and appointments; family must be compliant with the plan of care	Implanted by Neurosurgery and managed by Rehab MD Dosing in micrograms (mcg) versus milligrams (mg) Risk of infection is 10–19% Fewer side effects compared to oral baclofen If a baclofen pump alarm is sounding, this is an emergency To prevent withdrawal, pump needs to be interrogated Pump needs to be assessed with the programmer 1 h after MRI for proper function, as MRI can cause the pump to stall or pause—when scheduling MRI scans, the pump provider should be notified for availability Withdrawal symptoms include irritability, tachycardia, hypertension, pruritis, fever, seizures, increased spasticity, multi-organ failure, and death If baclofen withdrawal is suspected, consult with physiatry or neurology immediately for evaluation and adjustment of medications to assist with symptoms and prevent worsening of withdrawal symptoms	Parent to provide teach back to ensure understanding of: Reason for medication Side effects/withdrawal symptoms, when and who to notify for concerns of withdrawal
Surgical intervention: Selective Dorsal Rhizotomy (SDR)	Surgical procedure that *irreversibly* reduces spasticity by selectively cutting a proportion of abnormal sensory nerve roots Primarily used to treat lower extremity spasticity Functional vs Palliative	Functional SDR: Performed with a goal of improving ambulation Palliative SDR: Performed with aims to ease care burden on family by reducing tone without necessarily improving function. Aids in diaper changes, repositioning, activities of daily living, etc.	

    - Gabapentin (oral)
        - Side effects: Brain fog, drowsiness
    - Dantrolene
        - Side effects: Fatigue, dizziness, diarrhea, GI upset, flushing, shortness of breath, trouble swallowing
        - Caution: Can cause specific muscle weakness of the diaphragm and accessory respiratory muscles; requires liver enzyme levels every 6 months to monitor for hepatotoxicity
    - Benzodiazepines (oral)
        - Diazepam, clonazepam, lorazepam
        - Side effects: Drowsiness, fatigue, impaired cognition
        - Caution: Taper off; do not stop abruptly; Class 4 schedule medication can cause dependence or respiratory depression
        - Withdrawal symptoms: Tremors, anxiety, agitation, sweating, headache, confusion
    - Neurotoxin injections
        - Botulinum toxins: Botox, Dysport, Xeomin
        - Used in conjunction with oral medications or alone
        - Dosing based on weight
        - Used for severe focal limb spasticity, not general spasticity
        - Temporary; can be repeated every 12 weeks as needed
        - Not an acute treatment; therefore, usually performed out-patient
        - Commonly used in conjunction with serial casting for ankle spasticity
    - Nerve block (phenol or alcohol injection)
        - Used in conjunction with oral medications, botulinum toxin, or alone
        - Targets motor nerves
        - Used with electrical stimulation guidance
- *Surgical intervention:*
    - Consider spasticity refractory to oral medications, neurotoxin injections, and other conservative treatments.
    - *Baclofen Pump:*
        - Surgically implanted device (Medtronic Synchromed II and Flowonix Prometra II) with medication reservoir, implanted into the abdomen, with a catheter that delivers medication into cerebrospinal fluid (Fig. 1)
            - Programmable—Continuous dose with the ability to add custom boluses or variable rate of medication delivery based on specific patient needs
            - Candidacy typically determined by intrathecal baclofen trial (test dose)
            - Dosing in micrograms (mcg) versus milligrams (mg)
            - Risk of infection—10–19%
            - Fewer side effects compared to oral baclofen
            - Requires surgical replacement at the end of battery life (~7 years)

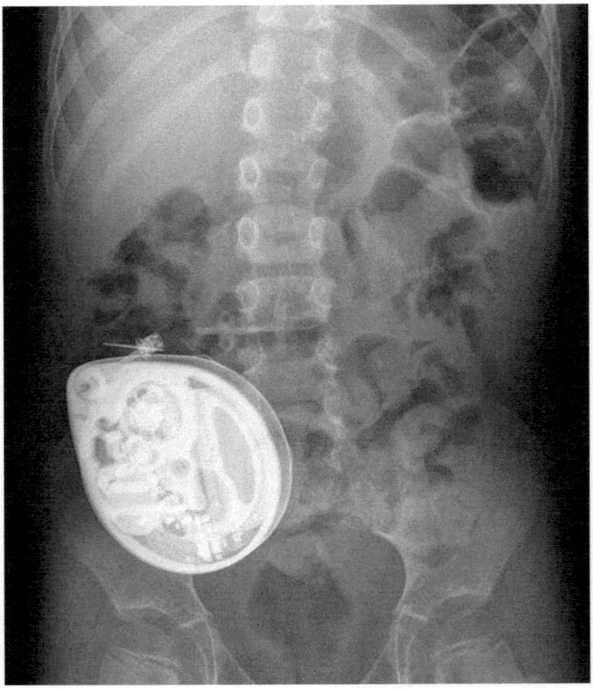

Fig. 1 Demonstration of a baclofen pump implanted into the abdominal wall and catheter placement into the spinal canal

- Alarms
  - Baclofen pumps all have an alarm date as a safeguard to remind family or patient their reservoir is getting low and they are due for a refill. This alarm date is determined by their rate and baclofen concentration. Most pumps are set to alarm when 2 mL of baclofen is remaining.
- Contraindications
  - Insufficient body mass or space
  - Spinal anomalies preventing catheter placement
  - Poor compliance—requires regular refills and appointments; family must be compliant with the plan of care

- *Selective Dorsal Rhizotomy (SDR):* (*see* Video 1)
  - Surgical procedure that irreversibly reduces spasticity by selectively cutting a proportion of abnormal sensory nerve roots
  - Primarily used to treat lower extremity spasticity
  - Functional vs palliative
    - Functional SDR performed with a goal of improving ambulation
      - Requires intensive rehabilitation
      - Recommend a detailed discussion with the patient and family prior to surgery date to allow postoperative planning and understanding of rehabilitation needs

        - Needs may include time in the hospital for initial surgical recovery, followed by inpatient rehab, followed by outpatient therapy.
        - Parents should also bring the patients' walking equipment (AFOs, wheelchair, walker, etc.) to the hospital to aid in early mobility postop.
        - Coordination and notification of rehab needs prior to surgery is helpful in a timely transition to outpatient therapy.
    - Palliative SDR aims to ease care burden on family by reducing tone without necessarily improving function. This aids in making diaper changes, position changes, and bathing easier.

Spasticity Patients Hospitalized for Other Illnesses

- *Patients with spasticity:*
  - Acute illness effects metabolic demands often causing acute increase in spasticity.
    - This may require short-term increase in spasticity medications.
    - May require consultation with a multidisciplinary team during an acute illness phase.
  - If appropriate due to illness severity, all assistive positioning devices and orthotics should be used while inpatient.
  - Patients should bring mobility devices with them during inpatient stays to maximize mobility.
- *Patients with a baclofen pump:*
  - If a Baclofen pump alarm is sounding, this is an emergency.
    - To prevent withdrawal, the pump needs to be interrogated .
  - Pump needs to be assessed with the programmer 1 h after MRI for proper function, as MRI can cause the pump to stall or pause—when scheduling MRI scans, the pump provider should be notified for availability.
  - Withdrawal symptoms—irritability, tachycardia, hypertension, pruritis, fever, seizures, increased spasticity, and death.
  - If baclofen withdrawal is suspected, consult with physiatry or neurology immediately for evaluation and adjustment of medications to assist with symptoms and prevent worsening withdrawal symptoms.
  - For a pump malfunction, an urgent revision may be required; consult with neurosurgery.

Inpatient Postoperative Care

- *Intrathecal Baclofen Pump:*
  - Implantation
    - Pump is implanted by neurosurgery.
    - Device representative initiates the pump and programs start dose: "Recommended initial total daily dose is double the screening dose that gave a positive effect" [5].
    - Initial medication concentration, 500 mcg/mL; medication changed to a higher concentration, 2000 mcg/mL, at first fill.
    - Dose titration can be adjusted inpatient or outpatient— dose increase by 5–15% every 24 h.
    - Keep site clean and dry, wash with soap and water daily, do not submerge incision underwater until cleared to do so by neurosurgery.
    - Evaluate for site complications.
      - Seroma, hematoma, dehiscence, skin breakdown, CSF leak
    - Evaluate for overdose of medication.
      - Signs/symptoms: Fatigue, lightheadedness, nausea, vomiting, low blood pressure, headaches, seizures, and muscle weakness
      - Very uncommon
    - Evaluate for signs of malfunction.
      - Catheter complications—disconnection, kinking, breakage, migration
      - Pump alarm
      - Withdrawal symptoms: High body temperature, mental confusion, rigid muscles, convulsions, death
    - Evaluate for signs of infection.
      - Redness, swelling, discomfort, fever, pus
      - May require removal of pump and prolonged IV antibiotic therapy along with transition to oral baclofen until the pump is able to be replaced
  - Explantation (removal of pump)
    - Target dose for safe removal should be <200 mcg/day.
    - Evaluate for signs of withdrawal.
    - Assure PO medications are on board to negate any withdrawal symptoms, which can include anti-spasticity medications (i.e., baclofen and diazepam) as well as management of pruritus (i.e., diphenhydramine or hydroxyzine).
    - Provide wound care instructions with return demonstration: Clean incision/s daily with soap and water, monitor site for signs of infection.
  - Baclofen pump management:
    - Patient should have a scheduled office visit for refill prior to low reservoir alarm date by the managing provider.
    - Provide postoperative site information to patient and family per hospital protocol.

- *Selective Dorsal Rhizotomy*
  - Postop complications include:
    - Neuropathy—Consider gabapentin if not already started preoperatively for surgically related neuropathy, typically foot tingling/discomfort.
    - Urinary retention or incontinence.
  - Consult with the case management and care team to ensure coordination of care for transition to inpatient rehab (if applicable) or outpatient therapies.
  - Activity restrictions if determined by surgeon or facility—remain flat postop for a period of time to reduce risk of CSF leak (24–72 h).
  - Ensure physical and occupational therapy disciplines are consulted for postop mobilization.
  - Consider surgical site instructions.

Outpatient Planning

- Multidisciplinary follow-up: Physical Medicine and Rehabilitation (PMR)/ Neurology, Neurosurgery, Orthopedics
- Rehab coordination (if applicable)–Inpatient or outpatient physical/occupational therapies
  - Postop therapy protocols for SDR patients may differ depending on selective dorsal rhizotomy vs palliative dorsal rhizotomy. SDR will need extensive outpatient therapies depending on the protocol at the facility.
- Case management
  - To assist with care coordination
  - Ongoing medication management and follow-up care
  - Equipment—any acute equipment needs for patient to safely discharge

Suggested Reading

Reynolds R, Ryan C, Akbari SHA. Management of spasticity. In: Shimony N, Jallo G, editors. Pediatric neurosurgery board review. Cham: Springer; 2023. https://doi.org/10.1007/978-3-031-23687-7_14.

Types of cerebral palsy. Cerebral Palsy Research Network. 2025. https://cprn.org/types-of-cerebral-palsy/.

https://nbiacure.org/learn/living-with-nbia/what-is-a-baclofen-pump/.

Verduzco-Gutierrez M, et al. AAPM&R consensus guidance on spasticity assessment and management. PM&R. 2024;16(8):864–87. https://doi.org/10.1002/pmrj.13211.

https://lioresal.com/hcp/dosing-and-administration/doing-long-term-management-recommended-practices/#risk.

Masrour M, Zare A, Presedo A, et al. Intrathecal baclofen efficacy for managing motor function and spasticity severity in patients with cerebral palsy: a systematic review and meta-analysis. BMC Neurol. 2024;24:143. https://doi-org.proxy1.library.jhu.edu/10.1186/s12883-024-03647-7.

Infections of the Central Nervous System

Elena Bertolino and David Hersh

Definitions

1. Meningitis: Inflammation of the meninges—the membranes surrounding the brain and spinal cord
2. Encephalitis: Inflammation of the brain parenchyma (brain tissue)
3. Myelitis: Inflammation of the spinal cord
4. Epidural abscess: Infection of the space between the inner table of the bone and the dura (the outermost membrane surrounding the brain and spinal cord)
5. Subdural empyema: Infection of the space between the dura and the arachnoid (the middle of the three membranes surrounding the brain and spinal cord)
6. Brain abscess: A localized pocket of infection within the brain parenchyma
7. Pott's puffy tumor: Osteomyelitis of the frontal bone with an associated subperiosteal abscess

Presenting Symptoms

1. Infants
   (a) Irritability
   (b) Poor feeding
   (c) Lethargy

E. Bertolino (✉)
Anesthesia and Critical Care Medicine, Johns Hopkins University, Baltimore, MD, USA
e-mail: ebertol1@jh.edu

D. Hersh
Division of Neurosurgery, Connecticut Children's, Hartford, CT, USA
e-mail: dhersh@connecticutchildrens.org

K. Battick et al. (eds.), *Nursing Guide for Pediatric Neuroscience Patients*,
https://doi.org/10.1007/978-3-032-22664-8_18

2. Older children
   (a) Altered mental status
   (b) Headache
   (c) Nausea and/or vomiting
   (d) Neck pain and/or stiffness
   (e) Photophobia
3. Seizures may occur in up to one-half of all neonates and up to one-third of all children presenting with bacterial meningitis [1–4]. Seizures may also occur in patients with viral encephalitis and are common among patients with a subdural empyema [5, 6].
4. Viral meningitis is usually associated with a less severe clinical course than acute bacterial meningitis, and systemic findings that are associated with specific viral infections may aid in the diagnosis (Table 1).

Table 1 Viral causes of meningitis and encephalitis

Virus	Specific viruses	Associated findings	Notes
Enterovirus	Poliovirus Coxsackie virus Echovirus Parechovirus	Exanthema Hand–foot–mouth disease	
Herpes viruses	HSV-1 HSV-2 EBV CMV HHV6	Herpetic gingivostomatitis (HSV-1) HSV keratitis	Neonatal transmission (HSV-2)
Arboviruses	St Louis encephalitis virus La Crosse encephalitis virus West Nile virus Eastern equine encephalitis virus Western equine encephalitis virus Powassan virus		Vector-borne illnesses spread by mosquito and tick bites
HIV		Neurodevelopmental delay Secondary opportunistic infections	Neonatal transmission from mother to child
Influenza		Flu-like prodrome	
Lymphocytic choriomeningitis virus (LCMV)		Biphasic presentation: 1. General febrile illness, followed by recovery 2. Progression to CNS involvement manifesting as meningitis or encephalitis	
Mumps		Parotitis	
Rabies		Encephalomyelitis, anxiety, nightmare, hallucinations, insomnia	

5. Concurrent hand, foot, and mouth disease may occur in patients with a viral encephalitis caused by an enterovirus [7–9].
6. Symptoms of a concurrent sinusitis or otitis media may occur in some patients with an epidural abscess, subdural empyema, intraparenchymal brain abscess, or Pott's puffy tumor.

Physical Examination

1. Infants
   (a) Hypotonia
   (b) Full or bulging anterior fontanelle
2. Older children
   (a) Altered mental status.
   (b) Papilledema.
   (c) Nuchal rigidity (sensitivity 64.5%, specificity 53.5%).
   (d) Kernig's sign—the patient lies on his or her back, with the hips and knees bent at a 90° angle, while the examiner straightens one knee at a time—resistance, lower back pain, or inability to fully extend the knee represents a positive sign (sensitivity 52.6%, specificity 77.5%) [10–12].
   (e) Brudzinski's sign—the patient lies on his or her back, while the examiner passively flexes the patient's neck—automatic flexion of the hips and knees in response to neck flexion represents a positive sign (sensitivity 51.4%, specificity 95%) [10–12].
3. Fever is common among both age groups.
4. Focal neurological signs might be present in children with a viral encephalitis or intraparenchymal brain abscess, depending on the regions of the brain that are involved.
5. Swelling of the frontal region and/or orbital region may occur in children with a frontal osteomyelitis/subperiosteal abscess and/or extension of the infection into the orbit.

Laboratory Studies

1. Serum
   (a) Complete blood count (especially white blood count with differential to determine the % of neutrophils, lymphocytes, and monocytes).
   (b) Inflammatory markers.
      (i) Erythrocyte Sedimentation Rate (ESR)—nonspecific inflammatory marker that remains elevated after surgery

Table 2 CSF studies in the setting of meningitis

Microbe	Protein content	Glucose	Pleocytosis	Other
Bacterial	High	Low	Neutrophilia	High lactate and ferritin
Viral	Normal to slightly elevated	Normal to slightly low	Lymphocytosis	Viral PCR of CSF
Fungal	High	Low	Neutrophilia	Beta-D glucan positive
Tuberculosis	High	Low	Lymphocytosis	High adenosine deaminase, acid-fast bacilli

(ii) C-Reactive Protein (CRP)—normalizes more quickly than the ESR after surgery and may be more reliable when trending the inflammatory markers over time

(iii) Procalcitonin level—more specific in the setting of a bacterial infection

(c) Blood cultures should be sent.

2. Cerebrospinal fluid (CSF; Table 2)
   (a) Note—a lumbar puncture should *not* be performed in the setting of an intracranial lesion (such as an epidural abscess, subdural empyema, or intraparenchymal abscess) with mass effect due to the potential risk of cerebral herniation.
   (b) Bacterial meningitis may be associated with [13, 14]:
      (i) Complete Blood Count (CBC) demonstrating pleocytosis with an elevated neutrophil count on the differential.
      (ii) Elevated protein concentration.
      (iii) Decreased glucose level.
      (iv) Presence of organisms on Gram stain and culture—interpret negative cultures with caution if empiric antibiotics had already been administered.
      (v) Polymerase Chain Reaction (PCR) can be considered.
   (c) Viral meningitis and/or encephalitis may be associated with [13]:
      (i) CBC demonstrating pleocytosis with lymphocyte predominance on the differential.
      (ii) Normal or mildly increased protein concentration.
      (iii) Normal or mildly decreased glucose level.
      (iv) PCR testing should be performed to identify the underlying virus.

Imaging

1. MRI brain with and without gadolinium

   (a) MRI Fluid Attenuated Inversion Recovery (FLAIR) sequences are sensitive but not specific for viral encephalitis [15], with white matter changes in the regions of the brain that are involved. Herpes viruses, the most common viruses to cause a primary viral encephalitis (HSV-2 in neonates and HSV-1 in older children) [16, 17], tend to migrate along the olfactory or trigeminal nerves [18] and often induce a focal encephalitis localized to the medial temporal and/or inferior frontal lobes.

(b) MRI Diffusion-Weighted Imaging (DWI) and Apparent Diffusion Coefficient (ADC) sequences should be used to assess for restricted diffusion (hyperintense on DWI and hypointense on ADC). Restricted diffusion is suggestive of an infection in the appropriate clinical context (it can also be seen in ischemic infarcts as well as in some hypercellular tumors).

(c) MRI T1 pre-gadolinium and post-gadolinium sequences should be compared to assess for contrast enhancement.

2. CT head and/or sinuses with contrast can be considered to assess for associated sinusitis, as well as to assess for osteomyelitis.
3. CT venogram or MR venogram can be considered to assess for a cerebral venous sinus thrombosis, particularly in the setting of an epidural abscess or subdural empyema (Fig. 1) [19].
4. Patterns of infection on imaging:
   (a) Epidural abscess (Fig. 2)
      (i) Often have a convex shape
      (ii) Do not cross the cranial sutures
      (iii) Demonstrate restricted diffusion and peripheral contrast enhancement
      (iv) Dural thickening and enhancement may be present
   (b) Subdural empyema (Fig. 3)
      (i) Crescentic shape
      (ii) Demonstrate restricted diffusion and peripheral contrast enhancement
   (c) Intraparenchymal brain abscess
      (i) Variable in size, number, and location.
      (ii) Dental X-rays and an echocardiogram should be considered to assess for the source of the infection.

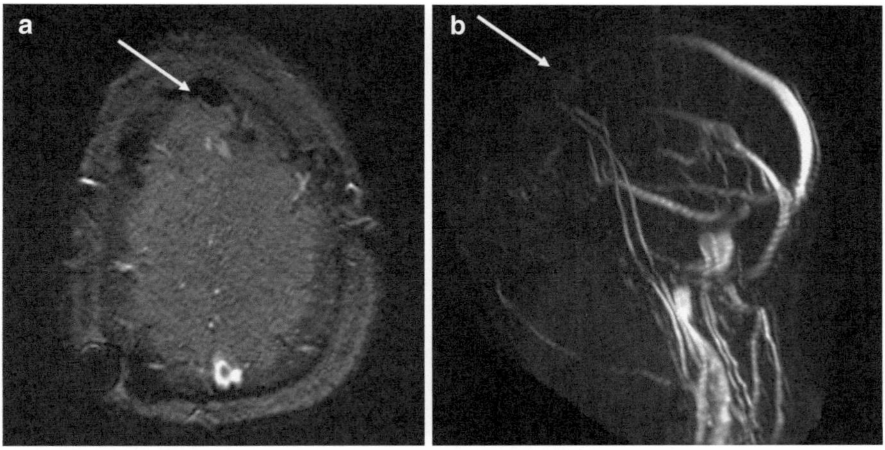

Fig. 1 MR venogram two-dimensional axial sequence (**a**) and three-dimensional reconstruction (**b**) demonstrating occlusion of the anterior half of the superior sagittal sinus (arrows), as well as a thrombosed cortical vein, in an 8-year-old boy presented with a sinogenic epidural abscess

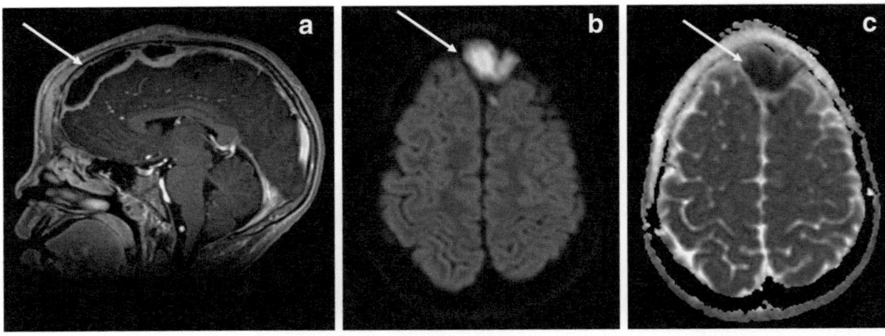

Fig. 2 Sagittal T1 post-gadolinium (**a**), diffusion-weighted imaging (**b**), and apparent diffusion coefficient map (**c**) MRI sequences demonstrating a sinogenic epidural abscess (arrows) in an 8-year-old boy presented with fever and frontal and right orbital swelling

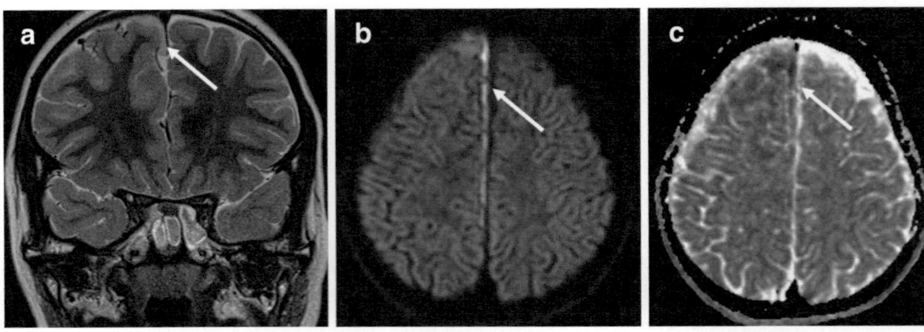

Fig. 3 Coronal T2-weighted imaging (**a**), diffusion-weighted imaging (**b**), and apparent diffusion coefficient map (**c**) MRI sequences demonstrating an interhemispheric subdural empyema (arrows) in a 5-year-old girl presented with fevers and a seizure in the setting of pan-sinusitis

(d) Pott's puffy tumor
    (i) Osteomyelitis of the frontal bone with an associated subperiosteal abscess [20].
    (ii) Imaging demonstrates bony resorption, bone edema, and a periosteal reaction [21].

Medical Management

1. Bacterial meningitis.
    (a) Bacterial meningitis score can be used to identify patients at risk for bacterial meningitis and may be used to guide empiric antibiotic administration while awaiting cultures [22].
    (b) Antibiotics should be administered empirically when bacterial meningitis is suspected [10, 23].
        (i) Neonates: Ampicillin and gentamicin

(ii) Children older than 1 month: Vancomycin and ceftriaxone

2. Viral meningitis.
   (a) Supportive treatment (self-limiting course).
   (b) Cases that occur in the context of HIV are treated with anti-retroviral therapy.
3. Viral encephalitis.
   (a) Supportive treatment.
   (b) Empiric treatment with intravenous acyclovir should be started immediately when viral encephalitis is suspected, until herpes encephalitis has been ruled out [24–26].
4. Epidural abscess, subdural empyema, intraparenchymal brain abscess, and Pott's puffy tumor.
   (a) Empiric treatment with vancomycin, a 3rd or 4th generation cephalosporin, and metronidazole (typically initiated in conjunction with surgical drainage).
   (b) Antibiotics are subsequently tailored to individual organisms following culture and susceptibility testing.
5. Anti-epileptic medication may be considered, particularly for patients with a bacterial meningitis, viral encephalitis, or subdural empyema.

Surgical Management

1. Surgical drainage is required for an epidural abscess, subdural empyema, or Pott's puffy tumor.
2. Surgical drainage of a subdural empyema, in particular, is considered a surgical emergency (Fig. 4).

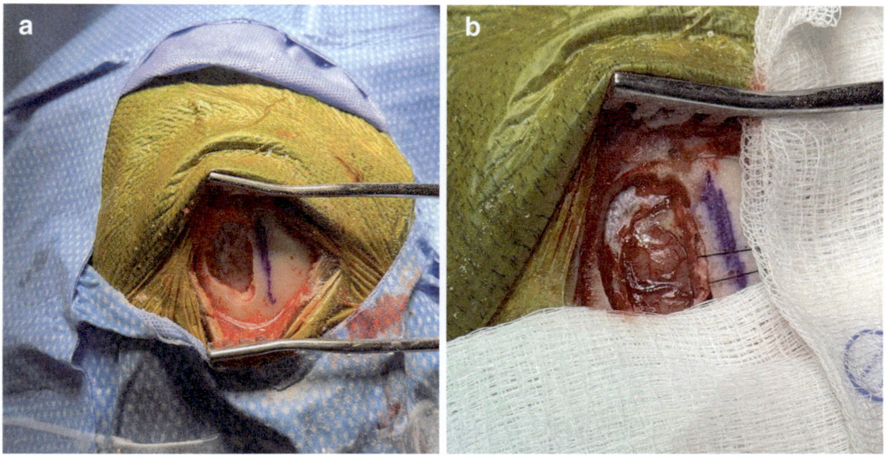

Fig. 4 Intraoperative photos and of subdural empyema. (**a**) Craniotomy has been performed and dura is visualized. (**b**) Dura is opened and brain is hyperemic but no visible purulent fluid is loculated

3. Options for the drainage of an epidural abscess or subdural empyema include the following:
   (a) Burr hole
   (b) Craniotomy
   (c) Craniectomy (in the setting of significant osteomyelitis)

   Craniotomies have been shown to be more effective than burr hole washouts and are associated with lower rates of re-operation [27].
4. A surgical drain (subgaleal, epidural, and/or subdural) is often left in place for a variable duration postoperatively.
5. Options for the drainage of an intraparenchymal brain abscess include the following:
   (a) Stereotactic needle aspiration—typically advocated for deep abscesses [28].
   (b) Surgical excision—typically performed for multiloculated abscesses, traumatic abscesses, fungal abscesses, or when the abscess has not responded to an initial aspiration. Primary excision is associated with a lower recurrence rate and shorter duration of antibiotics but carries increased risks [29].

   Primary goals of surgery include confirmation of the diagnosis, sampling of the purulent material for cultures to guide antibiotic treatment, and reduction of the mass effect of the abscess [30]. Small abscesses may sometimes be treated with antibiotics alone, particularly when an organism has already been obtained from an alternative source.
6. When associated with a concurrent sinus infection, endoscopic drainage of the sinuses by an otolaryngologist is often performed for primary source control in conjunction with the neurosurgical drainage.

Nursing Care and Management

Infections of the Central Nervous System (CNS) often cause abnormalities in neurologic status, including Level of Consciousness (LOC), vital sign changes, motor/sensory changes, and behavioral changes.

Refer to the hospital policy for institutional guidelines/policies for required communication of neurologic decline to medical providers.

1. Assessment
   (a) Subjective symptoms (patient or guardian reports):
      (i) Fever
      (ii) Headache, neck pain/stiffness
      (iii) Photophobia
      (iv) Dizziness
      (v) Nausea/vomiting
      (vi) Confusion
      (vii) Irritability
      (viii) Fatigue

   (ix) Seizures
   (x) In infants, decreased oral intake, fussiness, and decreased independent waking [31, 32]
 (b) Objective signs (observed or measured):
   (i) Altered LOC—lethargy, obtundation/delirium [decrease in Glasgow Coma Score or other evidence-based coma scores]
   (ii) Any new asymmetry—facial droop, one-sided weakness
   (iii) Gait disturbance
   (iv) Fever
   (v) Pain score >2
   (vi) Tachycardia or bradycardia
   (vii) Changes in pupillary exam: Anisocoria, nonreactive pupils
   (viii) Abnormal limb movements
   (ix) Decrease in motor strength/weakness
   (x) Sensory deficits: Vision or hearing changes, decreased verbal communication
   (xi) Emesis
   (xii) Signs of increased intracranial pressure (ICP): Bradycardia, hypertension, and apnea/bradypnea [8, 31]
   (xiii) Dysautonomia: Tachycardia, sweating, posturing, rigidity [8]
   (xiv) In infants, full or bulging fontanelle
 (c) NANDA-I Nursing Diagnoses:
   (i) Hyperthermia related to fever or dysautonomia, as evidenced by elevated body temperature
   (ii) Acute pain related to headache, neck pain, increased intracranial pressure, as evidenced by reported/assessed pain
   (iii) Disturbed sensory perception related to neurologic deficit, as evidenced by neurologic deficits, visual or sensory changes, or seizure activity [31]

2. Plan
 (a) Prepare/educate the patient and family about care needs: Blood draws, lumbar puncture, radiologic testing, postoperative course; engage child life team for developmentally appropriate patient preparation [8].
 (b) Encourage balance of stimulation and quiet time.
 (c) Provide a safe environment (lower bed, use of side rails, seizure precautions).
 (d) Anticipate patient and family stress/anxiety.
 (e) Anticipate cleaning and dressing supplies when planning surgical site cleaning and dressing changes [33].
 (f) Anticipate patient's intravenous (IV) access requirements and discuss with the medical team.
   (i) Peripherally Inserted Central Catheter (PICC) line may be indicated for long-term antimicrobial course in infants and/or children.
   (ii) Maintain aseptic technique and adhere to hospital policy for care and maintenance of peripheral IV or PICC line [34].

(g) NANDA-I Nursing Diagnoses:
    (i) Risk for injury related to altered LOC, seizure activity [31].

2. Interventions
   (a) Administer medications as ordered: Analgesics, anti-seizure medications, antimicrobials, IVFs. *Check with provider to coordinate timing of cultures, lumbar puncture, and antibiotic administration* [8].
   (b) Monitor patient: Vital signs, neurological exams/changes in consciousness, seizure activity, acute changes in physical exam, response to medications, medication side effects [35].
   (c) Recognize changes in consciousness affecting the maintenance of a patent airway and adequate breathing and circulation—provide immediate cardiorespiratory support and call for help [32, 35].
   (d) Report changes in assessment to medical provider including but not limited to: Decline in responsiveness/new changes in mental status or neurological exam, high and/or persistent fever, significant changes in HR, BP, oxygen saturation, new or prolonged seizures, severe headache.
   (e) Use age-related pediatric modifications to the GCS as appropriate [36].
   (f) Maintain activity and Head of Bed (HOB) restrictions as ordered. HOB at 30° and midline head positioning are generally indicated if an increase in intracranial pressure is present or suspected.
   (g) Provide nonpharmaceutical pain/comfort measures [31].
   (h) Postoperative care for ventricular drains, empyema evacuation—pain assessment and control, encourage OOB, mobility with activities, ambulation.
   (i) Maintain aseptic technique with surgical dressings, IVs and IV fluids, care/maintenance of closed drainage systems—utilize chlorhexidine or hospital-specific wound cleansers.
   (j) Maintain occlusive dressings [33].
   (k) Provide patient and family education on the need for peripheral IV and PICC line for stable and potentially prolonged IV access.
   (l) Maintain sinus precautions as ordered.
   (m) Assure IV access as indicated.
   (n) Monitor and document intake and output as ordered [35].
   (o) Assist with procedures: Blood draw, lumbar puncture, radiology testing.
   (p) Manage and monitor equipment in use: Extraventricular shunt, surgical drains.
   (q) Turn and position patients with altered LOC [31].
   (r) Advocate for early referral to rehabilitation needs assessment [8].

3. Evaluation
   (a) Reassess changes to patient's signs and symptoms, neurological assessment, vital signs, and pain scores. Report decline or improvement to medical providers and document [31].

4. Discharge teaching
   (a) Use of the teach-back method of patient–family education is associated with clients' attainment of new knowledge and understanding of medications and new information.
   (b) Assure patient/family can teach back or demonstrate:
      (i) Medication administration, use of medications, management of side effects.
      (ii) Adequate fluid and food intake [35].
      (iii) Seizure action plan.
      (iv) Any activity/school/daycare restrictions or home safety needs, especially if seizure activity is present.
      (v) Understanding of long-term convalescence from CNS infections—need for rehabilitation, school plan/learning problems, behavioral changes, motor weakness [32].
      (vi) Ability to care for a PICC line, including but not limited to aseptic technique, dressing change, flushing the line, protection from dislodgement, signs of infection or complications, i.e., breakage or leakage, and when to call a provider. *Provide written resources as able for this extensive and critical information* [34].
      (vii) When to call a provider:
         1. New or continuous fever
         2. Changes in appearance or drainage, pain at surgical site
         3. Change in behavior or alertness
         4. New or increased seizure activity [37]
         5. Uncontrolled headache or pain [31]
      (viii) Follow-up appointments and contact information of providers [37]

References

1. Pong A, Bradley JS. Bacterial meningitis and the newborn infant. Infect Dis Clin N Am. 1999;13(3):711–33.
2. Gaschignard J, Levy C, Romain O, Cohen R, Bingen E, Aujard Y, et al. Neonatal bacterial meningitis. Pediatr Infect Dis J [Internet]. 2011;30(3):212–7. Available from: https://journals.lww.com/pidj/Abstract/2011/03000/Neonatal_Bacterial_Meningitis__444_Cases_in_7.7.aspx.
3. Chang CJ, Chang HW, Chang WN, Huang LT, Huang SC, Chang YC, et al. Seizures complicating infantile and childhood bacterial meningitis. Pediatr Neurol. 2004;31(3):165–71.
4. Briand C, Levy C, Baumie F, Joao L, Béchet S, Carbonnelle E, et al. Outcomes of bacterial meningitis in children. Med Mal Infect. 2016;46(4):177–87.
5. De Bonis P, Anile C, Pompucci A, Labonia M, Lucantoni C, Mangiola A. Cranial and spinal subdural empyema. Br J Neurosurg [Internet]. 2009 [cited 2023 Jun 29];23(3):335–40. Available from: https://pubmed.ncbi.nlm.nih.gov/19533473/.
6. Banerjee A, Pandey P, Indira Devi B, Sampath S, Chandramouli BA. Pediatric supratentorial subdural empyemas: a retrospective analysis of 65 cases. Pediatr Neurosurg. 2009;45(1):11–8.
7. Koskiniemi M, Korppi M, Mustonen K, Rantala H, Muttilainen M, Herrgård E, et al. Epidemiology of encephalitis in children. A prospective multicentre study. Eur J Pediatr [Internet]. 1997 [cited 2024 Mar 2];156(7):541–5. Available from: https://pubmed.ncbi.nlm.nih.gov/9243237/.

8. Messacar K, Fischer M, Dominguez SR, Tyler KL, Abzug MJ. Encephalitis in US children. Infect Dis Clin N Am [Internet]. 2018;32(1):145–62. Available from: https://www.ncbi.nlm.nih.gov/pmc/articles/PMC5801071/#S17title.
9. Britton PN, Dale RC, Blyth CC, Clark JE, Crawford N, Marshall H, et al. Causes and clinical features of childhood encephalitis: a multicenter, prospective cohort study. Clin Infect Dis. 2019;70(12):2517–26.
10. Swanson D. Meningitis. Pediatr Rev. 2015;36(12):514–26.
11. Curtis S, Stobart K, Vandermeer B, Simel DL, Klassen T. Clinical features suggestive of meningitis in children: a systematic review of prospective data. Pediatrics. 2010;126(5):952–60.
12. Bilavsky E, Leibovitz E, Elkon-Tamir E, Fruchtman Y, Ifergan G, Greenberg D. The diagnostic accuracy of the "classic meningeal signs" in children with suspected bacterial meningitis. Eur J Emerg Med [Internet]. 2013;20(5):361–3. Available from: https://pubmed.ncbi.nlm.nih.gov/22914116/.
13. Sanaei Dashti A, Alizadeh S, Karimi A, Khalifeh M, Shoja SA. Diagnostic value of lactate, procalcitonin, ferritin, serum-C-reactive protein, and other biomarkers in bacterial and viral meningitis. Medicine. 2017;96(35):e7637.
14. Domingues RB, Bruniera G, Brunale F, Senne C. Performance of lactate in discriminating bacterial meningitis from enteroviral meningitis. Rev Inst Med Trop Sao Paulo. 2019;61:e24.
15. Misra UK, Kalita J, Phadke RV, Wadwekar V, Boruah DK, Srivastava A, et al. Usefulness of various MRI sequences in the diagnosis of viral encephalitis. Acta Trop. 2010;116(3):206–11.
16. Venkatesan A, Murphy OC. Viral encephalitis. Neurol Clin. 2018;36(4):705–24.
17. Kimberlin DW. Herpes simplex virus infections of the newborn. Semin Perinatol. 2007;31(1):19–25.
18. Bradshaw MJ, Venkatesan A. Herpes simplex virus-1 encephalitis in adults: pathophysiology, diagnosis, and management. Neurotherapeutics [Internet]. 2016;13(3):493–508. Available from: http://content.ebscohost.com/ContentServer.asp?T=P&P=AN&K=117066417&S=R&D=ccm&EbscoContent=dGJyMMTo50Sep7M4xNvgOLCmr1Gep65Srqa4TLCWxWXS&ContentCustomer=dGJyMOrl63nq3%2BxT69fnhrnb5ofx6gAA.
19. Muzumdar D, Biyani N, Deopujari C. Subdural empyema in children. Childs Nerv Syst. 2018;34(10):1881–7.
20. Koltsidopoulos P, Papageorgiou E, Skoulakis C. Pott's puffy tumor in children: a review of the literature. Laryngoscope. 2018;130(1):225–31.
21. Lee YJ, Sadigh S, Mankad K, Kapse N, Rajeswaran G. The imaging of osteomyelitis. Quant Imaging Med Surg [Internet]. 2016;6(2):184–98. Available from: https://www.ncbi.nlm.nih.gov/pmc/articles/PMC4858469/.
22. Nigrovic LE. Clinical prediction rule for identifying children with cerebrospinal fluid pleocytosis at very low risk of bacterial meningitis. JAMA. 2007;297(1):52.
23. van de Beek D, Cabellos C, Dzupova O, Esposito S, Klein M, Kloek AT, et al. ESCMID guideline: diagnosis and treatment of acute bacterial meningitis. Clin Microbiol Infect. 2016;22(3):S37–62.
24. Tyler KL. Acute viral encephalitis. Ropper AH, editor. N Engl J Med. 2018;379(6):557–66.
25. Whitley RJ, Alford CA, Hirsch MS, Schooley RT, Luby JP, Aoki FY, et al. Vidarabine versus acyclovir therapy in herpes simplex encephalitis. N Engl J Med. 1986;314(3):144–9.
26. Tunkel Allan R, Glaser Carol A, Bloch Karen C, Sejvar James J, Marra Christina M, Roos Karen L, et al. The management of encephalitis: clinical practice guidelines by the Infectious Diseases Society of America. Clin Infect Dis [Internet]. 2008;47(3):303–27. Available from: http://www.antimicrobe.org/h04c.files/history/CID-Guideline-Tunkel%20et%20al-Encephalitis-2008.pdf.
27. Nathoo N, Syed Sameer Nadvi, Gouws E, James. Craniotomy improves outcomes for cranial subdural empyemas: computed tomography-era experience with 699 patients. Neurosurgery. 2001;49(4):872–8.
28. Hall WA, Truwit CL. The surgical management of infections involving the cerebrum. Neurosurgery. 2008;62(Supplement 2):SHC-519-30; discussion 30–1.

29. Zhai Y, Wei X, Chen R, Guo Z, Raj Singh R, Zhang Y. Surgical outcome of encapsulated brain abscess in superficial non-eloquent area: a systematic review. Br J Neurosurg [Internet]. 2016 [cited 2021 Mar 30];30(1):29–34. Available from: https://pubmed.ncbi.nlm.nih.gov/26569628/.
30. de Louvois J, Brown ER, Bayston R, Lees PD, Pople IK. The rational use of antibiotics in the treatment of brain abscess. Br J Neurosurg. 2000;14(6):525–30.
31. Hersi K, Gonzalez FJ, Kondamudi NP, Sapkota R. Meningitis (nursing) [Internet]. Nih.gov. StatPearls Publishing; 2023 [cited 2024 Sep 16]. Available from: https://www.ncbi.nlm.nih.gov/books/NBK568762.
32. Lam A, Sanchez GM. In: Reuter-Rice K, Bolick BN, editors. Pediatric acute care : a guide for interprofessional practice. Burlington: Jones & Bartlett Learning; 2012.
33. Anjos L, Arraes S, Ohana A, Maria S, Dos K, Mery B. Nursing care in the prevention of infections related to cerebrospinal fluid shunting: an integrative review. J Nurs UFPE. 2023;17(1):e257285.
34. Moureau NL. In: Verger JT, Lebet RM, editors. AACN procedure manual for pediatric acute and critical care. St. Louis: Saunders Elsevier; 2008.
35. Irmak B, Gedik H. Nursing care in infectious diseases. Int J Pharm Infect Ther. 2022;5(1):1–8.
36. Kirschen MP, Snyder M, Winters M, Ichord R, Berg RA, Nadkarni V, et al. Survey of bedside clinical neurologic assessments in U.S. PICUs*. Pediatr Crit Care Med. 2018;19(4):339–44.
37. Marks L, O'Sullivan L, Pytel K, Parkosewich JA. Using a teach-back intervention significantly improves knowledge, perceptions, and satisfaction of patients with nurses' discharge medication education. Worldviews Evid-Based Nurs. 2022;19(6):458–66.

Neuroinflammatory Disorders

Amy M. Davis and Richard Kanoff

Etiologies of Neuroinflammation

I. Active infection of the nervous system
II. Post-infection immune system activation
III. Drug-related immune activation
IV. Primary neuroinflammatory demyelinating diseases
V. Systemic autoimmune diseases
VI. Mimics of neuroinflammatory disorders

Localization: Where Is the Lesion?

A good history is imperative to identify the constellation symptoms present. Together with a careful neurologic examination, we can characterize which areas of the nervous system are involved. See Table 1. Once we identify the areas of the nervous system involved, we can define the clinical syndrome, which will direct the work-up, such as imaging, blood tests, and the need for lumbar puncture. See Table 2. Time course for presentation (acute, hyperacute, or recurrent) further helps define the clinical syndrome and the approach to treatment. See Table 3.

A. M. Davis
Jane and John Justin Institute for Mind Health at Cook Children's, Fort Worth, TX, USA
e-mail: Amy.Davis@cookchildrens.org

R. Kanoff (✉)
Hough Family Institute for Brain Protection Services, Johns Hopkins All Children's Hospital, St. Petersburg, FL, USA
e-mail: Rkanoff1@jhmi.ed

K. Battick et al. (eds.), *Nursing Guide for Pediatric Neuroscience Patients*,
https://doi.org/10.1007/978-3-032-22664-8_19

Table 1 Symptom-based localization

Location of inflammation	Symptoms
Supratentorial/hemispheres and basal ganglia	Altered mental status, behavioral changes, focal deficits (i.e., hemiparesis, visual changes, and movement disorders
Cranial nerves	Optic neuritis, facial nerve palsy
Peripheral nerves	Weakness (commonly bilateral, but asymmetric at first), loss of all reflexes at the level of weakness Guillain-Barre syndrome: Pain
Cerebellum	Ataxia, nystagmus, tremor
Brain stem	Global weakness, swallowing difficulty, breathing difficulty Area Postrema syndrome: Lethargy, vomiting
Spinal cord (examination localizes the level—where the spinal column becomes involved)	Sensory loss Weakness is commonly bilateral—loss of deep tendon reflexes at the level of injury (lower motor neuron sign), brisk reflexes below the level of injury (upper motor neuron sign) Bowel and bladder dysfunction

Table 2 Approach to work-up

Procedure	Why?	Testing to order	
Imaging	Symptoms and neurologic exam determine where to image first	CT scan: Shows swelling and rules out hemorrhage MRI: Higher sensitivity to visualize lesions; better to show inflammation and demyelination	Contrast is given to help visualize the areas of involvement and help distinguish between new and old areas of involvement
Lumbar puncture	Evaluate for infection, inflammation, and specific causative agents	Routine labs: Cell count, glucose, protein, cultures, PCR Markers of inflammation: IgG index, oligoclonal bands, neuro filaments Specific antibodies: Autoimmune encephalitis panel, paraneoplastic antibody panel	
Blood tests		Markers of systemic inflammation Specific antibody testing	

Table 3 Approach to treatment

	Treatment	What It Does	
Acute	IV steroids (followed by oral taper)	Decreases inflammation by suppressing the immune system	Steroids make Guillain-Barre syndrome worse
	IVIG	Supports the immune system; adds "good" antibody in hopes of neutralizing "bad" antibodies	
	Plasma exchange	Reduces the amount of offending antibody	Dialysis-like treatment Requires special catheter placement
	Remove/reduce offending drug agent		If drug-related
	Surgery	Bolt—measures and monitors CSF pressure EVD—removes CSF to give the brain room to swell Craniectomy—allows more room to accommodate swelling	Skull bone "flap" removal; bone is replaced later
Long-term	IVIG	Supports the immune system; adds "good" antibody in hopes of neutralizing "bad" antibodies	Given on recurring basis
	IV medications (Rituximab, Tocilizumab, etc.)	More specific targeting of antibodies than IVIG	Given on recurring basis

Examples of Neuro-Inflammatory Syndromes

I. Active infection of the nervous system
   (a) Typically viral
   (b) Encephalitis: Can globally affect the brain
   (c) Myelitis: Spinal cord
II. Post-infection immune system activation
   (a) Most commonly a monophasic, one-time illness
   (b) Demyelinating, edema, and swelling:
      (i) Optic Neuritis: Vision loss, often color perception lost first
      (ii) Acute Demyelinating Encephalomyelitis (ADEM): Altered behavior, focal deficits, often seizures. Can involve brain and cord = encephalomyelitis
      (iii) Cerebellitis: Ataxia, nystagmus, tremor
      (iv) Transverse myelitis: Sensory loss, weakness, bowel, and bladder dysfunction
   (c) Limbic encephalitis
      (i) Behavior changes, movement disorders, seizures
      (ii) Commonly caused by NMDAr antibody which can be triggered by infections, most notably herpes (HSV)

(d) Guillain-Barre syndrome (GBS)
  (i) Extremity weakness with loss of reflexes, progressive pattern, may start in the legs but not always.
  (ii) Commonly affects cranial nerves as well: Eye movements, facial strength, speech, swallowing, breathing.
  (iii) Children commonly have associated extremity pain.
  (iv) Triggered by infections: Respiratory, GI (Campylobacter).
  (v) Rarely triggered by vaccines: Influenza.

III. Drug-related immune activation
  (a) CART therapy for cancer
    (i) Encephalopathy
    (ii) Focal deficits
  (b) Heroin—Myelopathy

IV. Recurrent primary neuroinflammatory demyelinating diseases
  (a) Multiple Sclerosis (MS): Typically relapsing–remitting disease with old and new lesions on MRI, requires a long-term immune suppressant to prevent acute attacks.
  (b) Myelin Oligodendrocyte Glycoprotein Antibody Disorder (MOGAD): Specific antibody disorder. Typically, a one-time illness. Can affect any part of the nervous system. Can be recurrent.
  (c) Neuromyelitis Optica Spectrum Disorder (NMOSD): Antibody that most notably attacks optic nerves and spinal cord. It can affect any part of the nervous system. Typically, a chronic recurrent illness that requires a long-term immunosuppressant to prevent acute attacks. See Fig. 1.

V. Systemic autoimmune disease
  (a) Lupus
  (b) Rheumatoid arthritis
  (c) Chron's disease

VI. Paraneoplastic
  (a) Neuroblastoma—Opsoclonus myoclonus syndrome
  (b) Stiff person syndrome

VII. Rare mimics of inflammatory disease
  (a) Mitochondrial disorders; POLG1
  (b) Aicardi-Goutières
  (c) Leukodystrophies

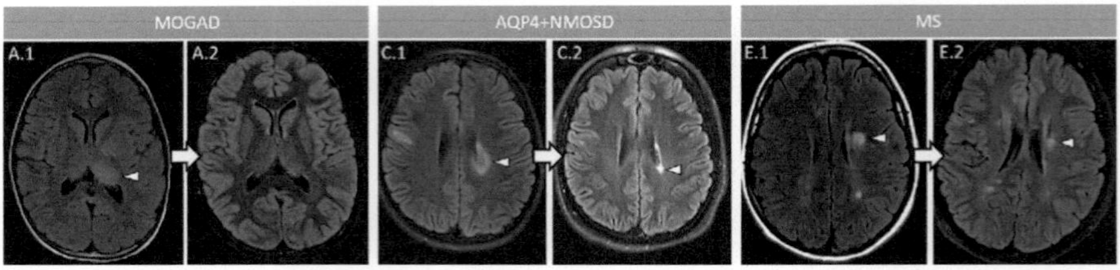

Fig. 1 Brain MRI T2-lesion evolution in MOGAD, AQP4 + NMOSD, and MS. Left thalamic lesion (A.1) demonstrated complete resolution at follow-up MRI (A.2). Periventricular lesion (C.1) shrinks but persisted at follow-up MRI (C.2). Periventricular lesion (E.1) improved slightly (E.2) at follow-up MRI [1]

Highlights of the More Common Disorders

Optic Neuritis Can begin with the loss of color vision, followed by a more global visual loss in one or both eyes. One of the more common causes of bilateral optic neuritis is MOGAD antibody. While optic neuritis can be a one-time occurrence, it can also be the first symptom of MS. It is treated urgently, typically with high-dose steroids. Treatment speeds up recovery, and it MIGHT reduce risk for recurrence. If failure to improve after 3 days of steroids, plasma exchange may be considered. MOGAD is treated with IVIG as well. May take 6 months to see ultimate recovery. NMOSD is a rare cause of optic neuritis in childhood [2].

ADEM 50% of cases may be due to MOGAD. It can affect any part of the nervous system. Typically involves altered mental status, seizures, and focal deficits. Treatment can include steroids, plasma exchange, and/or IVIG. While typically a one-time illness, patients are followed with clinical exam and imaging to see if it recurs over time. If there is recurrence, monthly IVIG or chronic immune suppression is the treatment option [3, 4].

Acute Ataxia of Childhood (AAC) AAC affects young children. There is acute onset of ataxia, unsteadiness, nystagmus, tremor—typically after a viral illness, classically, varicella. Except for the cerebellar features, the exam is normal and imaging is normal. LP can be deferred if clinically mild, stable, and normal imaging. In more severe cases, steroids can be given for the possibility of quicker improvement [5].

Cerebellitis Similar to ACC, but more severe presentation. Imaging shows cerebellar inflammation and swelling. May be LIFE-THREATENING due to swelling. Neurosurgery may be required to decompress the posterior fossa or provide a ventricular drain to allow more room for the swelling. Otherwise, treatment includes steroids, plasma exchange, and/or IVIG. LP is more commonly abnormal. Causative agents can be HSV, mycoplasma, among others. This can be a presentation for MOGAD, and there can be future demyelinating events elsewhere in the nervous system [6].

Area Postrema Syndrome Inflammation at the floor of the fourth ventricle, which affects our nausea center. Protracted emesis can be the predominant symptom, along with lethargy and weakness. This syndrome and characteristic MRI is classic for Neuro Myelitis Optica (NMOSD), a disorder that gets its name from its propensity to cause episodes of optic neuritis and myelitis. Steroids are often too little to help. The disorder is most commonly chronic and recurrent. IVIG, plasma exchange, and chronic immune suppressants are the treatments [7].

Transverse Myelitis Inflammation spanning across the spinal cord. May be a long or short segment. Affects motor and sensory function above and below the area involved, as well as bowel and bladder functions. This may be caused by acute infections, ADEM, antibodies like MOG, NMO, and systemic inflammatory disorders such as lupus, sarcoidosis, or a flair in MS [8].

MS A relapsing and remitting demyelinating disease. Although often associated with prior EBV infection, the exact cause is unknown and may be different for different individuals. More recent diagnostic criteria allow earlier diagnosis and therefore more prompt starting of disease-modifying medications. Acute attacks are still treated with high-dose steroids. Tumefactive MS refers to lesions of demyelination and edema that are large enough to result in mass effect and increased intracranial pressure. These lesions sometimes require neurosurgical approaches to manage the acute swelling (EVD, craniectomy) [9].

GBS An antibody attack on the myelin of peripheral and cranial nerves, particularly at the nerve roots near their entrance to the spinal cord and brain stem. Classically, the weakness begins in the legs, then "ascends" to involve the arms, and potentially the cranial nerves. However, there are variants in this presentation, sometimes affecting the cranial nerves more prominently. The sensory nerves become secondarily involved, producing pain. Children typically have more pain compared to adults, and pain may be their presenting complaint. Weakness with areflexia (lack of deep tendon reflexes), along with LP results that show an elevated protein without an increase in white blood cells, is the hallmark of this condition. However, the LP may be normal early in the course. Brain and spine MRI may be helpful to show enhancement of the nerve roots. GI illness caused by Campylobacter is an example of antigen mimicry. A protein on the bacteria is similar to myelin protein, which leads to the immune system attacking the nerves "by mistake". There is also a rare association with influenza vaccine. However, when GBS is not related to the vaccine, persons with a history of GBS are actually recommended to get the vaccine, as flu illness may worsen their residual symptoms. Treatment with steroids makes this condition WORSE! IVIG and plasma exchange are the primary acute therapies. Recovery can take 6 months to 2 years [10].

Nursing Care and Treatment

Assess for the following:

I. Fever, headache, nausea, vomiting
II. Seizures, confusion, drowsiness, agitation
III. Motor weakness, tremors, ataxia
IV. Abnormal sensations, numbness, visual problems
V. Nystagmus, dysarthria, dysphagia
VI. Movement disorders

VII. Bladder/bowel issues (constipation, urinary retention, etc.…)
VIII. Any deviation from previous assessment OR from patient's baseline assessment

Medication Administration and Side Effects

I. Steroids
  (a) Glucose assessment
  (b) Agitation, excitability, insomnia
II. IVIG
  (a) Infusion reaction (rash, fever, difficulty breathing, etc.…)
  (b) Headache, nausea, vomiting
III. Plasma exchange/plasmapheresis (done by dialysis)
  (a) Hypotension
  (b) Hypothermia
  (c) Electrolyte disturbances
  (d) Tiredness afterward is very common

Wound Prevention

I. Compression boots
II. Frequent change in positioning
III. PT/OT

Discharge Teaching

I. When to call Neurology
  (a) New signs/symptoms or worsening
  (b) F/u appt (if not already scheduled)
II. Outpatient PT/OT/ST referrals
III. Provide education on diagnosis
IV. Stress importance of keeping all appts

References

1. Redenbaugh V, Chia NH, Cacciaguerra L, Mccombe JA, Tillema J, Chen J, Lopez Chiriboga AS, Sechi E, Hacohen Y, Pittock SJ, Flanagan EP. Comparison of MRI T2-lesion evolution in pediatric MOGAD, NMOSD, and MS. Mult Scler J. 2023;29:799–808.
2. Jamali Dogahe S, Pakravan P, Pakravan M. Acute optic neuritis: an update on approach and management. J Ophthalmic Vis Res. 2023;18(4):433–40. https://doi.org/10.18502/jovr.v18i4.14556.
3. Kneen R. Acute disseminated encephalomyelitis (ADEM) in children. Encephalitis International; 2022. https://www.encephalitis.info/types-of-encephalitis/autoimmune-encephalitis/acute-disseminated-encephalomyelitis-adem-in-children/.
4. Gaillard F, Gajera J, Walizai T, et al. Acute disseminated encephalomyelitis (ADEM). Reference article. Radiopaedia.org. https://doi.org/10.53347/rID-852. Accessed on 17 Jan 2025.

5. Nussinovitch M, Prais D, Volovitz B, Shapiro R, Amir J. Post-infectious acute cerebellar ataxia in children. Clin Pediatr. 2003;42(7):581–4. https://doi.org/10.1177/000992280304200702.
6. Yildirim M, Gocmen R, Konuskan B, Parlak S, Yalnizoglu D, Anlar B. Acute cerebellitis or postinfectious cerebellar ataxia? Clinical and imaging features in acute cerebellitis. J Child Neurol. 2020;35(6):380–8. https://doi.org/10.1177/0883073820901407.
7. Ranjan A, Mudassir S, Sinha N, Panjwani A, Kumar A. Area postema syndrome: an initial presentation of double-seropositive AQP4 and MOG antibodies. Neurol Clin Pract. 2022;12(4):e82–4. https://doi.org/10.1212/CPJ.0000000000200065.
8. Sharma R, Walizai T, Verikios N, et al. Transverse myelitis. Reference article. Radiopaedia.org. https://doi.org/10.53347/rID-19537. Accessed on 17 Jan 2025.
9. Kaeser MA, Scali F, Lanzisera FP, Bub GA, Kettner NW. Tumefactive multiple sclerosis: an uncommon diagnostic challenge. J Chiropr Med. 2011;10(1):29–35. https://doi.org/10.1016/j.jcm.2010.08.002.
10. Leonhard SE, Mandarakas MR, Gondim FAA, Bateman K, Ferreira MLB, Cornblath DR, van Doorn PA, Dourado ME, Hughes RAC, Islam B, Kusunoki S, Pardo CA, Reisin R, Sejvar JJ, Shahrizaila N, Soares C, Umapathi T, Wang Y, Yiu EM, Willison HJ, et al. Diagnosis and management of Guillain-Barré syndrome in ten steps. Nat Rev Neurol. 2019;15(11):671–83. https://doi.org/10.1038/s41582-019-0250-9.

Determination of Neurologic Death in Infants and Children

Elisabeth Chinlund and Thomas A. Nakagawa

Introduction

Death has been traditionally declared following loss of circulation and respiration. With technology and medical advancements, the use of mechanical ventilation, mechanical circulatory devices, and anesthesia allowed individuals to remain in a state of unconsciousness while breathing and circulation were supported. This created difficulties determining when a person was alive or dead based upon an induced or irreversible coma.

A definition of irreversible coma was reported from the Ad Hoc Committee of the Harvard Medical School to examine the definition of death [1]. Irreversible coma and brain death were defined by this committee as unresponsiveness and lack of receptivity, absence of movement and breathing, absence of brain stem reflexes, and coma that had been identified. A confirmatory electroencephalogram could be obtained. Confusion continued to exist regarding the need for ancillary tests, exceptions to the stated criteria including if they applied to infants and children.

The Uniform Determination of Death Act (UDDA) was created by the Uniform Law Commission in 1981 to provide a consistent standard to determine death across all states. The UDDA provides two legal pathways to determine death and states that an individual who has sustained either (1) irreversible cessation of circulatory and respiratory functions (which is the traditional way people think of someone dying) or (2) irreversible cessation of all functions of the entire brain, including the

E. Chinlund (✉)
Pediatric Palliative Care, University of Florida Jacksonville, Wolfson Children's Hospital, Jacksonville, FL, USA
e-mail: Elisabeth.Chinlund@jax.ufl.edu

T. A. Nakagawa
Department of Pediatrics, University of Florida College of Medicine-Jacksonville, Jacksonville, FL, USA

Honorbridge, Chapel Hill, NC, USA

K. Battick et al. (eds.), *Nursing Guide for Pediatric Neuroscience Patients*,
https://doi.org/10.1007/978-3-032-22664-8_20

brain stem, is dead. A determination of death must be made in accordance with accepted medical standards. The United States (US) and many other countries around the world recognize both circulatory and respiratory and neurologic criteria to determine death for adults and children [2, 3].

The lack of definition and process to determine neurologic death in children remained, and in 1987, a Special Taskforce was established and created guidelines to determine brain death in children [4]. These separate pediatric guidelines provided physicians with a process to determine neurologic death in infants and children. Pediatric critical care medicine was further developing as a pediatric specialty and experience to determine brain death (BD) or death by neurologic death (DNC) at that time. These basic guidelines were updated in 2011 in a multisociety guideline from the Society of Critical Care Medicine (SCCM), American Academy of Pediatrics (AAP), and the Child Neurology Society (CNS) [4, 5]. The 2011 guidelines provided more specific information including what defined a child, specific criteria that must be determined prior to BD/DNC testing, components of the neurologic examination, apnea testing, and use of ancillary studies. These guidelines continued to recognize that BD/DNC was the irreversible cessation of all functions of the entire brain including the brainstem. This information was based on extensive literature reviews including information and experience gained to determine BD/DNC since the original publication in 1987. In 2023, a combined consensus guideline for adults and children was published by the American Academy of Neurology [6].

Neurologic death is a relatively rare occurrence in children [7]. The age of a pediatric patient in the US is defined as birth (term, newborn, 37 weeks gestational age) to 18 years of age. The exceptions are pediatric trauma patients who may be cared for in an adult intensive care unit after 16 years of age [5, 6, 8]. The vast age range results in anatomic and physiologic differences in children that must be considered when determining BD/DNC. The etiology of central nervous system (CNS) injury in children that results in BD/DNC differs from adults and is dependent on the age of the child. Hypoxic ischemic injury is the most common event in young children, while trauma accounts for a significant portion of injury in older children. Compared with adults, cerebrovascular injury is less common in children. Similar to adults, most children die following the withdrawal of life-sustaining medical therapies [9, 10]. Criteria to determine BD/DNC are the same for adults and children. However, the process to determine BD/DNC differs from adults because of the large age variation, significant anatomic and physiologic differences, and causes of central nervous system injury [5, 6, 8].

Prerequisite Criteria to Determine Neurologic Death

Eliminating factors that could affect the neurologic examination is crucial to avoid diagnostic error and a false determination of BD/DNC. Prerequisite criteria that must be fulfilled prior to determining BD/DNC include a known cause of coma, normal blood pressure for age, normal body temperature, euvolemia, correction of metabolic derangements, and allowing for metabolism of pharmacologic agents that could affect the neurologic examination [5, 6, 8].

1. Determining the cause of unconsciousness leading to coma
   (a) Imaging studies of the brain should be consistent with the cause of brain injury resulting in coma.
      (i) Normal brain imaging studies should prompt further investigation for the cause of coma.
   (b) Toxicology screens can be used to rule out drug ingestion.
   (c) Determination of unusual causes for coma including neurotoxins, envenomation, inborn errors of metabolism, chemical exposure.
   (d) Cervical spine injury can affect bodily reflexes and testing for apnea.
2. Waiting an appropriate time following a catastrophic neurologic event or cardiac arrest
   (a) A period of 24 h of observation or longer is suggested before BD/DNC testing is initiated.
   (b) A period of 48 h of observation or longer is suggested for children <2 years of age who suffered an anoxic injury before BD/DNC testing is initiated.
3. Normalizing blood pressure
   (a) Blood pressure must be normalized and maintained based on the age of the child.
   (b) Hypotension and shock must be treated and corrected with restoration of euvolemia.
   (c) Blood pressure should be monitored with invasive arterial blood pressure monitoring.
4. Normalizing core body temperature
   (a) The child must be normothermic before initiating testing for BD/DNC.
      (i) If therapeutic hypothermia is used, a period of 24 h of normothermia should be observed before initiating testing for BD/DNC.
5. Correction of metabolic, acid base, and endocrine disturbances capable of causing coma that could interfere with the neurologic examination must be corrected
   (a) Correction of metabolic factors including fluids and electrolytes
      (i) Serum sodium levels
         1. Normal serum sodium levels 130–160 mg/dL
      (ii) Serum glucose levels
         1. Euglycemia
      (iii) Serum blood urea nitrogen (BUN) and creatinine (Cr)
         1. If renal dysfunction or failure is present due to disease or hypoxia, blood urea nitrogen (BUN) and creatinine should be corrected, if possible.
      (iv) Serum ammonia levels
         1. If liver dysfunction or failure is present due to disease or hypoxia, serum ammonia levels should be determined and corrected, if possible.

6. Allowing for appropriate metabolism of medications that can interfere with the neurologic examination
   (a) Medications capable of affecting the neurologic examination should be discontinued, allowing for metabolism to eliminate these pharmacologic agents. These medications include sedatives, opioid analgesics, anti-seizure medications, alcohol, and neuromuscular blocking agents.
      (i) Total dose amount, duration of medication administration, and route of drug elimination should be considered.
      (ii) It is recommended that providers wait 5 half-lives of these pharmacologic agents prior to testing for BD/DNC.
      (iii) Drug metabolism can be affected by hypothermia and end-organ dysfunction or failure that must be considered when testing for BD/DNC.
      (iv) Drug levels should be obtained if possible to ensure these levels are in the low range of normal.
      (v) A nerve stimulator can test for residual neuromuscular blockade.

Process to Determine BD/DNC

Once criteria have been met to determine BD/DNC, the neurologic examination can be performed. Coma, apnea, and loss of brainstem reflexes must be present to determine DB/DNC [5, 6, 8]. The process to determine BD/DNC is examining evidence of brain activity that includes cortical and brainstem functions.

1. The neurologic examination assesses motor responses of the head, neck, and limbs. There should be complete loss of consciousness, vocalization, responsiveness, and purposeful movement:
   (a) Noxious central stimulation should not elicit any motor response or eye opening from the patient.
   (b) Spinal reflexes may be present and are not an indication of higher cortical function.
2. Loss of all brainstem reflexes
   (a) Pupils
      (i) The pupillary light reflex is controlled by cranial nerves II and III.
      (ii) A bright light is shined into the pupils.
      (iii) Fixed and dilated with no response to light.
      (iv) A pupillometer can be used to determine a neuropupillary index (NPI). The pupillometer is not indicated for children <6 months of age.
      (v) Smaller pupils in infants may require the use of a magnifying glass to determine if pupillary response is present or absent.
   (b) Loss of bulbar function that includes facial and oropharyngeal muscles with stimulation.
      (i) Bulbar reflexes are controlled by cranial nerves V and VII.
      (ii) Stimulation using pressure to the temporal mandibular joint or the supraorbital ridge should elicit no facial movement.

(c) Absent gag, cough, sucking and rooting reflexes.
  (i) Gag, cough, and sucking reflexes are controlled by cranial nerves IX and X.
  (ii) Gag reflex can be tested using a tongue depressor to stimulate the posterior pharynx.
  (iii) Cough reflex can be tested using a suction catheter advanced through the endotracheal tube to the level of the carina.
  (iv) Rooting reflex should be tested for children <6 months of age.

(d) Absent corneal reflex
  (i) The corneal reflex is controlled by cranial nerves V and VII.
  (ii) The corneal reflex can be tested using a cotton swab to gently touch the sclera, eye lashes, or gentle administration of saline to the cornea. No movement of the eyelid should occur.
  (iii) Care should be taken to avoid injuring the pupil with a cotton swab directly applied to the pupil.

(e) Absent oculovestibular reflex (cold calorics) or oculocephalic reflex (Doll's eyes).
  (i) The oculovestibular and oculocephalic reflexes are controlled by cranial nerves III, IV, VI, and VIII.
  (ii) The head should be elevated at 30°.
  (iii) Patency of the external auditory canal should be confirmed with direct visualization of the tympanic membrane. There should be no obstruction of the external auditory and no damage to the tympanic membrane.
  (iv) Each external auditory canal is irrigated with ice water using a small catheter inserted into the external auditory canal while exposing the eyes by holding the eyelids open.
    1. 10 mL of ice water is used for smaller children and 30 mL of ice water is used for irrigation in older children and adolescents.
    2. Each ear should be irrigated separately with an interval of 5 min between testing each ear.
  (v) Pupils should remain midline and nonreactive. There should be no movement or nystagmus of the eyes during 1–2 min of observation.
  (vi) Oculocephalic testing (Doll's eyes) can be performed if there is no contraindication to the movement of the neck. *This maneuver should not be performed for patients immobilized in a cervical collar or with suspected spinal cord injury.*
    1. The eyelids are held open and the head is turned from side to side while the eyes are monitored for any lateral movement within the orbit.
    2. Eyes that remain in a fixed position with no contralateral motion during side-to-side turning of the head are consistent with the loss of brainstem function.
  (vii) Determination of apnea.

Apnea Testing

Apnea testing is an essential component of the neurologic examination. The apnea test should only be attempted after the patient meets examination criteria and the neurologic examination is consistent with BD/DNC [5, 6, 8]. The apnea test evaluates the ability of the respiratory center located in the ventrolateral medulla oblongata to stimulate respiration with a rise in arterial CO_2. Prerequisite criteria must be maintained during apnea testing. This includes normotension, normothermia, correction of metabolic derangements, and absence of any pharmacologic agent that could affect the neurologic examination and apnea testing. There should be complete absence of documented respiratory effort with a measured arterial CO_2 ($PaCO_2$) $\geq$60 mm Hg and a $\geq$20 mm Hg increase above the baseline $PaCO_2$, and a pH < 7.30 [5, 6, 8].

Apnea testing must be performed safely. Testing for apnea in a patient that does not meet criteria can exacerbate CNS injury with the rise in carbon dioxide (CO_2), resulting in altered cerebral blood flow. Apnea testing should only be performed by a physician capable of resuscitating the patient if cardiorespiratory decompensation occurs. Apnea testing can be safely performed in children using established guidelines [11].

1. Preparing for apnea testing is essential to increase chances of successful testing [12].
   (a) Invasive arterial monitoring for blood gas analysis and continuous hemodynamic monitoring during the testing period is recommended.
   (b) The patient is preoxygenated with FiO_2 of 1.0 for 20 min.
   (c) The ventilator should be adjusted to obtain a normal $PaCO_2$ and pH.
   (d) Continuous cardiorespiratory and capnography with end-tidal CO_2 ($ETCO_2$) provide real-time monitoring and are required during apnea testing.
   (e) Transcutaneous CO_2 monitoring (TCOM) can be employed to noninvasively monitor CO_2 rise [13].
      (i) A baseline arterial blood gas is obtained.
         1. If a TCOM is used, the blood gas should be obtained to validate noninvasive monitoring.
2. Apnea testing
   (a) The patient is removed from the mechanical ventilator support.
      (i) If the patient is requiring high positive end expiratory pressure (PEEP), the endotracheal tube (ETT) should be clamped to avoid pulmonary decruitment.
      (ii) Capnography using $ETCO_2$ monitoring should remain in place.
      (iii) Oxygen should be provided to the patient during apnea testing (Fig. 1).
         1. A flow-inflating bag system (Mapleson circuit or anesthesia bag) with titration of PEEP.
         2. Oxygen flow and PEEP are adjusted to maintain bag inflation during apnea testing once connected to the ETT.

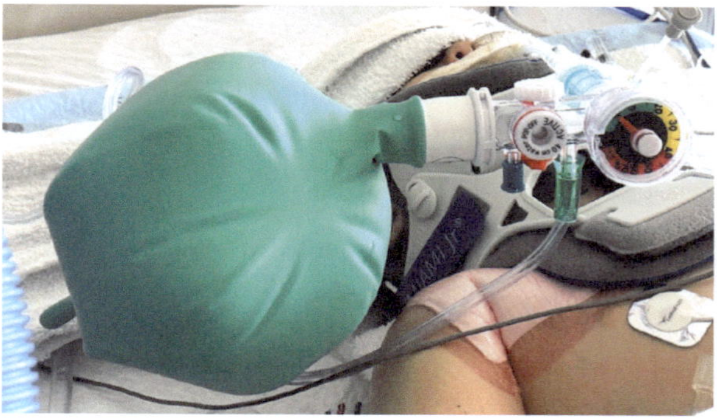

Fig. 1 Use of a flow-inflating bag system with a Positive End Expiratory Pressure (PEEP) valve to perform apnea testing. (Courtesy of Thomas Nakagawa)

3. Other methods to provide oxygen during apnea testing that are not recommended.
   (a) Continuous Positive Airway Pressure (CPAP) mode.
      (i) Modern ventilators will revert to a backup mode of ventilation when apnea is sensed.
      (ii) This feature can be disabled but can pose a safety issue if the feature is not restored after apnea testing.
      (iii) False triggering for the ventilator can occur simulating respiration if sensitivity of the ventilator is not adjusted appropriately.
   (b) Tracheal insufflation
      (i) Insertion of a small-bore tube into the ETT to provide a continuous flow of oxygen.
      (ii) This can result in barotrauma if there is not adequate excursion of inhaled gas.
      (iii) High oxygen flows can result in CO_2 washout and decrease the rise in $PaCO_2$ during apnea testing.
   (c) T-piece
      (i) This method provides oxygen without PEEP and can lead to pulmonary derecruitment if significant lung injury is present.
4. The patient is monitored during apnea testing for any respiratory effort.
   (a) Capnography waveform should be flat, reflecting apnea with no CO_2 exchange.
   (b) Arterial blood gas (ABG) analysis should occur 7–10 min to determine pH and $PaCO_2$.
      (i) CO_2 rises 3 mm Hg per min.
      (ii) Serial ABG analysis may be required to reach the pH and $PaCO_2$ threshold.
      (iii) TCO_2 monitoring correlates well with $PaCO_2$. TCO_2 monitoring can better estimate when an ABG should be obtained. TCO_2 monitoring may limit unnecessary blood gas analysis and apnea time [13].

    (iv) Use of venous blood gas for CO_2 analysis has not been validated and should not be used for apnea testing.
  (iv) Hemodynamic stability can be maintained with the titration of vasoactive or inotropic agents or fluid administration to support blood pressure.
  (v) If oxygen saturations fall <85% or the patient develops hemodynamic instability with hypotension, the apnea test should be terminated.
    1. The patient should be treated to restore normal oxygen saturations, normocarbia, and blood pressure hemodynamics parameters.
    2. The apnea test can be attempted at another time.
    3. If the apnea test cannot be completed, an ancillary study to determine BD/DNC is required.
  (vi) Any evidence of respiratory effort is inconsistent with apnea, and the apnea test should be stopped at that time.
  (vii) If no respiratory effort is noted during apnea testing and the arterial blood gas reflects a ($PaCO_2$) ≥60 mm Hg and a ≥20 mm Hg increase above the baseline $PaCO_2$, and a pH < 7.30, the apnea test is consistent with BD/DNC.
  (viii) Upon completion of the apnea test, the patient is placed back on mechanical ventilator support with continued medical management until death is declared.

3. Apnea testing for a patient supported with Extracorporeal Membranous Oxygen (ECMO) [8, 14]:
   (a) The procedure for a patient supported on ECMO is essentially the same as outlined above. Oxygen is controlled using the membrane oxygenation. Ventilation is controlled by adjusting the sweep gas. Membrane oxygenators are very efficient at gas exchange, and the rate of rise for CO_2 may be prolonged in this patient.
      (i) In-line ECMO continuous blood gas analyzer on the arterial limb of the ECMO circuit can alert the physician when $PaCO_2$ is 60 mm Hg, and an ABG should be obtained [13].
      (ii) Veno-veno, VV ECMO
         (a) Arterial blood gas sampling is obtained from the patient's arterial line in the same manner.
      (iii) Veno-arterial, VA ECMO
         1. Arterial blood gas sampling is obtained from the patient's arterial line and the post-oxygenator arterial limb of the ECMO circuit [8].
         2. Hemodynamic instability can be treated by increasing the ECMO circuit flow.
      (iv) $PaCO_2$ thresholds and pH remain the same for traditional apnea testing.

4. Apnea testing may not be successfully completed in patients requiring high ventilator settings or if hemodynamic instability requiring significant vasopressor or inotropic support is present. In these situations, an ancillary study is required to determine BD/DNC.

Ancillary/Neurodiagnostic Testing

Determination of BD/DNC is a clinical diagnosis [5, 6, 8, 12]. Ancillary studies are not required to determine death; however, there are situations when the neurologic examination and apnea testing cannot be completed. Facial or ocular injuries, cervical spine injury, uncertainty about the findings of the neurologic examination, spinal reflexes that interfere with the neurologic examination, or situations where an underlying medical condition or high ventilator settings or hemodynamic instability impedes completion of the neurologic examination or apnea testing. In these instances, an ancillary study is required to make a determination of BD/DNC. Prior to performing a neurodiagnostic study, normothermia, normotension should be established.

1. Neurodiagnostic studies that are used in conjunction with the neurologic examination to determine BD/DNC.
   (a) Four-vessel cerebral angiography.
      (i) This is considered the gold standard to determine the absence of cerebral blood flow (CBF).
      (ii) This study can be difficult to complete in smaller patients and may not be available at all institutions.
      (iii) Requires transport of the patient to the angiography suite.
      (iv) Requires a specialist to perform the angiographic study.
   (b) Nuclear medicine radionuclide cerebral blood flow or cerebral perfusion scan [5, 6, 8, 12] (Fig. 2).
      (i) Commonly used as an ancillary study
      (ii) Requires injection of a radiopharmaceutical agent to determine CBF
         1. Tc-99m hexamethylpropyleneamine oxime (HMPAO) Technetium 99 HMPAO is a lipophilic radiopharmaceutical that is preferred because it crosses the blood brain barrier and can provide dynamic and static images.
      (iii) Provides good visualization of the posterior fossa depending on the radiopharmaceutical agent used.
      (iv) Portable gamma cameras are available to perform this study at the bedside.
      (v) Requires a nuclear radiologist to interpret the study findings.
   (c) Altered intracranial pressure dynamics can affect neurodiagnostic studies.
      (i) Infants with open fontanels and nonfused sutures, patients with a decompression craniotomy, or open craniocerebral trauma may have altered intracranial pressure dynamics resulting in regional blood flow.

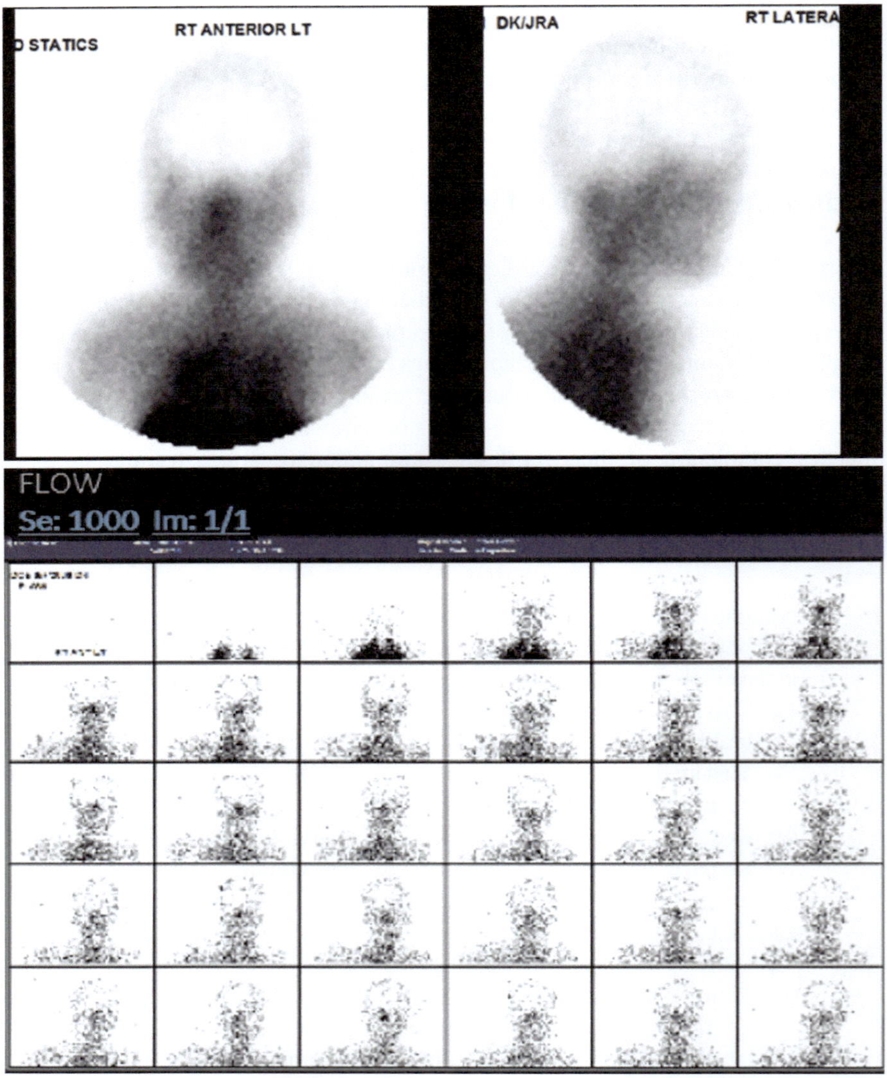

Fig. 2 Images of a CBF study showing dynamic (Left) and static imaging (Right). The "hollow skull" shows no update of the radiopharmaceutical agent in the brain. (Courtesy of Thomas Nakagawa)

2. Non-approved ancillary studies.
   (a) Electroencephalography (EEG) is no longer an accepted ancillary study [8].
      (i) EEG is affected by sedative agents, hypothermia, hypotension, and does not provide information about brain stem reflexes.
   (b) Magnetic resonance imaging.

   (c) Transcranial Doppler (TCD) ultrasonography.
   (d) Computed tomography (CT) angiography.
3. Repeating ancillary studies.
   (a) Radionuclide CBF study can be repeated in 24 h
      (i) Four half-lives of the radiopharmaceutical agent Technetium 99 HMPAO should elapse before the administration of another dose.

Requirements to Determine BD/DNC in Infants and Children

In the US and many other countries, two separate examinations by two separate physicians separated with a fixed observation period between examinations are required to determine BD/DNC in children [2, 3, 5, 6, 8]. The determination of BD/DNC is highly reliable when performed by skilled physicians trained to perform this examination [3, 5, 8]. Importantly, standardizing this process and use of a checklist are essential to prevent diagnostic error [15].

1. State and hospital policy may determine who is qualified to determine death.
2. In many states, pronouncement of the death of a child must be made by a licensed attending physician.
   (a) The death of a child by BD/DNC should be determined by experienced physicians and never relegated to inexperienced healthcare providers.
3. Documentation of the clinical examination, apnea test results including pre- and post-$PaCO_2$ levels, ancillary study results (if performed), date, and time of death using a standardized template to ensure all components have been completed should be appropriately documented in the child's medical record.

There are situations when the neurologic examination, apnea testing, and an ancillary study cannot be completed and the patient does not meet the criteria for BD/DNC. Situations may include the following:

1. A patient requiring high concentrations of oxygen, high ventilator settings, and advanced modes of ventilation may not tolerate apnea testing.
2. Hemodynamic lability requiring significant vasopressor or inotropic support may limit apnea testing.
3. The patient exhibits spontaneous respiratory effort during apnea testing.
4. Availability of ancillary studies, specialist availability, and transport for ancillary testing.
5. An ancillary study is not consistent with BD/DNC.

In these situations, repeat clinical testing for BD/DNC may be attempted at a later time if the patient's condition stabilizes. If BD/DNC cannot be declared, death can be determined by circulatory criteria.

Additional Considerations, Communication, and Unique Situations for Pediatric Patients

Determination of BD/DNC in neonates can be challenging. Infants must be term (37 weeks gestational age) to determine BD/DNC. There is no experience or guidance in determining BD/DNC in premature infants [5, 6, 8, 12]. Altered intracranial pressure dynamics can affect CBF and ancillary studies.

There are unique situations that can occur in pediatric patients [12]. Children with complex congenital heart disease with arterial and venous mixing lesions are desaturated. Apnea testing may be completed if the child has normal oxygen saturations in the 80 s. No guidance is provided for how low a chronically desaturated patient will be allowed to desaturate before terminating the apnea test. In these situations, an ancillary study should be used to assist with BD/DNC.

Suspicious deaths should be reported to the medical examiner per hospital and state policies. In these instances, investigation of events and preservation of evidence are crucial to ensure prosecution of cases can occur if intentional injury resulted in the death of the child.

Communication with families is essential to ensure families receive a consistent message to avoid confusion and development of mistrust of the medical team. Conversations about death and dying are difficult. Families should be made aware of the possibility of death in situations where severe brain injury has occurred. These conversations require family support. Involvement of chaplains, child life, and palliative care specialists [16, 17] can assist with providing care for not only the patient but also the family. Communication with terminology to discuss BD/DNC should be consistent [5, 6, 8, 12]. Brain death is a medical term used to describe the death of an organ. Death is not about an organ, it is about a person. The term brain death should be discouraged during family discussions. More appropriate language includes describing a severe brain injury with no hope for recovery and the person has died. Options for termination of artificial support should be avoided. Confusion can occur when terms such as life support are used in the context of artificial support for a decedent. Families should understand that medical therapies to help their child recover will be stopped since death has occurred.

Families may oppose testing for BD/DNC or termination of artificial support after death has been declared. Testing for BD/DNC is part of the normal examination process to determine if a patient is alive and if medical treatment should continue [8]. Many jurisdictions do not require parental or guardian consent; however, consent for BD/DNC testing may be required in some institutions. Termination of medical therapies used to support the living child is done when death has been declared. Hospital policy will dictate the time for families to spend with their child following death and before artificial support is stopped. There are some jurisdictions that make accommodations for families following the determination of BD/DNC. Only one state allows exemption to BD/DNC based on religious beliefs. More detailed ethical issues related to BD/DNNC are beyond the scope of this discussion and are addressed in a separate chapter.

Nursing Roles and Responsibilities

The bedside nurse plays a crucial role in the care of critically ill and injured patients. Communication with the family, the critical care team, and consultants is paramount to maintain the continuity of care for the patient and family. The primary role of the nurse caring for a child undergoing BD/DNC testing is to maintain the safety of the patient throughout the process [8, 18].

1. Perform and document ordered neurological examinations, notifying the medical provider of any changes in cerebral function.
2. Ensuring patient comfort, monitoring for pain, and providing safe sedation practices.
3. Attend to physiological management and maintain physiologic stability of the patient in collaboration with the multidisciplinary team.
   (a) Maintain normothermia, optimize blood pressure, titrate vasopressor and inotropic support, monitor urine output.
   (b) Obtain laboratory tests such as blood counts, chemistries, toxicology studies, drug levels, blood and urine cultures.
   (c) Medication administration including titration of continuous intravenous drips.
4. Provide compassionate family care, bridging the clinical and emotional aspects of the brain death workup, respecting cultural and religious backgrounds.
5. Coordinate the care of the patient and family with the interdisciplinary team including providers, subspecialists, social workers, pastoral care, child life, hospice, organ procurement organizations.
6. Preparing for BC/DNC testing
   (a) Obtain appropriate supplies for the examinations per provider preference and ensure they are readily available at the bedside.
   (b) Coordinate with the medical team, including the physician performing the examination, experienced nursing representation, and a respiratory therapist to assist with apnea testing.

Communication

The bedside nurse is intimately positioned to provide significant emotional support and plays a key role walking with families through the end-of-life process and establishing that their child has died. Families often find "BD/DNC" a difficult and confusing concept both before and after declaration of death. It is the responsibility and obligation of the medical team to support families by allowing them time to process information they have received as they grieve and progress toward accepting the finality of losing their child [19]. Families may ask the same questions repeatedly. Consistently reassuring and reinforcing information is essential to avoid confusion and mistrust of the medical team.

Grief is an individualized and longitudinal process. There is no "right way" to grieve, and it is experienced in an individually unique manner and timeline. Acknowledging and validating grief while recognizing emotions the family is experiencing is an important aspect of family care [20]. Identifying verbal and nonverbal communication is important to support families during difficult and stressful situations. Family emotions may range from disbelief, confusion, anger, and immense sadness, sometimes oscillating and changing as time progresses. Some family members may exhibit periods of happiness and hope, joyfully expressing memories of their child or speaking to them in the present-tense. Hopeful language is frequently used as a coping mechanism in an impossibly difficult scenario.

Therapeutic communication with families aids in clarifying misunderstandings, allowing space for acceptance of a devastating diagnosis, and can positively influence the bereavement process [16].

1. Communication should occur promptly and frequently.
2. Effective communication should be a consistent and longitudinal experience starting at the time of admission [21].
3. Medical team transparency regarding the severity of injury should be shared with the family starting from admission [19].
4. Family meetings with the multidisciplinary team may be helpful to prevent and correct miscommunications, gain clarification of family's understanding, and further explain the course of illness, and provide comfort and preparation for the family, promoting improved bereavement outcomes [17].
5. Therapeutic communication [22, 23].
   (a) Refer to the child by name and ask families what they prefer to call their child.
   (b) Acknowledge the presence of family or legal guardians, not just one parent or a single person.
   (c) Discussions should occur in a quiet space to limit distractions.
   (d) Sit with families and avoid standing over them.
   (e) Provide information in a way the family can understand, utilizing visual aids and interpreters as needed.
   (f) Speak with compassion and sensitivity, respecting familial and individual beliefs and cultural practices.
   (g) Use clear and consistent language [5, 6, 23, 24].
      1. Use simple, direct, and nonmedical terms that avoid ambiguity.
      2. Use the words "dying" or "death" instead of "passing away" or other nonspecific language.
      3. Maintain consistency in language between providers of the medical team as to avoid confusion.
   (h) Provide comfort and respect personal boundaries.
      1. Some individuals may not wish to be touched and prefer maintaining bodily autonomy over their personal space. Determine if providing physical contact (touching a knee, shoulder, or giving a hug) is acceptable.

Conclusions

The determination of BD/DNC requires a multidisciplinary team to care for the child and the family. Determination of death should be made in a timely manner and never be rushed to avoid diagnostic error. Determination of BD/DNC must be made in accordance with accepted guidelines and performed by experienced physicians with knowledge of neurologic injuries and management of critically ill and injured children. Communication is essential to provide consistent messaging to help families deal with the death of their child. The critical care nurse is an integral part of the multidisciplinary team caring for a critically ill or injured child and provides an essential role in helping families understand the death of their child.

References

1. A definition of irreversible coma: report of the ad hoc committee of the Harvard Medical School to examine the definition of brain death. JAMA. 1968;205(6):337–40. https://doi.org/10.1001/jama.1968.03140320031009.
2. Greer DM, Shemie SD, Lewis A, Torrance S, Panayiotis V, et al. Determination of brain death/death by neurologic criteria. The world brain death project. JAMA. 2020;324(11):1078–97. https://doi.org/10.1001/jama.2020.11586.
3. Nakagawa TA, Jacobe S. Pediatric and neonatal brain death. World brain death project. Determination of brain death/death by neurologic criteria. JAMA. 2020;324(11):1078–97. https://doi.org/10.1001/jama.2020.11586.
4. Report of Special Task Force. Guidelines for the determination of brain death in children. American Academy of Pediatrics Task Force on brain death in children. Pediatrics. 1987;80:298–300.
5. Nakagawa TA, Ashwal SA, Mathur M, Mysore M, and the Committee for Brain Death in Infants and Children. Guidelines for the determination of brain death in infants and children. An update of the 1987 task force recommendations. From the Pediatric Section of SCCM, American Academy of Pediatrics, Child Neurology Society. Crit Care Med. 2011;39:2139–55.
6. Nakagawa TA, Ashwal SA, Mathur M, Mysore M, and the Committee for Brain Death in Infants and Children. Clinical report – guidelines for the determination of brain death in infants and children. An update of the 1987 task force recommendations. Pediatrics. 2011;128(3):e720–40. https://doi.org/10.1542/peds.2011-1511.
7. Kirschen MP, Francoeur C, Murphy M, Traynor D, Zhang B, Mensinger JL, Ichord R, Topjian A, Berg RA, Nishisaki A, Morrison W. Epidemiology of brain death in pediatric intensive care units in the United States. JAMA Pediatr. 2019;173(5):469–76. https://doi.org/10.1001/jamapediatrics.2019.0249. PMID: 30882855; PMCID: PMC6503509.
8. Greer DM, Kirschen MP, Lewis A, Gronseth GS, et al. Pediatric and adult brain death/death by neurologic criteria consensus guideline. Neurology. 2023;101(24):1112–32. https://doi.org/10.1212/WNL.0000000000207740. Epub 2023 Oct 11. Erratum in: Neurology. 2024;102(3):e208108. https://doi.org/10.1212/WNL.0000000000208108. PMID: 37821233; PMCID: PMC10791061.
9. Burns JP, Seller DE, Meyer EC, Lewis-Newby M, et al. Epidemiology of death in the pediatric intensive care unit at five US teaching hospitals. Crit Care Med. 2014;42:2101–8.
10. Meert KL, Keele L, Morrison W, et al., Eunice Kennedy Shriver National Institute of Child Health and Human Development Collaborative Pediatric Critical Care Research Network. End-of-life practices among tertiary care PICUs in the United States: a multicenter study. Pediatr Crit Care Med. 2015;16(7):e231–8.

11. Puccetti DF, Morrison W, Francoeur C, Mai M, et al. Apnea testing using continuous positive airway pressure when determining death by neurologic criteria in children: retrospective analysis of potential adverse events. Pediatr Crit Care Med. 2020;21(12):e1152–6. https://doi.org/10.1097/PCC.0000000000002457. PMID: 32701745.
12. Nakagawa TA, Mathur M. The determination of brain death in infants and children. In: Nichols D, Shaffner H, editors. Rogers' textbook of pediatric intensive care. 6th ed. Philadelphia: Wolters Kluwer; 2023.
13. Sochet AA, Bingham L, Sreedhar S, Teppa B, et al. Transcutaneous carbon dioxide monitoring during apnea testing for determination of neurologic death in children: a retrospective case series. Pediatr Crit Care Med 2020;21:437–442.
14. Jarrah RJ, Ajizian SJ, Agarwal S, et al. Developing a standard method for apnea testing in the determination of brain death for patients on venoarterial extracorporeal membrane oxygenation: a pediatric case series. Pediatr Crit Care Med. 2014;15(2):e38–43.
15. Krawiec C, Mysore MR, Mathur M, Fang X, et al. Impact of the updated guideline for pediatric brain death determination on current practice. J Child Neurol. 2022. On line. https://doi.org/10.1177/08830738221104766 8.
16. Boss R, Nelson J, Weissman D, et al. Integrating palliative care into the PICU: a report from the Improving Palliative Care in the ICU Advisory Board. Pediatr Crit Care Med. 2014;15(8):762–7. https://doi.org/10.1097/PCC.0000000000000209.
17. Glajchen M, Goehring A, Johns H, Portenoy RK. Family meetings in palliative care: benefits and barriers. Curr Treat Options in Oncol. 2022;23(3):658–67. https://doi.org/10.1007/s11864-022-00957-1.
18. Starr R, Tadi P, Pfleghaar N, et al. Brain death (nursing). In: StatPearls [Internet]. StatPearls Publishing; 2024. Available from https://www.ncbi.nlm.nih.gov/books/NBK568811/.
19. Knihs NDS, Feisther LC, dos Santos J, da Silva RM, Schuantes Paim SM, Schirmer J, Pessoa JLE, dos Reis Bellaguarda ML. Brain death communication with parents of children and adolescents: care strategies. Rev Bras Enferm. 2022;75(3):e20210943. https://doi.org/10.1590/0034-7167-2021-0943.
20. Weaver MS, Nasir A, Lord BT, Starin A, Linebarger JS, Committee on Psychosocial Aspects of Child and Family Health, Section on Hospice and Palliative Medicine. Supporting the family after the death of a child or adolescent. Pediatrics. 2023;152(6):e2023064426. https://doi.org/10.1542/peds.2023-064426.
21. Martin DE, Nakagawa TA, Siebelink MJ, et al. Pediatric deceased donation—a report of the Transplantation Society meeting in Geneva. Transplantation. 2015;99(7):1403–9. https://doi.org/10.1097/TP.0000000000000758.
22. Lizotte M-H, Barrington KJ, Sultan S, Pennaforte T, Moussa A, Lachance C, Sureau M, Zao Y, Janvier A. Techniques to communicate better with parents during end-of-life scenarios in neonatology. Pediatrics. 2020;145(2):e20191925. https://doi.org/10.1542/peds.2019-1925.
23. Marie Curie. Communication needs in palliative care. Marie Curie. 2025. https://www.mariecurie.org.uk/professionals/palliative-care-knowledge-zone/communication-in-care.
24. Nakagawa TA. The determination of brain death in infants and children: a review of the updated brain death guidelines for infants and children. Clin Pulm Med. 2012;19(3):119–26. https://doi.org/10.1097/CPM.0b013e3182515420.

Ethics and Palliative Care

Lindsay Jones, Laura Drach, Mara DiBartolomeo, and Kristina Burger

In practice, when caring for medically complex pediatric neurosurgical patients, palliative care and ethical dilemmas often go hand in hand. In this chapter, we will discuss both palliative care and the role this discipline plays in the care of patients with neurological diagnoses as well as the ethical principles that are seen most often in this patient population.

Palliative care aims to improve the quality of life of patients by addressing the physical, psychological, social, or spiritual symptoms caused by a serious medical illness [13, 14]. Palliative care providers are specialty-trained medical professionals, composed of physicians, nurse practitioners, child life specialists, social workers, and pastoral care providers, who work with the patient's primary care team to address the needs of the patient from all aspects of care. This includes both the physical and emotional complexities of care, as well as assisting the primary care team with the coordination and communication of the patient and family's goals.

Clinical medical ethics is a specialized field within bioethics that focuses on the ethical issues and dilemmas that arise directly in the context of patient care. It

L. Jones (✉)
Cancer and Blood Disorders Institute, Johns Hopkins All Children's Hospital, Saint Petersburg, FL, USA
e-mail: ljones98@jhmi.edu

L. Drach
Division of Palliative Care, Johns Hopkins All Children's Hospital, Saint Petersburg, FL, USA
e-mail: ldrach1@jhmi.edu

M. DiBartolomeo
Maternal Fetal Neonatal Institute, Johns Hopkins All Children's Hospital, Saint Petersburg, FL, USA
e-mail: mdibart2@jhmi.edu

K. Burger
Johns Hopkins All Children's Hospital, Saint Petersburg, FL, USA

K. Battick et al. (eds.), *Nursing Guide for Pediatric Neuroscience Patients*,
https://doi.org/10.1007/978-3-032-22664-8_21

involves the application of ethical principles to clinical situations, aiming to resolve conflicts and guide decision-making. Health care providers are often faced with extremely complex situations that can result in ethical dilemmas among the care team, internally, and in interactions and decision-making with patients and their families. Patients and families may also experience ethical dilemmas due to family dynamics as well as cultural and spiritual beliefs. Generally, complex clinical cases often reveal these ethical concerns, which can lead to further discussion in the form of an ethics committee consultation.

In the majority of cases, the pediatric patient, as a minor, does not have the legal authority over their healthcare decision-making. The caregivers and healthcare team must work together to make decisions on behalf of the child. In Pediatric Neurosurgery, cases are often complex. With this complexity, conflicting opinions may arise regarding medical decisions, family wishes, and the desired outcomes for the patient. There are many factors that go into medical decisions, which can cause ethical conflicts, concerns, and/or dilemmas. Respect for autonomy, beneficence, non-maleficence, and justice are the four main pillars in medical ethics, and ethical dilemmas arise from conflicts among these principles. Members of the healthcare team should have a baseline working knowledge of these principles and know who to notify for consultation when a concern or dilemma occurs.

In medical ethics, autonomy is defined as respecting the patient's right to make their own informed decisions about their own healthcare [7]. When a patient is not competent to make medical decisions for him- or herself, a surrogate decision-maker is designated. In the case of pediatrics, this role nearly always falls to parents who are assumed to be making decisions in the patient's best interest [2, 8]. The principle of autonomy, or in pediatrics, "parental authority," ensures that the patient, and in this case the child's caregiver, have all of the necessary information related to the child's disease process and expected outcomes. This provides them the ability to make an autonomous decision for the treatment of the child. Often, other providers such as social workers or members of the Palliative Care Team participate in these difficult discussions and can help ensure caregivers understand the plan of care, answer questions, and discuss what is important to the caregivers regarding their child's medical journey.

Beneficence underscores the moral obligation to act for the benefit of others, including protecting the rights of and preventing harm to others, and helping those in danger. The principle of beneficence is often discussed in tandem with non-maleficence, meaning "do no harm". In medicine, the principle of beneficence can be seen as requiring the medical team to act in the patient's best interest [2, 8]. Applying the best interest standard leads to favoring interventions that are likely to provide greater benefit than burden for the child and discouraging the initiation or continuation of interventions that are likely to lead to greater burden than benefit [1, 8]. Pediatric medicine is constantly evolving, and treatment plans should not be without consideration of when treatment may no longer be of benefit. Treatments should have a clear rationale as to why they are being used, and this should be communicated to all members of the healthcare team as well as the caregivers.

As hinted at previously, non-maleficence focuses on avoiding harm to the patient. While this principle seems fairly straightforward, it is often at the root of many ethical concerns. This principle requires the medical team to weigh the risk versus benefit of specific interventions. When faced with difficult decisions such as withholding or withdrawing life-sustaining treatments, there may be discord among various providers and families. Deciding what constitutes a benefit to the patient's overall plan of care versus the risk of prolonging the patient's suffering must take a multifaceted approach.

The principle of justice focuses on the fair, equitable, and appropriate distribution of health care resources and implies that every child deserves the same treatment, surgery, therapy, or medical care. In the pediatric population, this principle is particularly important as it ensures that all children, regardless of their socioeconomic status, race, or geographic location, have equal access to necessary medical interventions. It also emphasizes the need for policies that address disparities in healthcare access and promote the well-being of vulnerable or underserved children. Unfortunately, there are still many known healthcare disparities occurring in pediatric healthcare today. It is up to the healthcare team to stay diligent to protect every pediatric patient from ethical injustice.

Pediatric neuroscience patients are often complex and are perceived as experiencing life-long comorbidities that require numerous and ongoing treatment decisions by their healthcare providers and caregivers. These decisions can be very straightforward or be life-saving and/or life-threatening. Children are often seen as having their whole lives ahead of them, making decision-making especially challenging as families and medical teams alike strive to ensure their long-term well-being. However, it is also of concern that the child's quality of life be preserved and that the caregivers weigh in on what they believe is the best quality for their child. All these factors can create ethical concerns or dilemmas that should be considered, discussed, and resolved in an objective manner for the best interest of the child.

Ethical principle	Key points	Example
Autonomy	Respecting the patient's right to make their own informed decisions about their healthcare	If the patient has to choose between two therapies, it is their right to choose which one they would want
Beneficence	The moral obligation to act for the benefit of others, including protecting the rights of and preventing harm to others, and helping those in danger	If a patient is using a therapy to treat themselves, which you know is harmful, it is your obligation to tell them
Non-maleficence	Avoiding harm to the patient	Do not give medications to patients just because they want it if there is no evidence that it would work
Justice	The fair, equitable, and appropriate distribution of health care resources and implies that every child deserves the same treatment, surgery, therapy, or medical care	If two patients show up to the ER, with the exact same diagnosis, you must offer them both the same treatment

In Ethics, case-based discussions are often helpful in assisting with education and application of the inherent ethical principles in medicine. Casuistry is a case-based method often used to apply these principles. The following case study highlights many of these principles in practice:

Emily is an 8-year-old girl with cerebral palsy, developmental delay, epilepsy, and hydrocephalus with a history of multiple brain surgeries for ventriculoperitoneal (VP) shunt placement. All of her VP shunt placements have come with known risks and complications including infection and malfunctions needing revision. Her last shunt malfunction was a year ago. Emily's parents brought her to the ER today as she was not acting like herself. An MRI is showing increased intracranial pressure. The neurosurgical team has recommended another revision given her clinical picture as Emily is also having associated symptoms including vomiting, irritability, and lethargy.

When you approach the parents for consent, the family questions whether another shunt replacement is in her best interest. They feel she has already suffered through multiple surgeries in the past. They have noticed that over the past year, since the last shunt revision, that she did not return to baseline. She does not smile, seems irritable, and is less interactive. She often has episodes of dysautonomia and crying which have been difficult to manage medically. They worry that she has a poor quality of life, and they are not sure that she would want to continue to live this way.

Ethical Dilemma

The family will need to make a decision regarding whether to proceed with another surgery. They know the surgery would relieve her current symptoms but know that it may not improve her overall quality of life. Her development has not progressed past that of a 2-year-old. They have seen her deteriorate medically over the last year. The family is torn, because they also are not sure they are ready to let her die.

Key Ethical Issues in This Case

Beneficence Versus Non-Maleficence

A key theme in the family's deliberations in this case is based on the ethical principles of beneficence versus non-maleficence. Beneficence dictates that the family and the medical team act in the best interest of Emily, making decisions that will most likely benefit both her health and her well-being. This has to be balanced with non-maleficence, and in this case, given Emily's history of shunt complications and ongoing developmental delays, the risk of surgery is significant. The family and the medical team must weigh potential benefits with potential burdens or harm.

Parental Autonomy/Authority

The parents in this case must be involved in the decision-making process. The medical team has recommended an additional surgery, but this requires the parents' consent prior to proceeding. The parents have the parental authority or "autonomy" to consent or not consent. The assumption is that the parents will act in Emily's best interest. When there are conflicting ideas of how to best proceed, the dilemma arises when discussing how much weight should be given to the family's wishes, as they have a personal understanding of Emily's quality of life and the impacts of an additional surgery, versus the clinical recommendations made by her medical team.

Quality of Life and Prognosis

Quality of life is truly in the eye of the beholder. What is an acceptable quality of life differs from person to person and family to family. In this case, how does the medical team assess the value of quality of life for a child who may not be able to experience the benefits of a surgery in the same way a neurotypical child would? Emily has limited developmental capabilities, and it is uncertain whether relieving the ICP will significantly improve her quality of life or simply prolong suffering. The team must balance the potential for prolonging life with the consideration that prolonged life with no meaningful improvement in quality of life may not be in her best interest.

Futility

At the crossroads of medical complex neurosurgical patients, pediatric palliative care, and ethics, there is often the question of medical futility. This often arises when discussing intensive care or interventions may be indicated, with the question of these interventions being done for the patient or to the patient. In this case, both the medical team and the family must weigh whether VP shunt revision will truly benefit Emily in the long term or whether continuing to perform surgeries might only prolong her suffering without improving her overall well-being.

Recommendations

1. Pediatric Palliative Care Consultation
   Pediatric Palliative Care can provide a layer of support to patients and families when making difficult decisions. Discussions regarding goals of care can often help the palliative care team assist the family with medical decisions that the team has asked the family to make. Understanding the family views on quality of life can also help guide the decision-making process. Using forms such as physician orders for life-sustaining treatment is often used in different states and

can assist. Consultation can also allow a more palliative approach if decided upon, with more of a focus on symptom management and comfort care rather than pursuing more aggressive treatments. Possibilities include measures to manage intracranial pressure without surgery, with medications, etc., avoiding potential risks associated with another shunt placement.

2. Ethics Committee Consultation
   Given the complexity of the case, the family and medical team could benefit from a consultation with an ethics committee to help guide decision-making. This would allow for a thorough discussion of the ethical principles involved and help ensure that the decision is made with a holistic understanding of Emily's medical, emotional, and familial contexts.

Most large hospitals and health care systems have Ethics Committees, and their main goal is to resolve ethical dilemmas for staff, patients, and family members. The committees are often available 24/7 for consultation requests and lead by medical ethicists or fellow peer staff with training in medical ethics. Placing an ethics consultation request should not be punitive but serve as a way to request help with a complex situation to ensure all of the ethical principles are adhered to and to protect the best interest of the child [16, 17].

Discussion

Palliative care and ethics are intertwined in most complex medical patients with serious illness. The technology we have today has pushed the limits of medicine and patient care. The question then becomes "Just because we can, should we"? Medical decisions that are being made can have long-lasting implications for patients and families. It is up to the medical community to assist the family on what the journey could look like based on the decisions that are being made, to the best of our ability. With every decision, there can be a long-lasting consequence. Only the family can judge whether it is beneficial for their loved one. Sometimes, these realizations happen in days or not for years to come. When we are asking whether a therapy is beneficial, we should also be considering the ethical implications that can follow it.

When an ethical concern or dilemma is present, it is important to acknowledge potential issues and create a multidisciplinary forum for concerns to be brought forward. Unresolved ethical dilemmas may lead to moral distress, compassion fatigue, and burnout over time. Both moral distress and ethical dilemmas require sensitive handling, clear communication, and support structures within healthcare environments to help providers navigate these challenges. Staff should be aware of who they can contact for reporting ethical concerns and requesting an objective resolution, as well as available resources to address their own moral distress before it progresses to compassion fatigue and eventually burnout.

Moral distress in pediatric healthcare occurs when healthcare professionals, such as doctors, nurses, and other caregivers, experience emotional discomfort or tension because they feel unable to act according to their moral beliefs [9, 10]. These feelings can be caused by differing opinions between members of the healthcare team and the patient and family, institutional and policy constraints, lack of inpatient and/or community resources, and other external factors. These feelings are often exacerbated as the patient nears the end of life.

The emotional tension caused by these feelings can lead to burnout, affect job satisfaction, and cause negative emotional repercussions not only professionally but also personally if not addressed. It further emphasizes the need for open communication, ethical decision-making frameworks, encouragement of self-care, and access to employee assistance programs within the pediatric healthcare setting.

Self-care in pediatric healthcare is essential for healthcare providers' overall well-being, job satisfaction, career longevity, and ability to deliver high-quality care. Nurses can have routine exposure to death, more so than any other health care provider. They are the ones who facilitate a dignified, comfortable death that honors both the child and the family. They are able to spend time getting to know the patient and family on a more personal level, which allows them to act as an advocate, companion, professional caregiver, educator, and supporter. As nurses, they also grieve the loss of the children they care for, but must put their own grief aside to provide care to the family. These situations are often emotionally challenging, and without proper self-care, burnout, compassion fatigue, and moral distress become more prevalent and can negatively affect both the individual and patient care.

There are many avenues to practice self-care, and there is not a one-size-fits-all approach. Self-care practices can take on many different forms; however, the goals remain the same—to remain engaged, compassionate members of the healthcare team, which in turn allows nurses to be effective in their many roles. Some self-care practices include taking of regular breaks (while on shift as well as practicing good work life balance), healthy eating, exercise, and sleep that have been shown to be effective [10].

As with any high-stress environment, this type of work can be extremely emotional and emotionally taxing for professional caregivers. Identifying a support system, whether it be professional counseling, a peer group, or trusted friend, is important to allow for the nurse to process the emotional challenges that working within this specialty brings. The earlier that the nurse identifies and institutes these supports, the easier it becomes to remain emotionally resilient as situations arise [11, 12].

Physical health is equally as important as emotional health. By participating in regular physical activity, including exercise, proper nutrition, hydration, and sleep, nurses are conditioned to endure the physical stamina needed to endure the long shifts. Physical activity has long been reported to stimulate the release of endorphins, which increases happiness, therefore reducing the feelings of anxiety and depression that can be associated with caring for complex patients [15].

When healthcare providers prioritize self-care, they are more likely to feel satisfied and motivated in their roles. This leads to greater professional fulfilment and a better sense of purpose. It allows for nurses and healthcare providers to remain engaged and connected to their work in especially challenging situations. This in turn not only benefits the nurse but also the patient and family experience. Nurses and healthcare providers who engage in self-care are better equipped to provide quality care to their patients. It has been shown that when providers feel physically and emotionally healthy, they can interact with more empathy with children and families, make more thoughtful decisions, and are able to manage work-related stress more effectively. This also helps to prevent medical errors and lapses in judgment that often occur as a result of being mentally exhausted or emotionally drained [11, 12].

Self-care is not just a personal benefit; it is a professional necessity in pediatric healthcare. It helps prevent burnout, enhances the quality of patient care, and fosters long-term career satisfaction and emotional well-being. By prioritizing self-care, pediatric healthcare providers are better equipped to handle the emotional, ethical, and physical challenges of their work, ensuring they remain healthy and effective in their roles.

Bibliography

1. American Academy of Pediatrics Committee on Bioethics. Guidelines on forgoing life-sustaining medical treatment. Pediatrics. 2000;106:1151–3.
2. Cummings CL, Mercurio MR. Ethics for the pediatrician: autonomy, beneficence, and rights. Pediatr Rev. 2010;31(6):252–5. https://doi.org/10.1542/pir.31-6-252.
3. Prince v. Massachusetts, 321 US 158 (1944) at: http://supreme.justia.com/us/321/158/case.html#170.
4. American Academy of Pediatrics Committee on Bioethics. Religious objections to medical care. Pediatrics. 1997;99:279–81.
5. Mercurio MR. The aftermath of Baby Doe and the evolution of newborn intensive care. Ga State Univ Law Rev. 2012;25:9.
6. Moon MR. The imperative of ethics in everyday clinical pediatrics. Pediatr Clin N Am. 2024;71(1):1–8. https://doi.org/10.1016/j.pcl.2023.09.001.
7. Carrese JA, Sugarman J. The inescapable relevance of bioethics for the practicing clinician. Chest. 2006;130(6):1864–72. https://doi.org/10.1378/chest.130.6.1864.
8. März JW. What does the best interests principle of the convention on the rights of the child mean for paediatric healthcare? Eur J Pediatr. 2022;181(11):3805–16. https://doi.org/10.1007/s00431-022-04609-2.
9. Prentice T, Janvier A, Gillam L, Davis PG. Moral distress within neonatal and paediatric intensive care units: a systematic review. Arch Dis Child. 2016;101(8):701–8. https://doi.org/10.1136/archdischild-2015-309410.
10. Chen J, Lin N, Ye X, et al. Coping strategies and interventions to alleviate moral distress among pediatric ICU nurses: a scoping review. Nurs Ethics. 2025;32(2):437–59. https://doi.org/10.1177/09697330241252875.
11. Helmers A, Palmer KD, Greenberg RA. Moral distress: developing strategies from experience. Nurs Ethics. 2020;27(4):1147–56. https://doi.org/10.1177/0969733020906593.
12. Morley G, Sankary LR. Nurturing moral community: a novel moral distress peer support navigator tool. Nurs Ethics. 2024;31(5):980–91. https://doi.org/10.1177/09697330231221220.
13. Kaye EC, Weaver MS, DeWitt LH, et al. The impact of specialty palliative care in pediatric oncology: a systematic review. J Pain Symptom Manag. 2021;61(5):1060–1079.e2. https://doi.org/10.1016/j.jpainsymman.2020.12.003.

14. Marcus KL, Santos G, Ciapponi A, et al. Impact of specialized pediatric palliative care: a systematic review. J Pain Symptom Manag. 2020;59(2):339–364.e10. https://doi.org/10.1016/j.jpainsymman.2019.08.005.
15. Singh B, Olds T, Curtis R, et al. Effectiveness of physical activity interventions for improving depression, anxiety and distress: an overview of systematic reviews. Br J Sports Med. 2023;57(18):1203–9. https://doi.org/10.1136/bjsports-2022-106195.
16. Aulisio MP, Arnold RM, Youngner SJ. Health care ethics consultation: nature, goals, and competencies. A position paper from the society for health and human values-society for bioethics consultation task force on standards for bioethics consultation. Ann Intern Med. 2000;133(1):59–69. https://doi.org/10.7326/0003-4819-133-1-200007040-00012.
17. Nathanson PG, Walter JK, McKlindon DD, Feudtner C. Relational, emotional, and pragmatic attributes of ethics consultations at a children's hospital. Pediatrics. 2021;147(4):e20201087. https://doi.org/10.1542/peds.2020-1087.

MIX
Papier aus verantwortungsvollen Quellen
Paper from responsible sources
FSC® C105338

If you have any concerns about our products,
you can contact us on
ProductSafety@springernature.com

In case Publisher is established outside the EU,
the EU authorized representative is:
Springer Nature Customer Service Center GmbH
Europaplatz 3, 69115 Heidelberg, Germany

Printed by Libri Plureos GmbH
in Hamburg, Germany